ADVANCES IN APPLIED ELECTROMYOGRAPHY

Edited by **Joseph Mizrahi**

Advances in Applied Electromyography
Edited by Joseph Mizrahi

Published by InTech
Janeza Trdine 9, 51000 Rijeka, Croatia

Publishing Process Manager Masa Vidovic

Technical Editor Teodora Smiljanic

Cover Designer InTech Design Team

Additional hard copies can be obtained from orders@intechopen.com

Advances in Applied Electromyography, Edited by Joseph Mizrahi
p. cm.
ISBN 978-953-307-382-8

For EU product safety concerns:
IN TECH d.o.o., Prolaz Marije Krucifikse Kozulić 3, 51000 Rijeka, Croatia,
info@intechopen.com or visit our website at intechopen.com.

Meet the editor

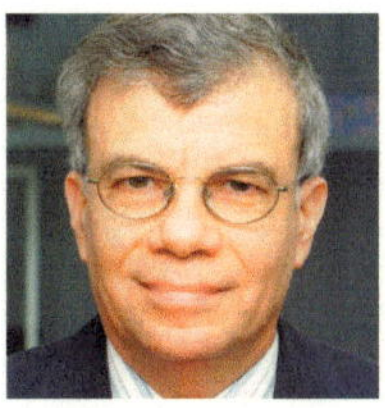

Professor Joseph Mizrahi received his BSc degree in aerospace engineering, the MSc degree in mechanics and the DSc degree in biomechanics, all from the Technion-Israel Institute of Technology, Haifa. He is a professor of biomedical engineering at the Faculty of Biomedical Engineering, Technion and is the incumbent of the Pearl Milch Chair of Biomedical Engineering Sciences and Fellow of the AIMBE. For 18 years, he also served as Head of the Biomechanics Laboratory at the Loewenstein Rehabilitation Center in Israel. He held visiting positions with several Universities, including Witwatersrand, Johannesburg, Harvard, Cape Town, Hong Kong Polytechnic and Drexel. During 2004-2009 he served as Dean of the Faculty of Biomedical Engineering at the Technion. Other academic responsibilities included memberships in the Technion Senate Steering and other committees. He is principal author of some 250 publications, including journal articles, books, book chapters and conference proceedings, and he holds several editorial responsibilities. His major research interests are in rehabilitation engineering and orthopedic biomechatronics.

Contents

Preface

The electrical activity of the muscles, as measured by means of electromyography (EMG), is a major expression of muscle contraction. Since the contracting skeletal muscles are greatly responsible for loading of the bones and joints, information about the muscle EMG is important to gain knowledge about musculo-skeletal biomechanics. Myoelectric signals can also demonstrate the development of loading imbalance and asymmetry, which in turn relate to physical disability. In smooth muscles, EMG may be used to indicate function of internal organs. EMG may thus be used clinically for the diagnosis of neuromuscular problems and for assessing biomechanical and motor control deficits and other functional disorders. It may also be used as a control signal for interfacing with orthotic and/or prosthetic devices or other rehabilitation assists. Apart from muscular activity, EMG may also be used to indicate and quantify the development of muscle fatigue.

EMG signals from whole muscles are generally stochastic in nature, thus requiring reference to methods of signal analysis in order to be characterized ad classified and to obtain quantitative information about muscle activity both in the time and the frequency domains. Exceptionally, EMG signals may exhibit a deterministic pattern when all the muscle fibers contract simultaneously. This takes place when the muscle's activation is being induced by means of electrical stimulation from a source external to the central nervous system. A synchronous compound muscle action potential (CMAP) then replaces the natural, somewhat random-like, signal produced by the asynchronous firing of the different motor units. Rather simple methods of signal processing are sufficient for characterizing the synchronous CMAP.

The EMG signal is usually accompanied by mechanical signals emerging from the contracting and vibrating muscles. Although these signals are measurable by means of microphones (acoustic myography, AMG) or accelerometers (mechano myography, MMG) the EMG is still the major and dominant source serving to monitor muscle activity. This is so because EMG signals are more reliable and reproducible compared to the AMG and MMG signals.

This book aims at providing an updated overview of the recent developments in electromyography from diverse aspects and various applications in clinical and experimental research. It consists of ten chapters arranged in four sections. The first section deals with EMG signals from skeletal muscles and their significance in assessing biomechanical and physiologic function and in applications in neuro-musculo-skeletal rehabilitation. The second section addresses methodologies for the treatment of the signal itself: noise removal and pattern recognition for the activation of artificial limbs. The third section deals with utilizing the EMG signals for inferring on the mechanical action of muscle, such as force, e.g., pinching force in humans or sucking pressure in the cibarial pump during feeding of the hematophagous hemiptera insect. The fourth and last section deals with the clinical role of electromyograms in studying the pelvic floor muscle function.

Prof. Joseph Mizrahi
Department of Biomedical Engineering
Technion Israel Institute of Technology, Haifa,
Israel

Part 1

Skeletal Muscles, Biomechanics and Rehabilitation

1

The Role of Electromyograms in Resolving Musculoskeletal Interactions in Able-Bodied and Disabled Human Individuals

J. Mizrahi
Department of Biomedical Engineering
Technion, Israel Institute of Technology, Haifa
Israel

1. Introduction

Electromyography (EMG) is a significant indicator of muscle activity and constitutes a fundamental and important tool in the fields of biomechanics, kinesiology and exercise physiology. Clinically, it serves for diagnosis and treatment monitoring. However, the raw signal obtained from the EMG of a muscle is difficult to interpret without the application of appropriate signal processing techniques. If processed in the time domain, the envelope of the rectified EMG signal may serve, with further processing, for several applications including: indication of muscle activity (Rakos et al, 1999), or estimation of force (Genadry et al, 1988). If processed in the frequency domain, EMG may point to the development of muscle fatigue (De Luca, 1997; Mizrahi et al, 2001). The electromyographic signal may also be used as a bio-control signal in conjunction with bio-assistive motion (Langzam et al 2006a, 2007; Mizrahi et al 1994; Peasgood et al, 2000; Saxena et al 1995; Thorsen et al, 1999). This Chapter deals with the role of electromyography in facilitating the biomechanical solutions of musculo-skeletal systems characterized by neuro-muscular indeterminacies.

2. Neuro-muscular redundancy and mechanical indeterminacy

A major and interesting question in human biomechanics and kinesiology is how many muscles are required for performing a given motor task? Not less intriguing is the question relating to the number of muscles actually engaged in performing this given motor task. Past work on human locomotion has demonstrated that, if we take level walking as an example, no less than 31 muscle groups are engaged in each leg. Electromyograms of the major muscles of the leg during locomotion have been used to show the sequence of muscle activation in the gait cycles (Bechtol 1975; Mizrahi 2004). The multi-muscle performance of the walking task involves patterns of timings and intensities necessitating central control to be provided by the central nervous system. For instance, the knee and ankle extensors must 'switch-on' their activity near heel-strike, and remain partly active in the mid-stance and swing phases, and much less so in the other phases of the gait cycle. It is the multi-muscle sequencing of this large-scale system that provides the smooth, graceful, motion of walking. In analogy, somewhat similar sequencing can be found in an orchestral score of a multi-instrument musical composition, such as a symphony or opera, assigning the temporal roles of the different musical instruments (Mizrahi, 2004). Here too, there is a need for a central control which in this case is provided by the orchestra's conductor.

It may be argued, though, that the involvement of all the muscles in the abovementioned walking task is not essential and that the locomotor system is neuro-muscularly redundant, with substantially more acting muscle groups than actually required. Mechanically, the consequence of this redundancy is that the number of unknown internal joint and muscle forces exceeds the number of mechanical equations, rendering the system mechanically indeterminate.

The origin of the abovementioned neuro-muscular redundancy can be found in the descending pathways from the central nervous system to the peripheral nervous system. As a matter of fact, there exist multiple pathways for the performance of a given motor task such that the same information may be processed in different ways. Thus, a given central command may result in different activations and, conversely, different commands can result in the same activation. A trivial example is presented in Figure 1, illustrating how a torque of required intensity at a joint can be provided. It is evident that this torque can be produced in an infinite number of ways, involving the possible co-activation of the antagonist muscles with various contraction intensities. From the purely mechanical aspect, such co-activation is actually undesirable because it results in an increased net joint force. Nevertheless, co-activation is physiologically beneficial because it facilitates stability and controllability of posture and motion.

In summary, indeterminacy occurs wherever the number of unknowns exceeds the number of available biomechanical equations. Indeterminacy is associated with a multitude of possible solutions of the available system of equations. Conventional methods of addressing mechanical indeterminacy usually refer to the implementation of optimization criteria (Patriarco et al, 1981) providing supplementary equations that allow eliminating inadequate solutions. The level of indeterminacy is expected to decrease with the reduction of redundancy. Particularly here information from electromyograms may become instrumental in resolving muscle and joint forces as well as other unknowns from the musculo-skeletal mechanical equations.

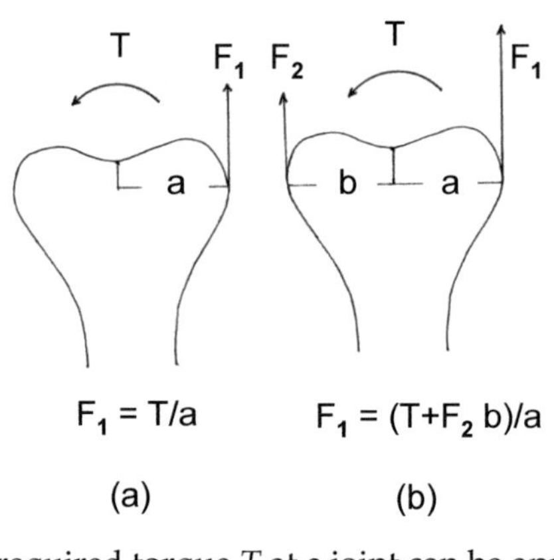

Fig. 1. Illustration of how a required torque T at a joint can be applied in multiple ways: (a) by means of the agonist only F_1; (b) by means of various co-activations of the agonist F_1 and the antagonist F_2. Note that in case (b) both F_1 and the resulting joint force are larger than in case (a).

3. Circumstances where neuro-muscular redundancy may diminish

Neuro-muscular redundancy may get reduced under several circumstances, including the following:
(a) Grouping together of neighboring muscles which share a cooperative action about a joint, referred to as Muscle Synergy. An example of muscle synergy can be seen in cycling motion, as shown in Figure 2, where the sequence of muscle activation of four of the major muscle groups of the lower leg is shown by means of their raw Electromyograms. Cycling motion has been acknowledged as a significant rehabilitation modality for neurologically impaired subjects (Peng et al, 2011). The sequence of muscle action, as well as the patterns of the timings and intensities of the muscles is clearly noticed. Cycling is a smaller-scale motion-system compared to walking and the musical analogy can be demonstrated here by the score of one of Mozart's string quartets, indicating the assignment of the temporal roles of each of the four string instruments (Figure 2). The role of electromyograms in resolving joint dynamics in the context of muscle synergy is elaborated in Section 4.

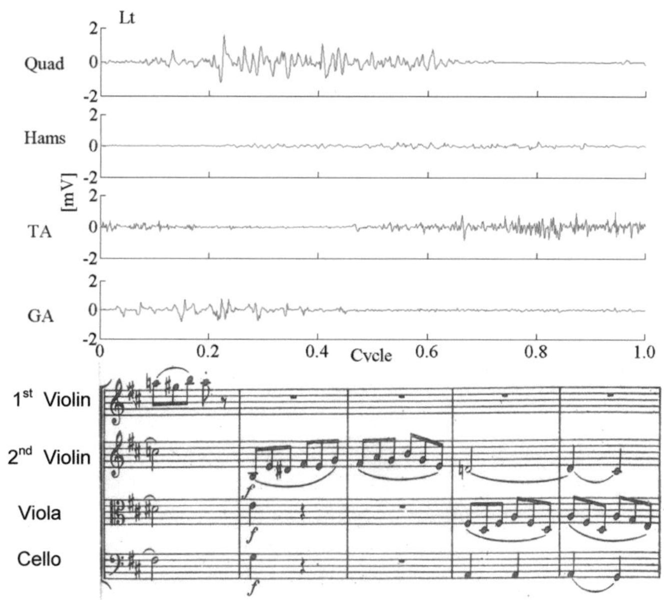

Fig. 2. Sequence of muscle activation during cycling motion of four of the major muscle groups of the left lower limb, including Quadriceps (Quad), Hamstrings (Hams), Tibialis Anterior (TA) and Gastrocnemius (GA). A musical analogy is shown in the lower part of the Figure by means of a line from one of Mozart's string quartets (in D major K 499, last movement). The analogy refers to the assignment of the temporal roles of each of the four string instruments versus sequencing of muscle action and patterns of timings and intensities of the muscle groups.

(b) Reducing redundancy through the volitional, deliberate, and selective exclusion of part of the musculo-skeletal system from being actively involved in the mechanical task. An example of the intentional abstention to utilize part of the body structures or actuators is noticed when standing on one leg only (as compared to two). This issue is further elaborated in Section 5.

(c) Short-term neuro-muscular deficiency, such as during muscle Fatigue. This issue is dealt with in Sections 4 & 5.
(d) Long-term, or permanent, neuro-musculo-skeletal deficiency, such as weakness, paralysis and the like. In the extreme case of paraplegia, when the fully paralyzed quadriceps muscle is activated by external electrical stimulation, this muscle becomes under conditions of low spasticity the only active muscle in the lower limb. Under these conditions redundancy is entirely eliminated and, consequently, the musculo-mechanical system becomes determinate allowing us to resolve the actual muscle force from the externally measured torque (Giat et al, 1993). However, in case of partial deficiency, although not entirely eliminated, redundancy becomes reduced. The issue of partial deficiency is elaborated in Section 6.

4. Muscle synergy

Under what conditions can one possibly correlate the torque about a joint, as indicated by the electromyograms of the actuating muscles, with the kinematics of that joint? This question was specifically dealt with by Russek (2002) in the Lab of the present author. The work focused on the utilization of the myoelectric signals from the Gastrocnemius and Tibialis Anterior antagonists to estimate ankle kinematics. These specific muscles were previously reported to adequately serve for the prediction of ankle torque (Cavanagh, 1990; Prilutsky et al 1998).
The paradigm used by Russek (2002).was of running on a level treadmill for a total period of 30 min at a running speed just exceeding the anaerobic threshold (average ~ 3.5 m/s). EMG data of the Tibialis Anterior and Gastrocnemius muscles were online collected, simultaneously with the kinematics of the lower limb, as obtained from video data. The above-selected values of running speed and duration allowed, in addition, monitoring the effect of progressing fatigue on the EMG/kinematics relations. The EMG signals were band-pass filtered with a 10th order Butterworth filter with a cut-off frequency of 10-500 Hz (De Luca 1997; Oppenheim & Schafer 1975), in order to eliminate noise and artifacts, due to leg movement and muscle contraction, and sampled at 1667 Hz. Since the EMG signal was non-stationary during long periods of data, it was segmented into short epochs of wide-stationary cycles (Bendat & Piersol, 1970), corresponding to the running cycle.
The foot-strike event points were obtained from the signals of an accelerometer attached at the tibial tuberosity of the running subjects. Since the exact timing of the foot strike point could not be estimated directly from the video data due to its low sampling rate (50 Hz), the accelerometer signal was taken to indicate the peak of the foot strike. The foot-strike point was set to precede the peak acceleration by 30 ms (Daily, 1998). The toe-off event points were obtained from the repetitive Gastrocnemius signal, using an algorithm that identifies the periods of muscular activity (Marple-Horvat & Gilbey, 1992). The kinematic data were smoothed with a 4th order Butterworth low-pass filter with a cut frequency of 10 Hz (Bourdin et al, 1995; Prilutsky et al, 1998). To address the problem of different sampling frequencies between EMG and kinematical data, low-pass interpolation was used by inserting zeros into the original sequence and then applying a special symmetric Finite Impulse Response low-pass filter (IEEE, 1979).

4.1 Analysis

The analysis presented is for general dynamic conditions, thus extending previous analyses done under either isokinetic or isotonic conditions (Colson et al, 1999; Kellis& Baltzopoulos,

1998; Tamaki et al 1997,). The foot segment is assumed to move under general plane motion in the sagittal plane. The moments about the center of gravity thus involve the reaction forces at the ankle joint and the foot-ground contact, as well as the net joint torque about the ankle due to the co-contraction of the Tibialis Anterior and Gastrocnemius muscles. At first, a proportionality relation between the net actuating ankle torque and the angular acceleration of the foot segment is sought. This may, however, involve an error, reflecting the absence of torques of the reactive forces; this error will be later dealt with. Since the torques of the muscles can be represented by their respective EMG signals, the proportionality relation will, after time-integration, read as follows:

$$K_G \cdot iEMG_G - K_T \cdot iEMG_T \propto \Delta\omega_A \qquad (1)$$

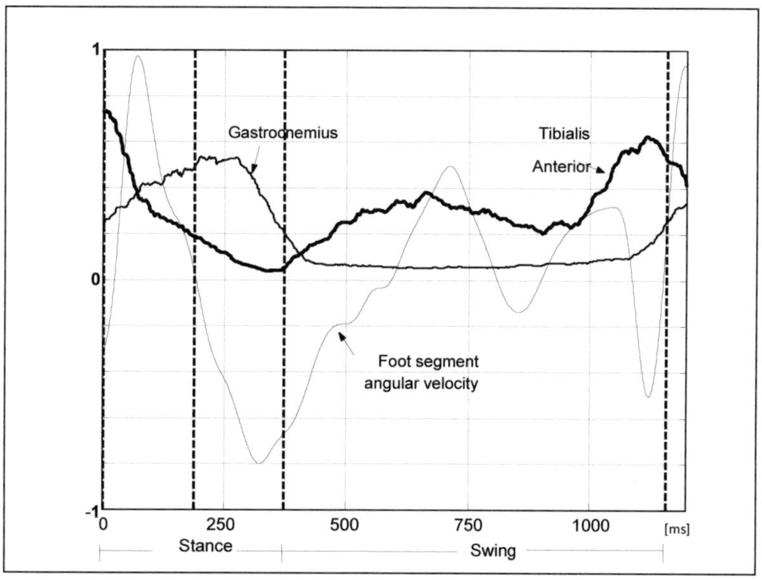

Fig. 3. One running-cycle illustration of the smoothed, rectified, EMG signals of the Gastrocnemius and Tibialis Anterior and of the ankle angular velocity (normalized units on vertical axis), segmented into three sections (separated by dashed vertical lines), namely: 1) first part of stance, 2) second part of stance, and 3) swing phase.

Where *iEMG* denotes the integrated EMG, with the subscript denoting the Gastrocnemius (*G*) or Tibialis Anterior (*T*) muscle, $\Delta\omega_A$ is the change of angular velocity of the foot segment and the *K*'s are respective coefficients. The proportionality (1) can be turned into an equation by modifying these coefficients as follows:

$$\hat{K}_G \cdot iEMG_G - \hat{K}_T \cdot iEMG_T \cong \Delta\omega_A \qquad (2)$$

Since the EMG signals of the Tibialis Anterior and Gastrocnemius muscles, as well as the angular velocity, are actually measured (as demonstrated in Figure 3), the coefficients $\hat{K}$'s in equation (2) can be obtained using parameter estimation methods. Rewriting, in a more general form, yields

$$\overline{\hat{K}} \cdot \overline{\overline{iEMG}} = \overline{\Delta\omega_A} \tag{3}$$

where $\overline{\Delta\omega_A} = [\Delta\omega_{A1}, \Delta\omega_{A2} ..... \Delta\omega_{Am}]$

and

$$\overline{\overline{iEMG}} = \begin{bmatrix} iEMG_{G1}, & -iEMG_{T1} \\ iEMG_{G2}, & -iEMG_{T2} \\ \vdots & \\ iEMG_{Gm}, & -iEMG_{Tm} \end{bmatrix} \tag{4}$$

$$\overline{\hat{K}} = [\hat{K}_G, \ \hat{K}_T] \tag{5}$$

m=1, 2..,number of running cycles during the time of data acquisition.
The earlier mentioned error $\bar{e}$ is

$$\bar{e} = \overline{\Delta\omega_A} - \overline{\hat{K}} \cdot \overline{\overline{iEMG}} \tag{6}$$

And the sum of the residual square is expressed as:

$$\varphi_{OLS} = \sum \bar{e}^2 = (\overline{\Delta\omega_A} - \overline{\hat{K}} \cdot \overline{\overline{iEMG}})^T (\overline{\Delta\omega_A} - \overline{\hat{K}} \cdot \overline{\overline{iEMG}}) \tag{7}$$

Using least-square methods, the vector $\overline{\hat{K}}$ can be calculated. It is convenient to express the separate coefficients as the respective co-activation ratios, as follows:

$$\hat{K}_G[\%] = \hat{K}_G \Big/ (\hat{K}_G + \hat{K}_T) \cdot 100\% \quad \text{and} \quad \hat{K}_T[\%] = \hat{K}_T \Big/ (\hat{K}_G + \hat{K}_T) \cdot 100\% \tag{8}$$

Substantial changes in the EMG signals take place within each running cycle. To account for these changes, the analysis was divided into segments. Previous studies used to divide the EMG signal into stance and swing phase of the entire stride cycle (Buczek & Cavanagh, 1990; Nilsson et al, 1985; Prilutsky et al, 1998). In view of the observed changes in muscular activity of both the Gastrocnemius and the Tibialis Anterior within the stance phase, it was decided to further divide the stance phase into two segments (corresponding to eccentric and concentric activities, respectively) giving altogether three segments for the running cycle. The weight coefficients $\hat{K}_G$ and $\hat{K}_T$ were estimated as indicators of muscular activity of the Gastrocnemius and Tibialis Anterior, respectively. Especially, they served as co-contraction indicators in the first part of the stance phase.

4.2 Coefficients of muscle activity and change in angular velocity

The estimation values, summarized in Table 1, indicate that in the first-stance section co-activation of the Gastrocnemius and Tibialis Anterior muscles prevails (57% and 43%, respectively). In the second-stance section the Gastrocnemius muscle becomes clearly dominant (79%, versus 21% for the T muscle) and in the swing section the opposite is seen, with nearly 90% for the Tibialis Anterior muscle and 10% for the Gastrocnemius muscle. It should be noted, though, that before the foot-strike, during the late part of the swing phase, the ankle performed dorsiflexion, preparing for the touch down to the ground, while the Tibialis Anterior muscle had the highest muscular activity.

$\hat{K}_G$ * [%]	Running time (min)		
	1	15	30
First-stance phase (Foot strike- Mid stance)	56.99 (12.48)	69.11 (11.53)	73.84** (15.43)
Second-stance phase (Mid stance - Toe off)	79.38 (12.53)	79.77 (13.18)	84.02 (12.62)
Swing phase Toe off - Foot strike	10.45 (5.89)	7.89 (4.92)	6.43 (5.38)

* $\hat{K}_T$ [%] =100 - $\hat{K}_G$ [%]; ** $p < 0.05$

Table 1. Summary of the estimated weight coefficients $\hat{K}_G$ and $\hat{K}_T$ * (expressed in %) for the three phases of the running cycle and for the 1st, 15th and 30th min of level running. Means (SD) are given. Double asterisks (**) denote a significant difference compared to the first minute of running ($p < 0.05$) as a result of fatigue.

The high Gastrocnemius muscular activity in the second part of the stance phase was accompanied by an elevated plantar-flexion, as the ankle joint decelerated until the final part of the second stance section, indicating a rapid generation of energy to propel the limb upward and forward (Winter & Scott, 1991). The significant increase in the Tibialis Anterior muscle activity during the swing phase is required for ankle dorsiflexion as this joint begins to accelerate. Later in the swing phase the Tibialis Anterior supports the foot against gravity and prepares for the heel contact.
Using the obtained EMG weight coefficients, the change in angular velocity $\Delta\omega_A$ was calculated and compared to that actually measured. The results of this comparison indicated that the two quantities were closely similar with a proximity coefficient (using Pearson correlation) of 0.998 and up for each of the three cycle sections.

4.3 Fatiguing effect

Following fatiguing after 30 min of running at a speed exceeding the anaerobic threshold, the coefficient $\hat{K}_{Gn}$ increased in the stance phase and decreased in the swing phase, although this change was significant ($p<0.05$) in the first-stance (eccentric) phase only. The effect of fatiguing was thus noticed in the first part of the stance phase, and as mentioned above; this phase is characterized by co-activation of the two antagonist muscles. However, due to progressing fatigue, there was a significant increase of the Gastrocnemius coefficient with a parallel decrease of the Tibialis Anterior coefficient from the first to the thirtieth minute of running ($p = 0.024$). The increasingly higher Gastrocnemius activity was required in order to change from dorsi- to plantar-flexion and to decelerate the angular ankle velocity.

5. Intentional reduction of redundancy

A fundamental difficulty in biomechanics is that the internal muscle and joint forces cannot be directly and non-invasively measured. More easily accessible measurements include the external loads and EMG's of the major limb muscles. However, as a consequence of the neuro-muscular redundancy and the resulting biomechanical indeterminacy, these EMG signals cannot be readily and simply correlated to the external loads acting on the human body. This Section demonstrates how, in cases where the neuro-muscular redundancy of the system can be reduced, the EMG signals may become more correlated to the externally measured reactive foot-ground forces. The paradigm used here is the regulation of balance during quiet standing in the upright position.

5.1 The regularly redundant case

Balance regulation while maintaining the standing-still posture is achieved by the interplay between body sway motion and the external forces acting on the swaying body. These include, apart from the gravitational force, the foot-ground reaction forces (Levin & Mizrahi 1996; Levin et al, 1998; Mizrahi et al, 2002; Mizrahi & Susak, 1982). Balance regulation is made possible by the continuous activity of the leg and lower trunk muscles. An obvious question, therefore, is whether the activity of these muscles, as monitored by their electromyograms (EMG), correlates to the external forces involved in the regulation of balance. If correlated, to what extent? An additional question is whether reduced redundancy modifies the extent of correlation and makes EMG and ground reaction forces become more correlated? With bi-pedal or double-stance standing as the reference posture, this question was studied by successively removing redundancies from the neuro-musculo-skeletal system.

5.2 Successive reduction of neuro-muscular redundancies

The first stage is to substitute the normal pi-pedal or double-stance case by single-stance standing. In single-leg standing, the musculo-skeletal system responsible for postural control has been reported to be less redundant than in double-leg standing (Levin et al, 2000a). In this posture, the standing body is acted upon by the reactive forces from one leg only and the task of balance regulation is performed by activation of the muscles of this leg, resulting in a smaller number of muscles actively engaged in stabilizing the standing posture. Further reduction of redundancy may be achieved by eliminating visual feedback, i.e. with the eyes closed, as opposed to eyes open.

Standing posture experiments, as reported from the lab of the present Author (Levin & Mizrahi, 1996; Levin et al, 1998; Levin et al, 2000a; Suponitsky et al, 2008), performed simultaneous on-line measurements of ground reaction forces and EMG's of the leg's major muscle groups for double- and single-stance standing. The double-stance standing experiments were for 30 s and the duration of the single-stance was for as long as the tested subject was able to maintain balance equilibrium.

The acquired force-plate and raw EMG signals were de-trended to compensate for long-term drift and their DC levels were set to zero. Each signal vector was then divided into epochs of 1 s for which the root mean square were calculated. The 1-s root mean square and values of the myoelectric activity were correlated with the corresponding root mean square values of the force plate data, using the Pearson's correlation coefficient with the significance level set at $p < 0.05$. Differences between the standing positions were tested for the mean values of the force plate and EMG results by using the student's t-test (statistical significance set at the 0.05 level).

The comparisons between double- and single-stance standing are demonstrated in Tables 2 & 3 which summarize, respectively, results for the foot-ground reactions forces and the myoelectric activity of the four major muscle groups. It is evident that in single-stance standing there is a substantial increase in force and muscle activity compared to double-stance standing. The reactive forces (Table 2) are described in terms of their three components: anterior-posterior, medial-lateral and vertical. The vertical values represent fluctuations ('ac' component) about the baseline ('dc' component) of the force beneath the supporting leg. An increased force activity and center-of-pressure (COP) excursion is noticed in single-stance compared to double-stance standing. The EMG signals of four of the major muscles are summarized in Table 3. Like with the reactive forces, an increased muscle activity is noticed in single-stance compared to double-stance standing.

		RMS	
		Double stance	Single stance
Force [N]	Anterior-posterior	0.6(0.2)	2.5(1.0)*
	Medial-lateral	0.6(0.2)	3.6(2.0)*
	Vertical	4.5(1.1)	6.3(3.5)*
Center of pressure [cm]	Anterior-posterior	0.3(0.1)	0.6(0.2)*
	Medial-lateral	0.2(0.3)	0.6(0.1)*

Table 2. Average (SD) of the root-mean-square (RMS, time domain) of the foot ground reaction forces. *significant differences ($p < 0.05$) between single stance and double stance

EMG	RMS [%MVC]	
	Double stance	Single stance
Tibialis Anterior	3.5(3.6)	26(20)*
Gastrocnemius	8.4(8.8)	58(32)*
Quadriceps	1.2(1.0)	8(3.5)*
Gluteus Maximus	3.4(2.0)	11(8)*

Table 3. EMG of the major leg muscles presented in Averages (SD) of the root mean square (RMS, time domain). The EMG RMS is expressed as percentage of the maximum voluntary contraction (%MVC). The asterisk *denotes significant differences ($p < 0.05$) between single stance and double stance.

5.3 Force/EMG correlations

Regarding the correlation between foot-ground reaction forces and muscle activity, Figure 4 displays a comparison of the occurrence of significant correlation between the foot-ground reaction forces and the EMG of three of the leg major muscles (both expressed by means of their root mean squares): Tibialis Anterior, Quadriceps and Gluteus Maximus. Each of these muscles is correlated with the foot-ground reaction forces and COP components, as indicated in the Figure. It is noticed that the correlation patterns between foot-ground reaction forces and EMG strongly depend on the standing conditions tested. Particularly, in single-stance with the eyes closed the occurrence of significant correlation is increased compared to the other conditions between the Tibialis Anterior and each of the vertical and medial-lateral force components and between each of the Quadriceps and Gluteus Maximus and the vertical force component. With regards to the center of pressure, the occurrence of significant correlation in single-stance with the eyes closed is increased compared to the other conditions between the Tibialis Anterior and the medial-lateral component and between the Quadriceps and each of the anterior-posterior and medial-lateral components. This suggests that in single-stance standing there is a stronger degree of synchronization between muscle activity and the external force.

The results thus indicate that in 2-leg standing EMG and foot-ground reaction forces signals correlate with each other to a very low extent, whereas under conditions of lower redundancy EMG & foot-ground reaction forces signals become more correlated together. It should be reminded, though, that the three ankle muscles treated here are not the sole actuators of postural sway. Posture models have dealt with both the ankle and hip joints, each as a two degree-of-freedom joint, thus presenting multi-joint, multi-actuator models. The models were represented by closed-chain and open-chain models for double (Levin and Mizrahi 1996, Levin et al 1998) and single-stance standing (Mizrahi et al 2002), respectively. On the other hand, the correlation between the medio–lateral component of the reaction force and the activity of the three shank muscles is higher than the correlation between the anterior–posterior component of the reaction force and the activity of these muscles. This can be explained by the higher postural sway in the medial–lateral direction compared to the anterior–posterior direction (Table 2).

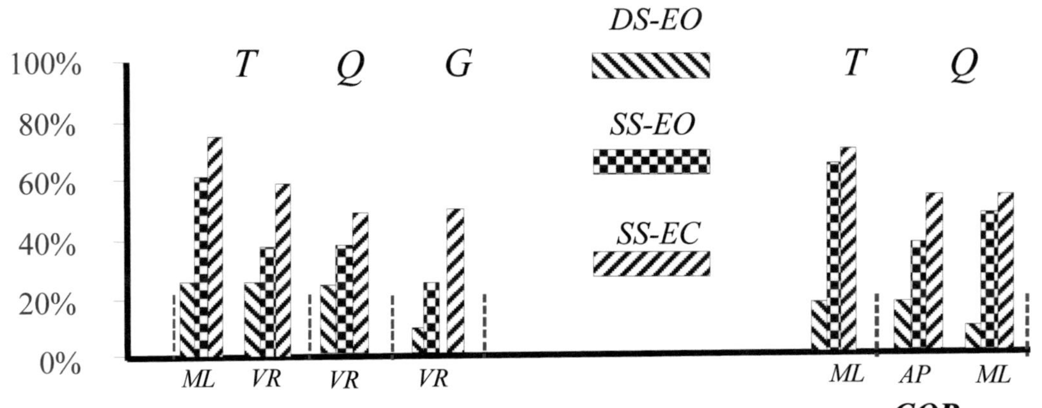

Fig. 4. Occurrence of significant correlation between the root mean square of the foot-ground reaction forces and root mean square of the EMG of three of the leg major muscles: Tibialis anterior (T), Quadriceps (Q) and Gluteus Maximus (G). Each of these muscles is correlated with the components of the foot-ground reaction forces and of the centre of pressure (COP). DS = double stance; SS = single stance; EO = eyes open; EC = eyes closed; ML = medial-lateral; VR = vertical; AP = anterior-posterior.

5.4 Effect of fatiguing of the shank muscles on single-leg-standing balance

Redundancy can be further reduced by temporarily incapacitating part of the lower leg muscles, through fatiguing. The fatiguing effect on single-stance standing sway dynamics was studied by means of two single-stance standing trials, separated by a quasi-isotonic sustained effort intended to induce fatigue of the Tibialis Anterior and Peroneus muscles (Suponitsky et al, 2008). In the standing trials the following quantities were on-line monitored: (a) force-plate data including ground reaction forces and center of pressure displacements to represent sway-related variables, and (b) EMG signals of the Tibialis Anterior, Peroneus and Gastrocnemius muscles, representing the muscular activity about the ankle joint.

Fatiguing of the dorsi-flexors (Tibialis Anterior and Peroneus) was induced by means of suspending a dead weight of 100 N on the dorsal aspect through a strap. The sustained effort consisted of holding this weight for 240s, while aiming to steadily maintain the ankle angle at 90 degrees, resulting in a quasi-isometric effort. To facilitate tracking of the ankle angle a goniometer was used to provide on-line visual feedback to the tested subject.

Force-plate and ankle angle data were low-pass filtered using an 8th order Butterworth digital filter with a cutoff frequency of 10 Hz. EMG data were filtered using a band-pass filter (5–500 Hz) with 8th order Butterworth digital filter. The traces were thereafter divided into equal segments and the root mean square of each segment was calculated and the obtained vectors were normalized by the total standing time. The obtained root mean square vectors were then interpolated by using cubic spline interpolation. To account for the individual variability in standing time, all vectors (EMG, Ground Reaction Forces and Center of Pressure displacements) were normalized by the total standing time and rescaled to the total number of points. The data collected during the standing trials were normalized as follows: EMG of the muscle signals by the respective maximal voluntary contractions of these muscles, reactive force data by the weight of the tested subject and center of pressure data by the subject's length or width of the foot, as appropriate. This allowed comparing the standing experiments among and between subjects, despite the differences in the standing duration.

During the fatiguing protocol the data obtained from the Tibialis Anterior and Peroneus muscles and from the goniometer were divided into equal segments of 6 s duration. Root mean square of the EMG and of the goniometer data and mean power frequency of the power spectral density function of the EMG signal for every segment were calculated. Muscle fatigue was determined from the following three parameters: (a) inability to steadily keep the ankle angle in the 90 deg position, i.e., significant drift towards plantar-flexion of the ankle, (b) a significant increase of the EMG root mean square, and (c) a significant decrease of the EMG mean power frequency. The fatigue trend was determined by simple linear regression for the goniometer and EMG data versus time.

The development of fatigue during the 240 s quasi-isometric effort is illustrated in Figure 5 for the Tibialis Anterior muscle. Linear regression of the root mean square of the EMG signal (time domain) and mean power frequency (frequency domain) indicate a statistically significant increase of EMG root mean square and decrease of EMG mean power frequency.

Simple and multiple linear regressions with standard least-squares procedures were used to evaluate the fatigue effects on the relationship between the muscles EMG and the sway-related parameters in the pre- and post-fatigue conditions. The results are presented in Table 4: Pearson's correlation r, pre- and post-load conditions; synergistic activity of the Tibialis Anterior and Gastrocnemius muscles. As the result of fatigue, Muscle/Force correlation increased and became higher in the medial-lateral direction compared to the anterior-posterior direction. The simple linear regression slope between root mean square of the reaction forces and the root mean square of the EMG of three shank muscles changed from an insignificant value in the preloading single stance standing trial, to a statistically significant value ($p < 0.05$) in the post-loading standing trial. Multiple correlations in the post-load trials gave moderate and high correlation levels, respectively, between reaction force in the medial-lateral and each of the pairs Tibialis Anterior and Peroneus, and Peroneus and Gastrocnemius muscles with statistically significant slopes ($p < 0.05$). High correlation levels were also obtained between the anterior-posterior force component and each of the following muscle combination: Peroneus and Gastrocnemius, and Tibialis Anterior and Gastrocnemius, with significant slopes ($p < 0.05$).

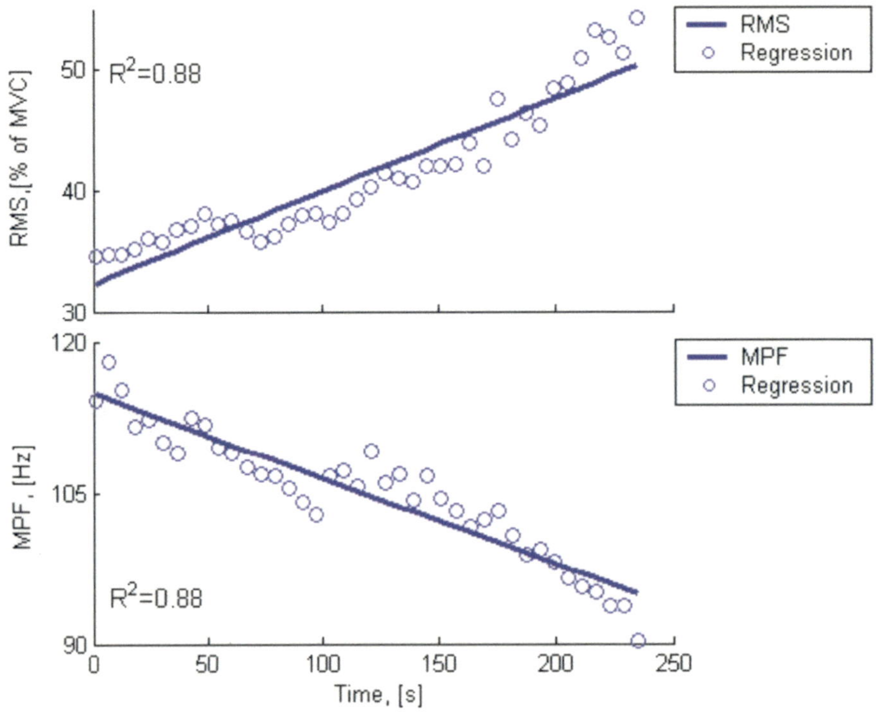

Fig. 5. Development of fatigue of the Tibialis Anterior muscle during the 240 s quasi-isometric effort. Root-mean square (RMS, top) and mean power frequency (MPF, bottom) of the EMG is averaged for five subjects.

6. Hybrid activation for muscle force enhancement

6.1 Partial, or incomplete, deficiency

Partial muscle force deficiency may be caused by a variety of reasons including, among others, incomplete spinal cord injury, stroke, cerebral palsy, muscle atrophy and ageing. Temporary deficiency may be the result of muscle fatigue [Mizrahi et al, 2000]. With partial deficiency, muscles can still be volitionally activated, although the resulting muscle force may be considerably lower as compared to those of healthy conditions.

Reaction Forces, vs	Pre/Post Fatigue	r	
		Medial-lateral	Anterior-posterior
Tibialis Anterior	Pre-Fatigue	0.17(0.03)	0.10(0.01)
	Post- Fatigue	0.69(0.05)*	0.62(0.02)*
Peroneal	Pre- Fatigue	0.03(0.01)	0.02(0.04)
	Post- Fatigue	0.82(0.09)**	0.73(0.04)**
Gastrocnemius	Pre- Fatigue	0.06(0.01)	0.17(0.03)
	Post- Fatigue	0.88(0.07)**	0.69(0.04)*
Tibialis Anterior & Gastrocnemius	Pre- Fatigue		0.31(0.09)
	Post- Fatigue		0.74(0.14)**

r = Pearson correlation coefficient
* medium correlation (r ~ 0.5-0.7)
** high correlation (r ~ 0.7-0.9)

Table 4. Linear regression between the EMG signal of the shank muscles and ground reaction forces, before and after fatigue (ML = medial–lateral component; AP = anterior–posterior component). All values are RMS [% MVC], normalized to the subject's weight and represent averages (SD) for all tested subjects

6.2 The concept of hybrid activation

Electrical Stimulation (ES) of muscles is a well-known and common technique for the management of muscle force deficiency. While in complete paralysis muscle activation is the result of ES only, in incomplete paralysis muscle activation may generally result from the combined volitional and ES-induced activations. In these latter cases ES is being used for the enhancement of muscle force and for improvement of function and motion of human populations with muscle disabilities [Katz et al 2003, 2008; Langzam et al, 2006a, 2006b, 2007). This modality of muscle activation has been termed hybrid activation (Langzam et al, 2006b), whereby the muscle force results from the combined volitional and electrically-induced components.

The mechanisms of hybrid activation are not clear. Although the components of this modality were separately investigated and reported, the physiological and mathematical patterns of this added effect are not entirely understood and the question of specific partition of the total muscle torque between these components is recently gaining increasing interest.

6.3 The partition of total torque into volitional and induced components

For one thing, hybrid activation can not be considered a simple summation of its components due to possible interactions between them. These interactions may be of the following types: (a) short-term, including reflex inhibition of the antagonistic muscles due to electrical stimulation of the agonistic muscles (Shoji et al, 2005), catch-like effects (Binder-Macleod et al, 2002), and stimulus rate modulation (if synchronized with the volitional pulse trains); (b) medium-term effects that can last for minutes after the ES pulse train was stopped, e.g., increased twitch forces (Eom et al, 2002), or enhanced cortico-spinal excitability (Thompson & Stein, 2004); (c) long-term changes following prolonged training involving strengthening of the muscle and remodulation of its fibers (Katz et al, 2003, 2008).

Apart from the better understanding of the mechanisms of hybrid activation, a major question of practical nature thus relates to the partition between the volitional and induced torques, within the overall torque. On the practical level, knowledge about the torque components can be readily utilized for muscle contraction manipulation.
In the presence of ES alone, the muscle is known to exhibit a typical recruitment curve (Levy et al, 1990), relating the stimulating current intensity to muscle force. However, when electrical stimulation is applied in addition to volitional activation of the muscle, the ES-induced component may not necessarily obey the recruitment curve displayed under ES alone. Thus, depending on the level of stimulation, the proportion between volitional and induced activations may vary.

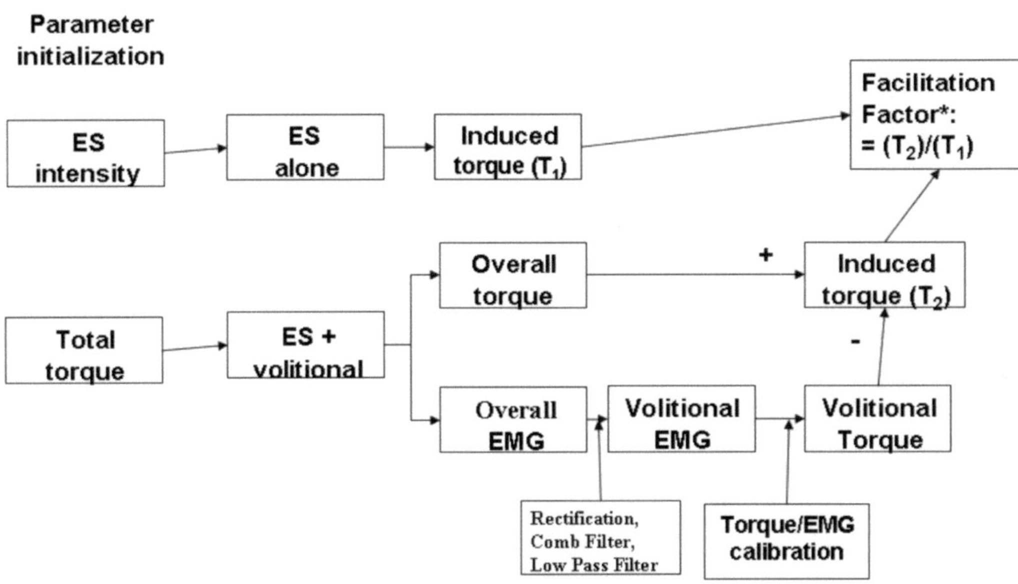

Fig. 6. Procedure for processing the monitored torque and EMG signals and definition of the facilitation factor. More details about the EMG processing are given in Fig. 7.

6.4 Past and recent works related to hybrid activation

Characterization of the sharing between the volitional and induced parts of activation has in the past been partly addressed. Early works evaluated the augmentation effect, though without addressing the hybrid operation mode of the muscle (Johnston et al, 2004; Pierce et al, 2004; Thorsen et al, 1999). Additional studies focused on the facilitation of the volitional force due to the accumulated training effect with ES, but did not address the effect of facilitation during stimulation (Katz et al, 2003; Knash et al, 2003; Liron-Keshet et al, 2001; Thompson & Stein, 2004).
The more recent studies dealing with the actual hybrid modality of activation [Langzam et al, 2006a, 2006b, 2007] go well beyond the previous ones, where the volitional EMG is used solely as a bio-trigger for the external stimulator in a hybrid contraction system (Peasgood et al, 2000; Rakos et al, 1999; Thorsen et al, 1999, 2002). In those recent studies the myoelectric signal assumes a key role.

6.5 The role of electromyograms in hybrid activation

In the recent studies dealing with hybrid activation [Langzam et al, 2006a, 2006b, 2007], the tested subjects were requested to track in real-time a visually displayed torque-time profile by activating the Tibialis Anterior muscle through the application of a dorsi-flexion torque at the ankle. Tracking was made in two modes of activation: 1) purely volitional activation, for calibration and system identification of the volitional component, and 2) hybrid activation, where volitional and ES-induced activations took place simultaneously. The general features of the target torque that the subjects were required to track mimicked different activities the Tibialis Anterior torque, such as observed during human gait. While performing the task, the subject was asked to maintain the torque trace within displayed limits on the feedback screen in front of them. During tracking, the applied ankle torque and the EMG of the Tibialis Anterior muscle were on-line monitored.

The myoelectric signal assumes a major role in dissociating between the volitional and induced torque components. It should be emphasized, however, that apart from specially designed signal processing, signal acquisition necessitates appropriate apparatus and stimulus artifact elimination (Minzly et al, 1993a, 1993b). The monitored signals were thus processed using the procedure outlined in Figure 6. The torque signals were first filtered (4th order Butterworth, cutoff frequency 100 Hz). For the EMG signals (Figure 7) a comb-filter was used to extract the volitional EMG from the overall raw EMG signals. A comb filter is a simple finite response filter, with adjustable parameters to match the stimulus frequency and to remove the ES component from the compound EMG signal. A more complete description of the filter is given elsewhere (Langzam et al 2006b; Thorsen et al 1999). The volitional EMG was rectified and filtered (4th order Butterworth low pass filter, cutoff frequency 5 Hz) to generate the voluntary EMG envelope. Using EMG values (envelope of the rectified signal) in the EMG–torque calibration curve yielded the volitional part of the torque within the total torque.

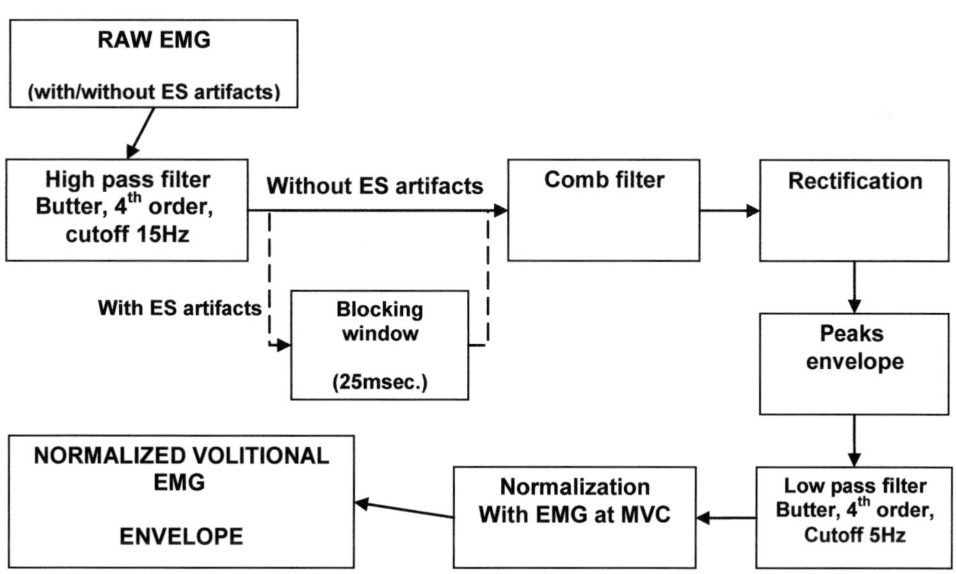

Fig. 7. Procedure used for dissociating between the induced and volitional components of the EMG signal in Hybrid Activation of the muscle.

The induced torque during hybrid activation was calculated as the difference between the total applied torque and the volitional torque. The obtained induced torque was then converted to current intensity by means of a pre-prepared recruitment calibration curve. This gave the equivalent current intensity, i.e., the intensity that would have produced the same torque during the muscle calibration process. The Facilitation Factor was defined as the ratio between this equivalent intensity and the actual current intensity during the hybrid activation experiment. Facilitation factor values can be greater than, equal, or smaller than one. When greater than one, this means that the equivalent current is greater than the actual stimulation current, therefore the produced induced torque is higher than expected. When the facilitation factor equals one, this means that both equivalent and actual currents are equal; therefore the expected induced torque is actually obtained, and that the electrical stimulation recruitment curve remains unchanged in hybrid compared to isolated stimulation. Facilitation factor lesser than one means that the equivalent current is lower than the actual stimulation current; therefore the produced induced torque is lower than expected. It should be noted that facilitation factors greater or smaller than one indicate that under the hybrid mode of activation, compared to the isolated conditions, changes in the actual stimulation recruitment curves take place.

6.6 Facilitation factor

Figure 8 exhibits typical results of the Facilitation Factor. A power regression curve was used to mathematically describe the facilitation factor versus current intensity. Initially, the facilitation factor value starts off at the lower intensity values of 3–6 mA with values greater than unity. Following a gradual decrease, the facilitation factor crosses the unity value termed as unity-crossing which is in this case at the current intensity of 6.5 mA, after which the facilitation factor values become smaller than unity. From this intensity onward, the combined torque effect in hybrid activation is smaller than the algebraic sum of the volitional and the ES-induced, as would have obtained from the recruitment curve. A facilitation factor greater than unity in the lower current range, indicates that muscle force augmentation is cost-effective. Conversely, a facilitation factor smaller than unity at the higher range of current intensity, indicates that augmentation becomes less effective. The results presented in Figure 8 indicate that although the hybrid torque is a linear combination of its volitional and induced components, it is not the simple summation of these components when acting alone. Clearly, the existence of an ES intensity range where the induced torque is enhanced compared to its expected contribution is of practical significance.

Summary of all tested subjects of Facilitation Factor versus ES intensity and of unity crossing is given in Table 5. This summary confirms that the effectiveness of the electrically-induced contribution in hybrid activation is highly dependent on the stimulation intensity. The facilitation factor parameter sheds light on the intensity ranges in which the effectiveness of the augmentation phenomenon is higher or lower. An increased effectiveness is indicated when torque augmentation exceeds the torque value resulting from the facilitation factor recruitment curve. Such a situation takes place at the lower intensity values.

6.7 Possible reasons for altered effectiveness of the activation components in Hybrid activation

Although the reasons for the changed effectiveness of the electrical activation are not clear, several possibilities can be suggested.

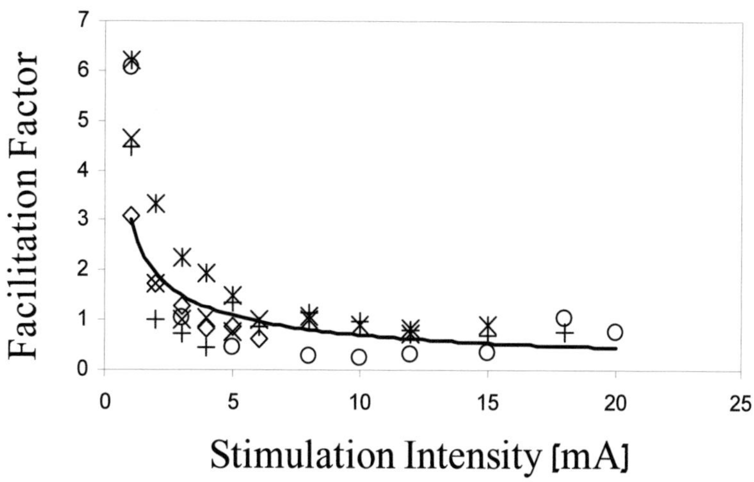

Fig. 8. Typical Facilitation Factor (defined in Fig. 6) as obtained from one subject. The solid curve represents regression of data ($y = ax^b$). The symbols indicate different testing days of the same subject.

Intensity (mA)	Average (SD)
1	3.52 (1.33)
5	1.41 (0.48)
10	0.96 (0.32)
15	0.77 (0.25)
30	0.52 (0.18)
Unity Crossing	9.83 (5.95)

Table 5. Summary for tested subjects of Facilitation Factor (defined in Fig. 6) versus stimulation intensity (mA), and of unity crossing.

(a) Mechanical redundancy of the musculo-skeletal system that enables the body to generate a given torque by several different activation patterns.

(b) Lack of specificity of the transcutaneous stimulation technique that may result in possible additional activation of nearby muscles to the Tibialis Anterior muscle itself or co-activation of the antagonistic muscles (Levin et al, 2000b).

(c) Recruitment pattern of an excited muscle that suggests that when both volitional and induced excitations act on the same part of the muscle, the fibers will respond to one excitation only. In hybrid activation mode, part of the muscle fibers may become inactive. Thus, during simultaneous excitation, the torque generated is expected to be lower than the summation of torques obtained when each excitation is performed alone, as there might be a disruption of the volitional excitation of some fibers by the presence of ES. Thus, the excitation preference may well be re-directed in hybrid activation. Besides, the effectiveness of the induced ES contribution is highly dependent on stimulation intensity. A counter-acting effect may be facilitation of volitional activation, due to the presence of the induced component. This effect has also been reported in the excitation of common peroneal nerve during transcranial magnetic stimulation (Thompson & Stein, 2004).

(d) Sensory effects of ES: it is likely that the hybrid activation not only directly elicited action potentials in motor axons, but also influenced the discharge of the motor neurons due to the sensory feedback associated with the ES-reflex response (Knash et al, 2003; Thompson & Stein, 2004).

The above-mentioned factors may thus provide an explanation to the non-additive properties between the volitional and induced torque components under hybrid muscle contraction, i.e., the torque is not the simple summation of its components (when each is acting alone).

Hybrid activation of muscles, combining volitional and ES-assisted excitations, introduces a powerful rehabilitation tool for populations suffering from deficiencies and requiring muscle force augmentation, enabling dynamic enhancement of their muscles. Understanding the interactions between the factors involved in Hybrid muscle activation is crucial to determine the intensity ranges where the ES component is more effective for force enhancement and to indicate the optimal mode of hybrid activation. The computational method presented demonstrates the key role of the myoelectric signals in partitioning the overall total torque obtained in hybrid activation into its two activation components, volitional and ES-induced. The induced torque component was calculated as the difference between overall and volitional torque and, together with the ES intensity-torque calibration data, determined the required intensity profile of the stimulation required for muscle force augmentation.

While the concept of hybrid activation was illustrated on the Tibialis Anterior muscle, it may be generalized to any other muscle. From the measured EMG it has been demonstrated how augmentation of the volitional torque can be computed at any given stimulation level. Conversely, the stimulation level can be indicated for a required force enhancement. The relationships between volitional, induced and overall torques provide the 'torque-lines' that can be used for the quantitative assessment of force enhancement in hybrid stimulation. The ability to predict the stimulation level required to achieve a given force augmentation enables us to better control, track, and analyze behavior and to provide the subject with a more customized, thus effective, treatment.

7. Conclusion

The role of electromyography in biomechanics and kinesiology was presented here in the context of redundancies of the neuro-muscular system. These redundancies introduce indeterminacies in the dynamic system, whereby the number of unknowns exceeds the number of available equations, hindering the possibilities to reach the actual physiological solution. It was shown that when redundancies are reduced, the system becomes less indeterminate and at cases it may become unequivocally soluble. It is in these cases where electromyographic data assume a crucial role.

Within the examples given to demonstrate the effects of reduced redundancy, it was shown that EMG data may resolve segment kinematics of the lower limb. This was demonstrated for the ankle joint through the combined activation of the ankle antagonist muscles. Further, the electromyograms were shown to provide indication about posture regulation through increased correlation with the externally measurable reactive forces, in cases of reduced redundancy through single stance standing or through fatiguing of part of the muscles.

Particularly, the results obtained have demonstrated that muscle fatigue evokes an increased correlation between the activity of the major muscles of the ankle and the sway related parameters, implying that higher levels in the nervous system become more unequivocally related to lower levels. The results thus obtained can serve for the detection of posture disorders in elderly populations or following spinal or lower limb injuries. The resulting activation modes of the muscles can serve as feasible activation modes in cases where functional electrical stimulation is used for the enhancement of muscle forces. The last example dealt with the information that EMG may provide to determine the effectiveness of hybrid activation of handicapped muscles.

8. Acknowledgement

This Chapter is partly based on results obtained in the Author's Biomechatronics Laboraory, Department of Biomedical Engineering, Technion - Israel Institute of Technology. The Author acknowledges the contribution of his former collaborators and graduate students, particularly O. Brion, D. Daily, A. Katz, E. Langzam, O. Levin, M. Levy, S. Liron-Keshet, D. Russek and Y. Suponitsky. The study was supported in part by the Israel Ministry of Science and Technology.

9. References

Bechtol, C.O. (1975). Normal Human Gait, In: *Atlas of Orthotics*, J.H. Bowker & C.B. Hall, (Eds.), pp. 133-143, Mosby, St. Louis.

Bendat, J.S. & Piersol, A.G. (1970). *Random Data: Analysis and Measurement Procedures*, Wiley & sons, Hoboken, NJ, USA.

Binder-Macleod, S. A.; Dean, J. C. & Ding, J. (2002). Electrical Stimulation Factors in Potentiation of Human Quadriceps Femoris. *Muscle Nerve*, vol. 25, pp. 271–279.

Bourdin, M.; Belli, A.; Arsac, L.M.; Bosco, C. & Lacour, J.R. (1995). Effect of vertical loading on energy cost and kinematics of running in trained male subjects. *Journal of Applied Physiology*, Vol. 79:6, pp. 2078-2085.

Buczek, F.L. & Cavanagh, P.R. (1990). Stance Phase Knee and Ankle Kinematics and Kinetics during Level and Downhill Running, *Med. Sci. Sports Exerc*, Vol 22:5, pp. 669-677.

Cavanagh, P.R. (1990). *Biomechanics of Distance Running*, Human Kinetics Books, Champaign, IL, USA, pp. 165-188.

Colson, S.; Pousson, M.; Martin, A. & Van Hoecke, J. (1999). Isokinetic Elbow Flexion and Coactivation Following Eccentric Training, *J. Electromyography & Kinesiology*, Vol. 9 pp. 13-20.

Daily, D. (1998). *Mechanical Factors in Shock Transmission in the Human Body: Effect of Muscle Fatigue*". Research Thesis for the Degree of Master of Science (J. Mizrahi and Y. Ben-Haim supervisors),, Technion, Israel Institute of Technology, Haifa, Israel.

De Luca, C. (1997). The Use of Surface Electromyography in Biomechanics, *J. of Applied Biomechanics*, Vol. 13, pp. 135-163.

Eom, G. M.; Watanabe, T.; Hoshimiya, N.& Khang, G. (2002). Gradual Potentiation of Isometric Muscle Force during Constant Electrical Stimulation, *Med. Biol. Eng. Comput.*, Vol. 40, pp. 137–143.

Genadry, W.F.; Kearney, R.E. & Hunter, I.W. (1988). Dynamic Relationship Between EMG and Torque at the Human Ankle: Variation with Contraction Level and Modulation, *Med Biol Eng Comput*, Vol. 26, pp. 489-493.

Giat, Y.; Mizrahi, J. & Levy, M. (1993). A Muscolutendon Model of the Fatigue Profiles of Paralyzed Quadriceps Muscle under FES, *IEEE Trans. Biomed. Eng.*, Vol. 40, no. 7, pp. 664-674.

IEEE. *Programs for Digital Signal Processing*. (1979) IEEE Press, John Wiley & Sons, ISBN-13: 978-0471059622, New York.

Johnston, T. E.; Finson, R. L.; McCarthy, J. J.; Smith, B. T.; Betz, R. R.; & Mulcahey, M. J. (2004). Use of Functional Electrical Stimulation to Augment Traditional Orthopedic Surgery in Children with Cerebral Palsy, *J. Pediatr. Orthop.*, Vol. 24, pp. 283–291.

Katz, A.; Tirosh, E.; Isakov, E. & Mizrahi, J. (2003). Below-Threshold FES in CP: Long-Term Training versus Orthosis Effect, *7th Terme Euganee Meeting Rehabil.*, pp. 233–233, Padova, Italy, June 14–15, 2003.

Katz, A.; Tirosh, E.; Marmur, R. & Mizrahi, J. (2008). Enhancement of Muscle Activity by Electrical Stimulation in Cerebral Palsy - a Case Control Study. *J. Child Neurology*, Vol.23, pp. 259-267.

Kellis, E. & Baltzopoulos, V. (1998). Muscle Activation Differences between Eccentric and Concentric Isokinetic Exercise, *Med & Science in Sports and Exercise*, Vol.30(11), pp. 1616-1623.

Knash, M. E.; Kido, A.; Gorassini, M.; Chan, K. M. & Stein, R. (2003). Electrical Stimulation of the Human Common Peroneal Nerve Elicits Lasting Facilitation of Cortical Motor-Evoked Potential, *Exp. Brain Res.*, Vol. 153, pp. 366–377.

Langzam, E., Nemirovsky, Y., Isakov, E., & Mizrahi, J. (2006a). Partition Between Volitional and Induced Forces in Electrically Augmented Dynamic Muscle Contractions. *IEEE Trans. on Neural Systems & Rehabilitation Engineering*, Vol.14, pp, 322-335.

Langzam, E.; Isakov, E. & Mizrahi J. (2006b). Evaluation of Methods for Extraction of the Volitional EMG in Dynamic Hybrid Muscle Activation, *Journal of NeuroEngineering and Rehabilitation*, Vol.3, 27.

Langzam, E., Nemirovsky, Y., Isakov, E. & Mizrahi, J. (2007). Muscle Enhancement Using Closed-Loop Electrical Stimulation: Volitional Versus Induced Torque. *J Electromyogr Kinesiol.*, Vol.17, pp.275-284.

Levin, O. & Mizrahi, J. (1996). An Iterative Model for the Estimation of the Trajectory of Center of Gravity from Bilateral Reactive Force Measurements in Standing Sway. *Gait & Posture*, Vol.4, pp. 89–99.

Levin, O.; Mizrahi, J. & Shoham, M. (1998). Standing Sway: Iterative Estimation of the Kinematics and Dynamics of the Lower Extremities from Force-Plate Measurements. *Biol Cybern*, Vol.78, pp. 319–27.

Levin, O.; Mizrahi, J.; Adam, D., Verbitsky, O. & Isakov, E. (2000a). On the Correlation Between Force Plate Data and EMG in Various Standing Conditions, In: *Proceedings of the Fifth Annual Conference of the International Functional Electrical Stimulation Society*, T. Sinkjaer, D. Popovic & J.J. Struijk (Eds), pp. 47–50, Center for Sensory-Motor Interaction, Aalborg University, Denmark,. June 18–24, 2000.

Levin, O.; Mizrahi, J. & Isakov, E. (2000b). Transcutaneous FES of Paralyzed Quadriceps: Is Knee Torque Affected by Unintended Activation of the Hamstrings? *J. Electromyogr. Kinesiol*, Vol.10, pp. 47–58.

Levy, M.; Mizrahi, J. & Suzak, Z. (1990). Recruitment, Force and Fatigue Characteristics of Quadriceps Muscles of Paraplegics, Isometrically Activated by Surface FES. *J. Biomed. Eng.*, Vol.12, pp. 150–156.

Liron-Keshet, S.; Tirosh, E.; Mizrahi, J.; Verbitsky, O.; Isakov, E.; Marmur, R. & Rabino, S. (2001). The Effect of Therapeutic Electrical Stimulation in Children with Diplegic Cerebral Palsy as Measured by Gait Analysis. *Basic Appl. Myol.*, Vol. 11, pp. 127–132.

Marple-Horvat, D.E. & Gilbey, S.L. (1992). A Method for Automatic Identification of Periods of Muscular Activity from EMG Recordings. *J. of Neuroscience Methods*, Vol. 42, pp. 163-167.

Minzly, J.; Mizrahi, J.; Hakim, N. & Liberson, A. (1993a). Stimulus Artifact Suppressor for EMG Recordings during FES by Constant-Current Stimulator. *Med Biol Eng Comput*, Vol.31(1), pp. 72-75.

Minzly, J.; Mizrahi, J.; Isakov, E.; Susak, Z., & Verbeke, M. (1993b). Computer-Controlled Portable Stimulator for Paraplegic Patients. *J Biomed Eng*, Vol.15(4), pp. 333-338.

Mizrahi, J. (2004). *Muscle/Bone Interactions in the Musculo-Skeletal System*. Published by the Center of Excellence for Applied Biomedical Modelling and Diagnostics, Warsaw, ISSN 1733-0874.

Mizrahi, J., Brion, O. and Adam, D. (2002) Open-Chain analysis of single stance. *J. Automatic Control*, 12: 46-55.

Mizrahi, J.; Levy, M.; Ring, H.; Isakov, E. & Liberson, A. (1994). EMG as an Indicator of Fatigue of Isometrically FES-Activated Paralyzed Muscles. *IEEE Trans. Rehab. Eng.*, Vol.2, pp. 57-65.

Mizrahi, J.; Verbitsky, O.; Isakov, E. & Daily, D. (2000). Effect of Fatigue on Leg Kinematics and Impact Acceleration in Long Distance Running. *Human Movement Science*, Vol.19 (2), pp. 139-151.

Mizrahi, J.; Verbitsky, O. & Isakov, E. (2001). Fatigue-Induced Changes in Decline Running, *Clin Biomech*, Vol.16 (3), pp. 207-212.

Mizrahi, J. & Susak, Z. (1989). Bilateral Reactive Force Patterns in Postural Sway Activity of Normal Subjects. *Biol Cybern*, Vol.60, pp. 297–305.

Nardone, A.; Tarantola, J.; Giordano, A. & Schieppati, M. (1997). Fatigue Effects on Body Balance. *Electroen Clin Neuro*, Vol.105, pp. 309–20.

Nilsson, J.; Thorstensson, A. & Halbertsma, J (1985). Changes in the Leg Movements and Muscle Activity with Speed of Locomotion and Mode of Progression in Humans. *Acta Physiol. Scand*, Vol.123 (4), pp. 457-475.

Oppenheim, A.V. & Schafer, R.W. (1975). *Digital Signal Processing*, Prentice-Hall, Saddle River, NJ.

Peasgood, W.; Whitlock, T.; Baman, A.; Fry, M.E.; Jones, R.S. & Davis-Smith, A. (2000). EMG-Controlled Closed Loop Electrical Stimulation Using Digital Signal Processor. *Electron Lett*, Vol.36(22), pp.1832-1833.

Patriarco, A.G.; Mann, R.W.; Simon, S.R.; & Mansour, J.M. (1981). An Evaluation of the Approaches of Optimization Models in the Prediction of Muscle Forces During Human Gait. *J Biomech.*, Vol.14, pp. 513-525.

Peng, C.W.; Chen, S.C.; Lai, C.H.; Chen, C.J.; Chen, C.C.; Mizrahi, J. & Handa, Y. (2011). Clinical Benefits of Functional Electrical Stimulation Cycling Exercise for Subjects with Central Neurological Impairments: Review, *Journal of Medical and Biological Engineering*, 31(1), pp. 1-11.

Pierce, S. R.; Laughton, C. A.; Smith, B. T.; Orlin, M. N.; Johnston, T. E. & McCarthy, J. J. (2004). Direct Effect of Percutaneous Electrical Stimulation During Gait in Children with Hemiplegic Cerebral Palsy: A Report of 2 Cases. *Arch. Phys. Med. Rehabil.*, Vol.85, pp. 339–343.

Prilutsky, B.I.; Gregor, R.J. & Ryan, M.M. (1998). Coordination of Two-Joint Rectus Femoris and Hamstrings during the Swing Phase of Human Walking and Running. *Exp. Brain Res.*, Vol.120, pp. 479-486.

Rakos, M.; Freudenschuss, B.; Girsch, W.; Hofer, C.; Kaus, J.; Meiners, T.; Paternostro, T. & Mayr, W. (1999). Electromyogram-Controlled Functional Electrical Stimulation for Treatment of Paralyzed Upper Extremity. *Artif Organs*, Vol.23(5), pp. 466-469.

Russek, D. (2002). *The Relation between EMG and Kinematics in Running Fatigue*, MSc Thesis (J. Mizrahi supervisor), Library System No. 002246490, Technion, Israel Institute of Technology, Haifa, Israel.

Saxena, S.; Nikolic, S. & Popovic, D. (1995). An EMG-Controlled System for Tetraplegics. *J Rehabil Res Dev*, Vol.32 (1), pp. 17-24.

Shoji, J.; Kobayashi, K.; Ushiba, J.; Kagamihara, Y. & Masakado, Y. (2005). Inhibition from the Plantar Nerve to Soleus Muscle during the Stance Phase of Walking. *Brain Res.*, Vol.1048, pp. 48–58.

Shumway-Cook, A.; & Woollacott, M. (1995). Motor Control: Theory and Practical Applications, Williams & Wilkins, Baltimore, MD.

Suponitsky, Y., Verbitsky, O., Peled, E., and Mizrahi J. (2008) Effect of Force Imbalance of the Shank Muscles, due to Selective Fatiguing, on Single-Leg-Standing Control, *J. Electromyography and Kinesiology*, 18:682-689.

Tamaki, H.; Kitada, K. & Akamine, T. (1997). Electromyogram Patterns during Plantarflexions at Various Angular Velocities and Knee Angles in Human Triceps Surae Muscles. *Eur. J. Appl. Physiology*, Vol.75, pp. 1-6.

Thompson, K. & Stein, R. B. (2004). Short-term effects of functional electrical stimulation on motor-evoked potentials in ankle flexor and extensor muscles. *Exp. Brain Res.*, Vol.159, pp 491–500.

Thorsen, R.; Ferrarin, M.; Spadone, R. & Frigo, C. (1999). Functional Control of the Hand in Tetraplegics Based on Residual Synergistic EMG Activity. *Artif Organs*, Vol.23(5), pp. 470-473.

Thorsen, R.; Spandone, R. & Ferrarin, M. (2001). A Pilot Study of Myoelectrically Controlled FES of Upper Extremity. *IEEE Trans Neural Syst Rehabil Eng*, Vol.9 (2), pp. 161-168.

Thorsen, R.; Ferrarin, M. & Veltink, P. (2002). Enhancement of Isometric Ankle Dorsiflexion by Automyoelectrically Controlled Functional Electrical Stimulation on Subjects with Upper Motor Neuron Lesions. *Neuromodulation*, Vol.5 (4), pp. 256-263.

Tropp H, Odenrick P. Postural control in single-limb stance. J Orthopedic Res 1988;6:833–9.

Vuillerme, N.; Danion, F.; Forestier, N. & Nougier, V. (2002). Postural Sway Under Muscle Vibration and Muscle Fatigue in Humans. *Neurosci Lett*, Vol.333, pp. 131–5.

Winter, D.; Prince, F.; Frank, J.; Powell, C. & Zabjek, K. (1996). Unified Theory Regarding A/P and M/L Balance in Quiet Stance. *J Neurophysiol*, vol.75, pp. 2334–43.

Winter, D.A. & Scott, S.H. (1991). *Technique for Interpretation of Electromyography for Concentric and Eccentric Contractions in Gait. J. of Electromyog. and Kinesiol.*, Vol.1(4), pp. 263-269.

Yaggie, J. & McGregor, S. (2002). Effects of Isokinetic Ankle Fatigue on the Maintenance of Balance and Postural Limits. *Arch Phys Med Rehabil*, Vol.83, pp. 224–8.

2

Electromyography Assessment of Muscle Recruitment Strategies During High-Intensity Exercise

François Billaut
School of Sport and Exercise Science, Institute of Sport Exercise and Active Living (ISEAL), Victoria University, Melbourne Australia

1. Introduction

Electromyography (EMG) is an experimental technique concerned with the recording and analysis of myoelectric signals. Since the EMG signal detected on the surface of the skin directly reflects the recruitment and firing characteristics of the detected motor units within an area, EMG activity can be used to study the neuromuscular activation of muscles within postural tasks, functional movements, work conditions and treatment/training regimes (Basmajian and De Luca 1985). Furthermore, EMG activity has been correlated on multiple occasions with fatigue-related events occurring within the muscle (Bigland-Ritchie et al. 1986a; Bigland-Ritchie and Woods 1984; Moritani et al. 1986; Nordlund et al. 2004). Other chapters in this book describe the use of EMG for various applications. In the exercise sciences, EMG activity is typically used to explore muscle recruitment strategies (*i.e.*, time-dependent, internal, physiological modifications) and, thereby, understand the complex relationship between the development of locomotor muscle fatigue and the cortical regulation of exercise intensity (Billaut et al. 2010; Marino 2004). Neuromuscular fatigue can be induced by sustained muscular contractions. It is essentially accompanied by external manifestations such as the inability to maintain a desired force output, muscular tremor, and localized pain. The effects of this fatigue are localized to the muscle or group of synergistic muscles performing the contraction. According to several authors (Bigland-Ritchie 1984; Fitts 1994; Gandevia 2001; Merton 1954; Szubski et al. 2007), this fatigue may have its source peripherally (within the muscle tissue or neuromuscular junction) and/or centrally (within the brain and spinal cord). During fatigue the EMG activity may display two typical characteristics. The first is a change in amplitude (Figure 1), whereby additional motor units are recruited or already-active motor units are de-recruited. The second characteristic is a shift of the EMG power frequency spectrum (Figure 2), which shows the relative electrical activity contributed by slow (on the left) or fast (on the right) motor units. A leftward shift suggests increased stimulation of smaller, slow, fatigue-resistant motor units.

However, studies have mainly explored constant work-rate tests, along with incremental tests to maximum effort. In these examples, ecological validity has been limited due to work rate being either fully or partly dictated by the protocol; this excludes the individual subjective assessment of the task. Because performance in competitive events depends largely upon pacing strategies (Figure 3) (Billaut et al. 2011; Hettinga et al. 2006; Palmer et al. 1997; Paterson and Marino 2004; St Clair Gibson et al. 2006), it is necessary to investigate the neuromuscular responses to self-paced exercise to further understand the role of the central nervous system (CNS) in the regulation of exercise performance. Thus, a more realistic paradigm for future research in the exercise sciences is one that would permit the individual to use sensory cues to adjust the effort along with the fatigue process. In fact, Marino and colleagues (2011) recently re-emphasised that bringing the brain (and subsequent muscle recruitment strategies) into modern fatigue research represents the next phase in the unravelling of the fatigue process.

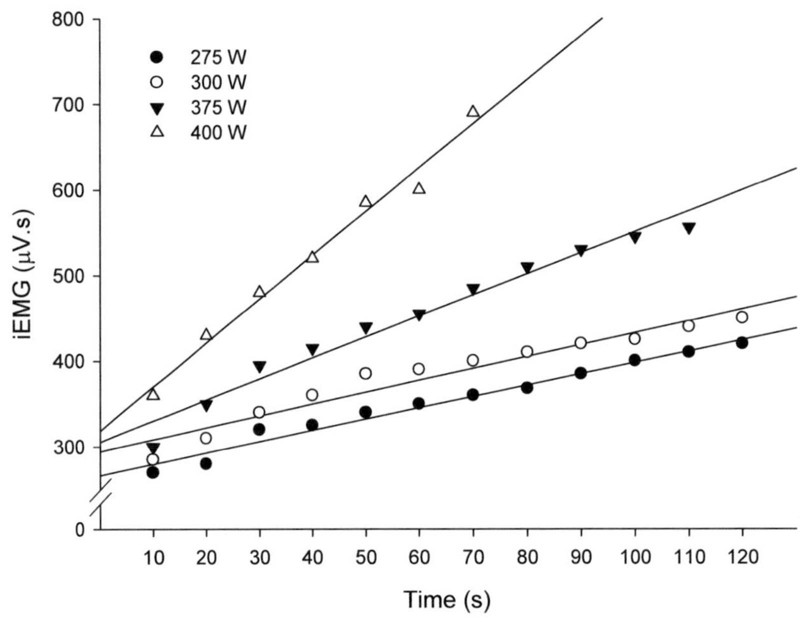

Fig. 1. Typical increase in EMG amplitude (represented on the y axis as integrated EMG, μV.s) with time (s) at constant intensities (275, 300, 350 and 400 watts). The increase in iEMG indicates the recruitment of additional motor units by the central nervous system to maintain the required power output as time (and fatigue) goes on. It can be seen that the slope of the linear regression (rate of rise in iEMG as a function of time) is higher at higher intensities because fatigue occurs more quickly. It was therefore suggested that the non-invasive analysis of iEMG slope coefficient could provide a sensitive measure of motor unit fatigability. Modified from Moritani et al. (1993).

Traditionally, endurance exercise has been researched extensively but our understanding of the factors that regulate muscle recruitment during very high-intensity exercise is much poorer. This is surprising since 1) many sports (*e.g.*, team and court sports, athletics) involved burst of "all-out" activity (Billaut and Bishop 2009; Spencer et al. 2005), and 2) newly-developed training regimes targeted at improving health include repetitions of sprint exercise (Gibala 2007). Certainly, a greater understanding of neural recruitment strategies during high-intensity tasks would lead to better training programs to enhance fitness in athletes and patient populations.

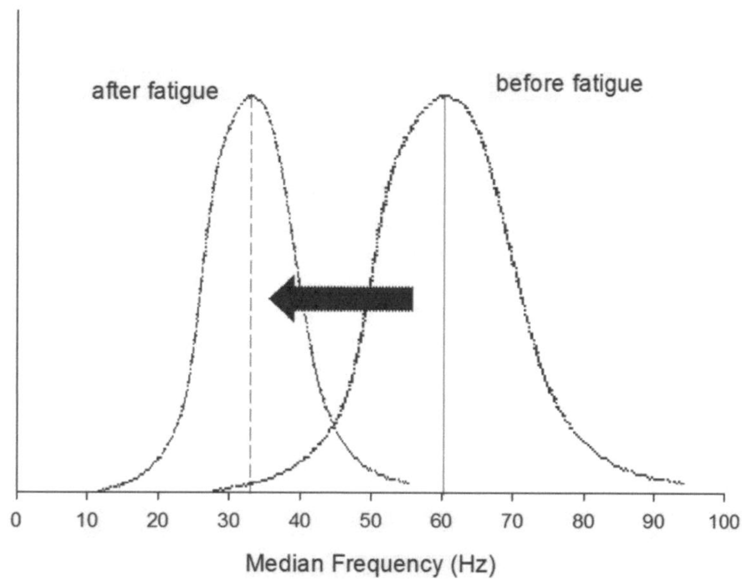

Fig. 2. Typical changes in EMG power frequency spectrum (Hz) of a muscle during a fatiguing contraction. The solid line indicates the pre-fatigue state, and the dash line indicates the fatigued state. The leftward shift in the EMG power frequency spectrum indicates the recruitment of more fatigue-resistant motor units (with lower firing frequency) to cope with the task constraint. The non-invasive analysis of the power spectra could provide a sensitive measure of motor unit fatigability that may reflect the activities of different types of muscle fibers.

Performing a sprint at "all-out" intensity requires very high levels of neural drive (typically +/- 5000 μV in elite sprinters) (Ross et al. 2001); therefore failure to activate fully the contracting musculature can theoretically decrease force and power production and, thereby, impair the ability to sprint. Whilst not a well-studied mode of exercise, several studies have demonstrated that the fatigue that develops during single and repeated sprints is associated with changes in muscle recruitment strategies which ultimately originate within the CNS. The aims of this chapter are 1) to use most recent data to describe the behaviour of the EMG signal (serving as a surrogate for muscle recruitment) during sprint exercise using traditional and innovative analysis techniques, and 2) to give some insights into the main mechanisms thought to contribute to the regulation of muscle recruitment and the fatigue process during sprint exercise.

2. A contemporary view of the fatigue phenomenon

For over a century, neuromuscular fatigue has been viewed and researched as a finite quantity of essential (metabolic and/or cardiovascular) resources causing exhaustion, independent of any regulation by the CNS (Allen et al. 1995; Bassett and Howley 2000; Fitts 1994; Hill 1924; Shephard 2009). This view has encouraged the interpretation that exercise results in linear changes in metabolism, in energy provision, and in the cardiovascular, respiratory, thermoregulatory, and hormonal responses, among many others. Ultimately, demand exceeds capacity in one or more systems, which causes them to fail. As a result, this failure to maintain homeostasis in the active muscles causes the termination of exercise. Overall, this has produced a "brainless" physiology (Marino 2004; Marino et al. 2011; Noakes 2011; Noakes et al. 2001) that is still currently taught in most exercise science classes throughout the world. In contrast, increasing evidence has accumulated in the last few years suggesting an anticipatory regulation of exercise intensity (Billaut et al. 2011; Kayser 2003; Marino 2004; Noakes 2011; Noakes et al. 2001; Noakes and St Clair Gibson 2004; St Clair Gibson et al. 2006; St Clair Gibson and Noakes 2004; Tucker et al. 2004). This mechanism allows feedback from varied sources to influence the magnitude of the feed-forward neural drive that determines the quantity of muscle mass recruited (*i.e.*, the number of motor units recruited in the exercising limbs). In this model, therefore, an athlete's pace is continuously regulated via the action of varied physiological and psychological inputs before and during exercise (Noakes 2011; Noakes and Tucker 2008; St Clair Gibson and Noakes 2004). In other words, the brain is able to anticipate a future failure and modify accordingly and in "real time" muscle recruitment and, hence, exercise intensity to ensure homeostasis is protected.

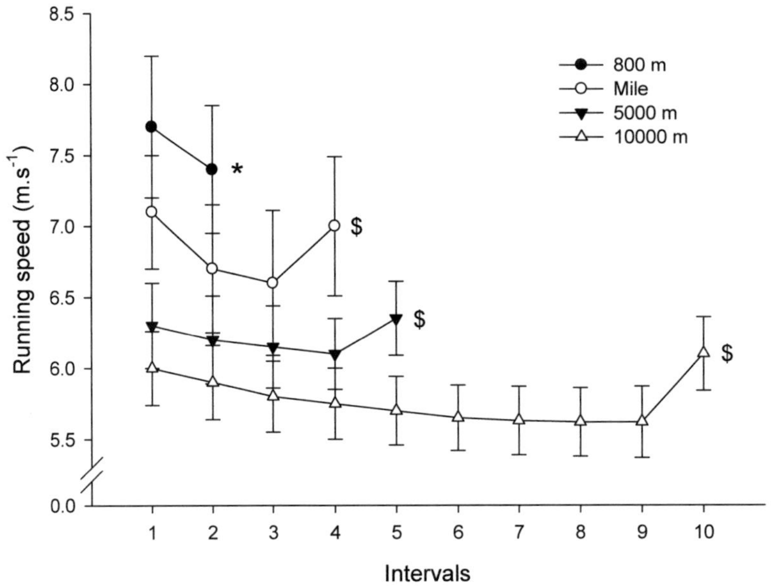

Fig. 3. Average running speed (meter.s^{-1}) for each interval during world-record performances in 800-m, 1-mile, 5000-m and 10000-m events. * Significantly slower than the first lap ($P < 0.05$). $ Significantly faster than the preceding interval ($P < 0.05$). This figure clearly shows different paces selected by athletes at the beginning of every race that depends upon the distance to run. The presence of an end-spurt is also shown in "endurance-type" events. Modified from Tucker et al. (2006a).

In this perspective, the results from several recent studies conducted on well-trained athletes and patient populations reveal that during high-intensity, constant-load and self-paced exercises participants terminate the task with a given level of severe locomotor muscle fatigue (assessed via quadriceps twitch force) that appears to be never exceeded under 'normal' exercise conditions, despite manipulations of exercise performance (Amann

2011; Amann et al. 2006a; Duffield et al. 2010; Romer et al. 2007; Saey et al. 2003). This end-exercise level of peripheral muscle fatigue has been purported to be task specific and to vary across participants (for review see (Amann 2011)). So, overall, in the early years of the 21st century, several scientists worldwide agree that the CNS constantly monitors and deliberately regulates and limits the development of peripheral fatigue in the exercising limbs (via changes in the extent of muscle recruitment). This may presumably be to avoid overtraining / overexertion and potentially long-lasting harmful consequences to critical organs (Amann 2011; Calbet 2006; Kayser 2003; Marino et al. 2011; Noakes 2011; Nybo and Secher 2004). Several physiological variables (*e.g.*, afferent feedback from exercising, fatiguing muscles (Amann et al. 2008; Amann et al. 2009), cerebral oxygenation (Billaut et al. 2010; Nielsen et al. 1999), rate of heat storage (Marino 2004; Marino et al. 2004; Tucker et al. 2006b)) would potentially be closely monitored depending upon the exercise conditions, and would influence more or less the CNS to attenuate muscle recruitment.

To the author's best knowledge, the presence of pacing during short and "all-out" sprints has been examined in one study. The authors (Billaut et al. 2011) deceived the participants to evaluate the degree of pacing depending upon the number of sprints to be performed. Astonishingly, the anticipation of performing fewer sprints (*i.e.*, 5 instead of 10) resulted in enhanced muscle recruitment (as evidenced by higher EMG activity in the lower limb), which was associated, in turn, with a higher mechanical output during the first 5 sprints. On the other hand, when participants were not informed of the actual sprint number they recruited less muscle and, hence, exhibited a lower mechanical output profile, despite similar levels of encouragement and similar perceived exertion. These results demonstrated that pacing occurs during short repeated-sprint efforts in anticipation of the number of sprints that are included in the trial (Billaut et al. 2011). Furthermore, it may be speculated from these findings that the pacing strategy adopted by these athletes has been mostly subconscious, because it is not clear how athletes can consciously regulate their muscle recruitment and power output precisely enough to account for such variations at this very high intensity and in this short time frame. Importantly, a key measure in all these experiments has been the central motor drive, namely muscle recruitment, which is directly assessed via EMG activity. Therefore, the investigation of EMG events holds a critical role in understanding humans' ability to cope with physical challenges.

3. Electromyographic events during single-sprint exercise

Although not extensively studied, changes in skeletal muscle recruitment may contribute to performance decrement during maximal sprint exercise. Vandewalle and colleagues (1991) observed a parallel decline in power output and integrated EMG of the *vastus lateralis* (average values not reported by the authors) during a 45-second cycle sprint, and suggested a progressive attenuation of spatial and/or temporal recruitment of motor units during the exercise. These findings are supported by another study that reported a ~15% ($P < 0.05$) decline in the integrated EMG of the plantar flexors and a ~15–19% ($P < 0.05$) reduction in the median frequency of the EMG power spectrum of the plantar flexors and the knee extensors during a 30-s Wingate anaerobic cycle sprint (Greer et al. 2006). While Hunter et al. (2003) did not observe any change in the EMG amplitude of the *vastus lateralis* muscle during a 30-second cycle sprint (whereas power output declined), the authors reported a shift of the mean power frequency towards lower values (–14.7%; $P < 0.05$). These acute frequency changes may be caused by an accumulation of metabolites and a consequent decrease in muscle pH, and/or some form of neural control through reflex regulation of muscle force to prevent excessive metabolic perturbations (De Luca 1997; Juel 1988; Noakes 2011; Noakes et al. 2004; St Clair Gibson et al. 2001). Unfortunately, skeletal muscle function was not examined in these studies (via maximal voluntary contraction and twitch technique), which precludes from drawing firm conclusions about the (maximal allowed) level of peripheral muscle fatigue at the end of these tasks. Clearly, more studies using electrically- or magnetically-evoked stimulation need to be conducted to clarify whether central motor drive parallels the power output decline observed during a single maximal effort and whether it is regulated in an anticipatory manner to limit development of excessive limb muscle fatigue.

4. Electromyographic events during repeated-sprint exercise

4.1 Muscle recruitment strategies

The first investigations of the changes of the EMG signal (serving as surrogate for muscle recruitment) provoked by "all-out" repeated sprints have only been conducted recently (Billaut and Basset 2007; Billaut et al. 2006; Giacomoni et al. 2006). These studies have examined the EMG activity of the quadriceps muscles during brief, maximal, isometric voluntary contractions of the knee extensors performed before and immediately after the ten 6-s sprints separated by 30 s of passive rest. In every case, the maximal knee extensors force was reduced after the sprints (average: ~12%; $P < 0.05$) and this was accompanied by a higher EMG activity (average: ~15%; $P < 0.05$). The authors also observed a concomitant decrease in frequency components, which suggests a modification in the pattern of muscle fibre recruitment and a decrease in conduction velocity of active fibres (Basmajian and De Luca 1985; De Luca 1997; Gerdle and Fugl-Meyer 1992; Linnamo et al. 2000; Moritani et al. 1986). In fact, during the final sprints, the relative contribution of less-powerful type I muscle fibres involved in the production of power may have increased as a result of the greater fatigability of type II muscle fibres, highly solicited during this type of exercise (Casey et al. 1996; Gerdle and Fugl-Meyer 1992; Komi and Tesch 1979; Ross et al. 2001). However, the conclusions from these studies may have been confounded by methodological factors. Indeed, while investigating EMG activity during isometric contractions may greatly reduce muscle movements underneath EMG electrodes and artefacts due to wire movements, and thus ease signal processing (Farina et al. 2004; Merletti and Lo Conte 1997), it is now well accepted that physiological responses and neuromuscular fatigue are highly task specific (Hunter 2009; Maluf and Enoka 2005). Accordingly, results and conclusions would be highly specific to the task performed, hence, the isometric contraction, with less relevance to the actual fatigue that develops during the repeated sprints.

More recently, muscle recruitment strategies have been investigated during sprints, and authors have reported a concurrent decline in mechanical performances and the amplitude of the EMG signal in primer-mover muscles (Billaut and Smith 2009; Billaut and Smith 2010; Mendez-Villanueva et al. 2007, 2008; Racinais et al. 2007; Smith and Billaut 2010). For example, Billaut and Smith (2010) demonstrated a ~15% decline ($P < 0.05$) in the quadriceps muscles EMG activity from the first to the twentieth cycle sprint of 5 s separated by 25 s of rest. Importantly, such a reduction in agonist muscle recruitment during repeated cycle sprints has been strongly correlated ($r = 0.91$ to 0.98, $P < 0.05$, Figure 4) with the decline in mechanical output (Billaut and Smith 2009; Billaut and Smith 2010; Mendez-Villanueva et al. 2008). That being said, it is interesting to note that when fatigue is moderate (*e.g.*, fatigue index or sprint decrement score is ~10% or lower), studies have typically reported a steady level of muscle recruitment during repeated-sprint exercise (Billaut and Basset 2007; Billaut et al. 2005; Girard et al. 2008; Hautier et al. 2000; Matsuura et al. 2007). However, when the neuromuscular fatigue level is more substantial (> 20%), a concurrent decline in mechanical performance and the amplitude of EMG signals has consistently been reported across sprint repetitions (Billaut et al. 2011; Billaut and Smith 2010; Mendez-Villanueva et al. 2007, 2008; Racinais et al. 2007; Smith and Billaut 2010). Furthermore, a reduction in the knee flexor EMG amplitude (*i.e.*, antagonist muscle) has been observed during fifteen cycle sprints of 5 s separated by 25 s of rest (Hautier et al. 2000). Overall, these data suggest that under conditions of considerable neuromuscular fatigue development the failure to fully activate the contracting musculature may become an important factor limiting performance during "all-out" sprint repetitions.

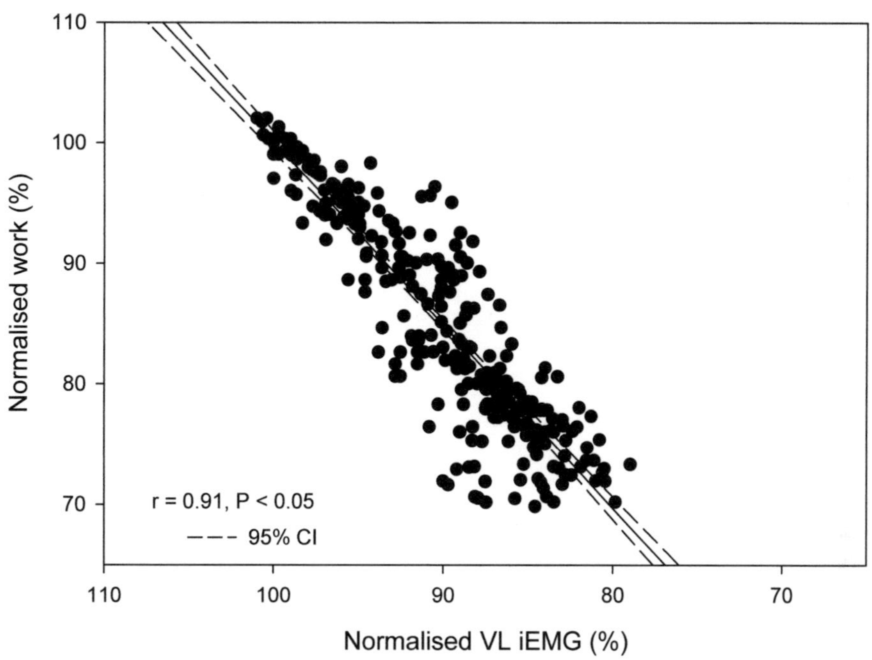

Fig. 4. Relationship of EMG amplitude (integrated EMG) of the *vastus lateralis* muscle (expressed as a percentage of initial-sprint value) to mechanical work (expressed as a percentage of initial-sprint value) performed over twenty 5-s cycle sprints interspersed by 25 s of rest. The correlation shows that the greater the drop in EMG amplitude the greater the drop in mechanical work [r = 0.91 (95% Confidence Interval, 0.75;0.97)]. The short-dashed lines represent 95% confident intervals. Reproduced from Billaut and Smith (2010) with permission.

4.2 Timing of muscle activation

Thus far, the above sections have particularly highlighted the importance of the "quantity" of EMG activity or muscle recruitment in the production of maximal power. During "all-out" actions, the timing of muscle activity also comes into play in determining neuromuscular performance. In fact, during sprint exercises maximal power production requires muscles to be fully activated during shortening and fully relaxed during lengthening phases (Neptune and Kautz 2001). Thus, when studying sprint exercises, the inter-muscle coordination patterns (*i.e.,* the kinematics of muscle activation and deactivation) should also be taken into account when analysing the fatigue process (Neptune and Kautz 2001; Prilutsky and Gregor 2000; Van Ingen Schenau et al. 1992). Muscle coordination is defined as a "distribution of muscle activation or force among individual muscles to produce a given combination of joint moments" (Prilutsky and Gregor 2000), and, therefore, can be studied from both EMG and force patterns of individual muscles. The appropriateness of using EMG recordings for studying muscle coordination has been discussed on several occasions and the reader is referred to the following detailed reviews (Hug 2011; Hug and Dorel 2009). Studies that focus on muscle coordination usually report muscle activity profiles (*i.e.,* EMG patterns; Figure 5). Typically, a linear envelope of the EMG signal is first computed by rectification (Hug and Dorel 2009). Then, the EMG is related to mechanical events (*e.g.,* foot switches, force signal), and is time normalized. Finally, a representative EMG profile is obtained for every muscle by averaging the linear envelopes for a number of consecutive cycles or trials. EMG profiles are characterised by bursts of activity. Muscle coordination is presumably modulated by the neural command in order to generate an appropriate neural control strategy or more simply reflects task constraints (Hug 2011; Tresch and Jarc 2009). Thus, it provides an attractive simplifying strategy to study the control of complex movements in sports and daily activities. Because this approach allows describing multiple patterns of muscle activity in an integrative fashion, it is believed to be a useful way of examining muscle coordination.

As this is a rather innovative approach of using EMG signals to study the brain regulation of exercise capacity, very few data are available during sprint exercise. To the author's best knowledge, the only study on coordination patterns in sprints has demonstrated that the agonist–antagonist activation strategy is altered during ten 6-s cycle sprints. The *biceps femoris* muscle was activated earlier within a pedaling cycle presumably to account for the loss of force of the prime movers in order to maintain the transfer of force to the pedal. Importantly, this locomotor alteration occurred before any changes in the "quantity" of muscle recruitment (*i.e.,* EMG amplitude), which suggests that muscle activation sequence is an important parameter in the regulation of exercise intensity (Billaut et al. 2005). Admittedly, much work lies ahead to substantiate this hypothesis and fully comprehend the neural processes behind the complex regulation of muscle actions. Future studies devoted at challenging muscle coordination and investigating how the brain copes with task constraints are warranted.

4.3 At least two potential causes for down-regulation of muscle recruitment

While it is suspected that multiple feedback originating from various locations within the body alter the output of the spinal motor neuron pool, and therefore muscle recruitment, research into neuromuscular fatigue during "all-out" sprints has defined at least two potential influences. The mechanisms that lead to a decreased output of the spinal motor neuron pool are still not well understood, especially during repeated sprints. Nevertheless, it is now clear that the CNS receives sensory input from muscle afferents (*e.g.,* muscle spindles, Golgi tendon organs, group III and IV fibres) which are integrated into the determination of central motor drive. Evidence is accumulating that the purpose of this reflex mechanism may be to limit the development of excessive peripheral muscle fatigue (Amann 2011; Kayser 2003; Marino et al. 2011; Noakes 2011). This consensus is supported by experimental studies showing that pre-existing locomotor muscle fatigue has a dose-

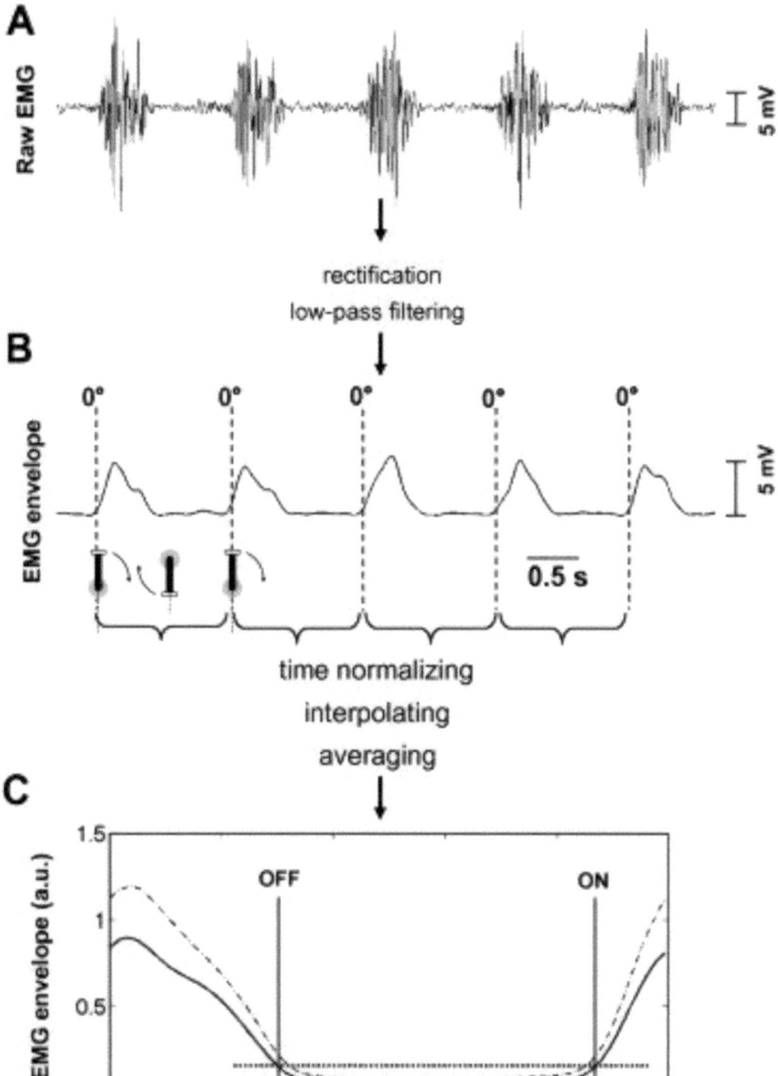

Fig. 5. Example of surface electromyographic signal processing to examine muscle coordination strategies. Panel A displays a raw EMG signal recorded from the *vastus lateralis* muscle during pedalling. The linear envelope is first computed by rectification and low-pass filtering (9 Hz in this example). All cycles are then extracted using a trigger pulse that is delivered at the top dead centre (crank angle = 0°; Panel B) and time normalised. Finally, a representative EMG profile is obtained for every muscle by averaging the linear envelopes for a number of consecutive cycles (Panel C). Onset and offset values are then determined from this averaged pattern using an EMG threshold (fixed at 20% of the peak EMG recorded during the cycle in this example; horizontal dashed line). Reproduced from Hug (2011) with permission.

dependent, inverse effect on muscle recruitment and power output during a 5-km time trial (Amann and Dempsey 2008). Specifically, the higher the level of pre-existing fatigue, the lower the muscle recruitment and power output during the trial. Furthermore, in a nicely-designed series of studies Amann and colleagues (2008; 2009) presented convincing results that sensory feedback from fatiguing muscles restrict muscle recruitment and, therefore, the exercise-induced development of peripheral fatigue during whole-body endurance exercise. However, whether the central projection of afferent feedbacks from fatigued muscles changes according to the continuous vs. intermittent nature of the exercise task remains unknown. It is intuitive that the dramatic metabolic disturbances that occur within the exercising muscle during "all-out" and repeated sprints (for review see (Billaut and Bishop 2009)) influence the central projection of these feedbacks and thus affect the central neural drive during such intense tasks (Billaut et al. 2005; Billaut and Smith 2010; Mendez-Villanueva et al. 2008; Racinais et al. 2007). That being said, the manipulation of intramuscular pH, for example, by oral administration of sodium bicarbonate does not influence EMG activity and mechanical performance during repeated cycling sprints (Matsuura et al. 2007). Further studies manipulating the metabolic "milieu interieur" during sprint repetitions to examine the effects on centrally-regulated muscle recruitment are needed.
A second potential line of inquiry for fatigue research during "all-out" activity is the influence of oxygenation on motor neuron activity. Recently, studies have been performed to further unravel changes in muscle activation. In this perspective, it is worth noting that the drop in EMG amplitude observed during repeated sprints has been shown to be strongly correlated ($r = 0.80$ to 0.95, $P < 0.05$) with a decline in arterial blood oxygen (O_2) saturation (Billaut and Smith 2009; Billaut and Smith 2010). This relationship is also very similar in men and women, suggesting that there is no sex dimorphism in this phenomenon (Billaut and Smith 2009) and demonstrating the strong recurrence of this phenomenon. So, is it simply coincidence that muscle recruitment falls concomitantly with arterial saturation? One may interpret existing correlative evidence (Billaut et al. 2010; Billaut and Smith 2009; Billaut and Smith 2010) to mean that the CNS deliberately down-regulates muscle activity to keep peripheral fatigue within "tolerable" limits. We further tested this hypothesis and used a hypoxia paradigm to alter O_2 delivery to tissues and evaluate its impact on muscle recruitment. The reduction in prefrontal cortex oxygenation induced by acute hypoxia was correlated ($r = 0.89$ to 0.92, $P < 0.05$) with the changes in EMG amplitude of active muscles during ten 10-s cycle sprints (Smith and Billaut 2010). This shows that the larger the brain deoxygenation, the lower the muscle recruitment. At this point however, it is important to acknowledge that the use of surface EMG as a sole determinant of the neural response is questionable and requires caution, even though its rate of change throughout the exercise may be used as an index of the rate of motor unit recruitment (Amann et al. 2008; Amann et al. 2006b; Amann et al. 2007; Romer et al. 2007). Taken as it is (*i.e.,* without neuromuscular stimulation technique), our EMG data are compatible with the general finding that hypoxia has an effect on cortical and subcortical functions of the CNS, and thereby, on motor neuron excitability and synaptic neurotransmission. This hypothesis is consistent with the findings that systemic hypoxaemia and insufficient brain oxygenation depress central neural drive (Amann et al. 2006a; Amann and Kayser 2009; Bigland-Ritchie et al. 1986b; Dillon and Waldrop 1992; Dousset et al. 2003). The latest research has strengthened this consensus by showing that scalp-recorded brain cortical activity (as assessed via electroencephalography combined with localized electromagnetic tomography) is affected during whole-body

exercise at high intensity (Brummer et al. 2011; Schneider et al. 2010) and in a hypoxic environment (Schneider and Struder 2009). The use of electromagnetic tomography during supra-maximal exercise is restricted by head movement artifacts, but remains a powerful tool to shed light on muscle recruitment strategies in future years.

5. Conclusion

It is becoming clear that the CNS modulates muscle recruitment (both quantity of muscle mass and coordination strategies) to cope with task constraints during high-intensity exercise. It may do so presumably to counteract the increasing fatigue process and limit the development of peripheral muscle fatigue to a non-harmful level. Exercise physiologists and sport scientists can no longer pretend that conscious or subconscious decision making plays no role in the fatigue process and, ultimately, in the regulation of exercise intensity. Perhaps, as Marino and colleagues wrote, "*this means that studying fatigue as a closed feedback loop will no longer suffice. At this stage in our understanding of the brain, bringing feed-forward mechanisms of the brain into fatigue process*" is necessary to promote greater understanding of human physiology (Marino et al. 2011). Now is an appropriate time to move the field of exercise physiology forward and acknowledge the controlling role of the brain. Understanding these complex neural strategies during sprint exercise constitutes a necessary step if we want to implement such tasks in interventions designed to enhance performance and health. And in this quest, the recording of surface EMG activity holds potential.

6. References

Allen DG, Westerblad H, Lännergren J (1995) The role of intracellular acidosis in muscle fatigue. Adv Exp Med Biol 384: 57-68

Amann M (2011) Central and Peripheral Fatigue: Interaction during Cycling Exercise in Humans. Medicine and science in sports and exercise

Amann M, Dempsey JA (2008) Locomotor muscle fatigue modifies central motor drive in healthy humans and imposes a limitation to exercise performance. J Physiol 586: 161-173

Amann M, Eldridge MW, Lovering AT, Stickland MK, Pegelow DF, Dempsey JA (2006a) Arterial oxygenation influences central motor output and exercise performance via effects on peripheral locomotor muscle fatigue in humans. J Physiol 575: 937-952

Amann M, Kayser B (2009) Nervous system function during exercise in hypoxia. High Alt Med Biol 10: 149-164

Amann M, Proctor LT, Sebranek JJ, Eldridge MW, Pegelow DF, Dempsey JA (2008) Somatosensory feedback from the limbs exerts inhibitory influences on central neural drive during whole body endurance exercise. Journal of applied physiology 105: 1714-1724

Amann M, Proctor LT, Sebranek JJ, Pegelow DF, Dempsey JA (2009) Opioid-mediated muscle afferents inhibit central motor drive and limit peripheral muscle fatigue development in humans. J Physiol 587: 271-283

Amann M, Romer LM, Pegelow DF, Jacques AJ, Hess CJ, Dempsey JA (2006b) Effects of arterial oxygen content on peripheral locomotor muscle fatigue. J Appl Physiol 101: 119-127

Amann M, Romer LM, Subudhi AW, Pegelow DF, Dempsey JA (2007) Severity of arterial hypoxaemia affects the relative contributions of peripheral muscle fatigue to exercise performance in healthy humans. J Physiol 581: 389-403

Basmajian JV, De Luca CJ (1985) Muscle fatigue and time-dependent parameters of the surface EMG signal. Muscles alive Their functions revealed by electromyography. Williams and Wilkins, pp. 201-222

Bassett DR, Jr., Howley ET (2000) Limiting factors for maximum oxygen uptake and determinants of endurance performance. Med Sci Sports Exerc 32: 70-84

Bigland-Ritchie B (1984) Muscle fatigue and the influence of changing neural drive. Clin Chest Med 5: 21-34

Bigland-Ritchie B, Cafarelli E, Vollestad NK (1986a) Fatigue of submaximal static contractions. Acta Physiol Scand Suppl 556: 137-148

Bigland-Ritchie B, Woods JJ (1984) Changes in muscle contractile properties and neural control during human muscular fatigue. Muscle Nerve 7: 691-699

Bigland-Ritchie BR, Dawson NJ, Johansson RS, Lippold OC (1986b) Reflex origin for the slowing of motoneurone firing rates in fatigue of human voluntary contractions. J Physiol 379: 451-459

Billaut F, Basset FA (2007) Effect of different recovery patterns on repeated-sprint ability and neuromuscular responses. J Sports Sci 25: 905-913

Billaut F, Basset FA, Falgairette G (2005) Muscle coordination changes during intermittent cycling sprints. Neurosci Lett 380: 265-269

Billaut F, Basset FA, Giacomoni M, Lemaître F, Tricot V, Falgairette G (2006) Effect of high-intensity intermittent cycling sprints on neuromuscular activity. Int J Sports Med 27: 25-30

Billaut F, Bishop D (2009) Muscle fatigue in males and females during multiple-sprint exercise. Sports Med 39: 257-278

Billaut F, Bishop DJ, Schaerz S, Noakes TD (2011) Influence of Knowledge of Sprint Number on Pacing During Repeated-Sprint Exercise. Med Sci Sports Exerc 43: 665-672

Billaut F, Davis JM, Smith KJ, Marino FE, Noakes TD (2010) Cerebral oxygenation decreases but does not impair performance during self-paced, strenuous exercise. Acta Physiol (Oxf) 198: 477-489

Billaut F, Smith K (2009) Sex alters impact of repeated bouts of sprint exercise on neuromuscular activity in trained athletes. Appl Physiol Nutr Metab 34: 689-699

Billaut F, Smith KJ (2010) Prolonged repeated-sprint ability is related to arterial O2 desaturation in man. Int J Sports Physiol Perform 5: 197-209

Brummer V, Schneider S, Struder HK, Askew CD (2011) Primary motor cortex activity is elevated with incremental exercise intensity. Neuroscience 181: 150-162

Calbet JA (2006) The rate of fatigue accumulation as a sensed variable. The Journal of physiology 575: 688-689

Casey A, Constantin-Teodosiu D, Howell S, Hultman E, Greenhaff PL (1996) Metabolic response of type I and II muscle fibers during repeated bouts of maximal exercise in humans. Am J Physiol 271: E38-43

De Luca CJ (1997) The use of surface electromyography in biomechanics. J Appl Biomechanics 13: 135-163

Dillon GH, Waldrop TG (1992) In vitro responses of caudal hypothalamic neurons to hypoxia and hypercapnia. Neuroscience 51: 941-950

Dousset E, Decherchi P, Grelot L, Jammes Y (2003) Comparison between the effects of chronic and acute hypoxemia on muscle afferent activities from the tibialis anterior muscle. Exp Brain Res 148: 320-327

Duffield R, Green R, Castle P, Maxwell N (2010) Precooling can prevent the reduction of self-paced exercise intensity in the heat. Medicine and science in sports and exercise 42: 577-584

Farina D, Merletti R, Enoka RM (2004) The extraction of neural strategies from the surface EMG. J Appl Physiol 96: 1486-1495

Fitts R (1994) Cellular mechanisms of muscle fatigue. Physiological Reviews 74: 49-94

Gandevia S (2001) Spinal and supraspinal factors in human muscle fatigue. Physiological Reviews 81: 1725-1789

Gerdle B, Fugl-Meyer AR (1992) Is the mean power frequency shift of the EMG a selective indicator of fatigue of the fast twitch motor units? Acta Physiol Scand 145: 129-138

Giacomoni M, Billaut F, Falgairette G (2006) Effects of the time of day on repeated all-out cycle performance and short-term recovery patterns. Int J Sports Med 27: 468-474

Gibala MJ (2007) High-intensity interval training: a time-efficient strategy for health promotion? Curr Sports Med Rep 6: 211-213

Girard O, Lattier G, Maffiuletti NA, Micallef JP, Millet GP (2008) Neuromuscular fatigue during a prolonged intermittent exercise: Application to tennis. J Electromyogr Kinesiol 18: 1038-1046

Greer F, Morales J, Coles M (2006) Wingate performance and surface EMG frequency variables are not affected by caffeine ingestion. Applied physiology, nutrition, and metabolism = Physiologie appliquee, nutrition et metabolisme 31: 597-603

Hautier C, Arsac L, Deghdegh K, Souquet J, Belli A, Lacour J (2000) Influence of fatigue on EMG/force ratio and cocontraction in cycling. Med Sci Sports Exerc 32: 839-843

Hettinga FJ, De Koning JJ, Broersen FT, Van Geffen P, Foster C (2006) Pacing strategy and the occurrence of fatigue in 4000-m cycling time trials. Med Sci Sports Exerc 38: 1484-1491

Hill AV (1924) Muscular Activity and Carbohydrate Metabolism. Science 60: 505-514

Hug F (2011) Can muscle coordination be precisely studied by surface electromyography? J Electromyogr Kinesiol 21: 1-12

Hug F, Dorel S (2009) Electromyographic analysis of pedaling: a review. J Electromyogr Kinesiol 19: 182-198

Hunter AM, St Clair Gibson A, Lambert MI, Nobbs L, Noakes TD (2003) Effects of supramaximal exercise on the electromyographic signal. Br J Sports Med 37: 296-299

Hunter SK (2009) Sex differences and mechanisms of task-specific muscle fatigue. Exerc Sport Sci Rev 37: 113-122

Juel C (1988) Muscle action potential propagation velocity changes during activity. Muscle Nerve 11: 714-719

Kayser B (2003) Exercise starts and ends in the brain. Eur J Appl Physiol 90: 411-419

Komi PV, Tesch PA (1979) EMG frequency spectrum, muscle structure, and fatigue during dynamic contractions in man. Eur J Appl Physiol 42: 41-50

Linnamo V, Bottas R, Komi PV (2000) Force and EMG power spectrum during and after eccentric and concentric fatigue. J Electromyogr Kinesiol 10: 293-300

Maluf KS, Enoka RM (2005) Task failure during fatiguing contractions performed by humans. J Appl Physiol 99: 389-396

Marino FE (2004) Anticipatory regulation and avoidance of catastrophe during exercise-induced hyperthermia. Comp Biochem Physiol B Biochem Mol Biol 139: 561-569

Marino FE, Gard M, Drinkwater EJ (2011) The limits to exercise performance and the future of fatigue research. British journal of sports medicine 45: 65-67

Marino FE, Lambert MI, Noakes TD (2004) Superior performance of African runners in warm humid but not in cool environmental conditions. J Appl Physiol 96: 124-130

Matsuura R, Arimitsu T, Kimura T, Yunoki T, Yano T (2007) Effect of oral administration of sodium bicarbonate on surface EMG activity during repeated cycling sprints. Eur J Appl Physiol 101: 409-417

Mendez-Villanueva A, Hamer P, Bishop D (2007) Fatigue responses during repeated sprints matched for initial mechanical output. Med Sci Sports Exerc 39: 2219-2225

Mendez-Villanueva A, Hamer P, Bishop D (2008) Fatigue in repeated-sprint exercise is related to muscle power factors and reduced neuromuscular activity. Eur J Appl Physiol 103: 411-419

Merletti R, Lo Conte LR (1997) Surface EMG signal processing during isometric contrations. J Electromyogr Kinesiol 7: 241-250

Merton P (1954) Voluntary strength and fatigue. J Physiol 123: 553-564

Moritani T, Muro M, Nagata A (1986) Intramuscular and surface electromyogram changes during muscle fatigue. J Appl Physiol 60: 1179-1185

Moritani T, Takaishi T, Matsumoto T (1993) Determination of maximal power output at neuromuscular fatigue threshold. J Appl Physiol 74: 1729-1734

Neptune R, Kautz S (2001) Muscle activation and deactivation dynamics: the governing properties in fast cyclical human movement performance? Exerc Sport Sci Rev 29: 76-81

Nielsen HB, Boushel R, Madsen P, Secher NH (1999) Cerebral desaturation during exercise reversed by O2 supplementation. Am J Physiol 277: H1045-1052

Noakes TD (2011) Time to move beyond a brainless exercise physiology: the evidence for complex regulation of human exercise performance. Applied physiology, nutrition, and metabolism = Physiologie appliquee, nutrition et metabolisme 36: 23-35

Noakes TD, Peltonen JE, Rusko HK (2001) Evidence that a central governor regulates exercise performance during acute hypoxia and hyperoxia. J Exp Biol 204: 3225-3234

Noakes TD, St Clair Gibson A (2004) Logical limitations to the "catastrophe" models of fatigue during exercise in humans. Br J Sports Med 38: 648-649

Noakes TD, St Clair Gibson A, Lambert EV (2004) From catastrophe to complexity: a novel model of integrative central neural regulation of effort and fatigue during exercise in humans. Br J Sports Med 38: 511-514

Noakes TD, Tucker R (2008) Do we really need a central governor to explain brain regulation of exercise performance? A response to the letter of Dr. Marcora. Eur J Appl Physiol

Nordlund MM, Thorstensson A, Cresswell AG (2004) Central and peripheral contributions to fatigue in relation to level of activation during repeated maximal voluntary isometric plantar flexions. J Appl Physiol 96: 218-225

Nybo L, Secher NH (2004) Cerebral perturbations provoked by prolonged exercise. Prog Neurobiol 72: 223-261

Palmer GS, Noakes TD, Hawley JA (1997) Effects of steady-state versus stochastic exercise on subsequent cycling performance. Med Sci Sports Exerc 29: 684-687

Paterson S, Marino FE (2004) Effect of deception of distance on prolonged cycling performance. Percept Mot Skills 98: 1017-1026

Prilutsky BI, Gregor RJ (2000) Analysis of muscle coordination strategies in cycling. IEEE Transactions on Rehabilitation Engineering 8: 362-370

Racinais S, Bishop D, Denis R, Lattier G, Mendez-Villaneuva A, Perrey S (2007) Muscle Deoxygenation and Neural Drive to the Muscle during Repeated Sprint Cycling. Med Sci Sports Exerc 39: 268-274

Romer LM, Haverkamp HC, Amann M, Lovering AT, Pegelow DF, Dempsey JA (2007) Effect of acute severe hypoxia on peripheral fatigue and endurance capacity in healthy humans. Am J Physiol Regul Integr Comp Physiol 292: R598-606

Ross A, Leveritt M, Riek S (2001) Neural influences on sprint running: training adaptations and acute responses. Sports Med 31: 409-425

Saey D, Debigare R, LeBlanc P, Mador MJ, Cote CH, Jobin J, Maltais F (2003) Contractile leg fatigue after cycle exercise: a factor limiting exercise in patients with chronic obstructive pulmonary disease. American journal of respiratory and critical care medicine 168: 425-430

Schneider S, Askew CD, Abel T, Mierau A, Struder HK (2010) Brain and exercise: a first approach using electrotomography. Medicine and science in sports and exercise 42: 600-607

Schneider S, Struder HK (2009) Monitoring effects of acute hypoxia on brain cortical activity by using electromagnetic tomography. Behav Brain Res 197: 476-480

Shephard RJ (2009) Is it Time to Retire the 'Central Governor'? Sports Med 39: 709-721

Smith KJ, Billaut F (2010) Influence of cerebral and muscle oxygenation on repeated-sprint ability. Eur J Appl Physiol 109: 989-999

Spencer M, Bishop D, Dawson B, Goodman C (2005) Physiological and metabolic responses of repeated-sprint activities:specific to field-based team sports. Sports Med 35: 1025-1044

St Clair Gibson A, Lambert EV, Rauch LH, Tucker R, Baden DA, Foster C, Noakes TD (2006) The role of information processing between the brain and peripheral physiological systems in pacing and perception of effort. Sports Med 36: 705-722

St Clair Gibson A, Lambert MI, Noakes TD (2001) Neural control of force output during maximal and submaximal exercise. Sports Med 31: 637-650

St Clair Gibson A, Noakes TD (2004) Evidence for complex system integration and dynamic neural regulation of skeletal muscle recruitment during exercise in humans. Br J Sp Med 38: 797-806

Szubski C, Burtscher M, Loscher WN (2007) Neuromuscular fatigue during sustained contractions performed in short-term hypoxia. Med Sci Sports Exerc 39: 948-954

Tresch MC, Jarc A (2009) The case for and against muscle synergies. Curr Opin Neurobiol 19: 601-607

Tucker R, Lambert MI, Noakes TD (2006a) An analysis of pacing strategies during men's world-record performances in track athletics. International journal of sports physiology and performance 1: 233-245

Tucker R, Marle T, Lambert EV, Noakes TD (2006b) The rate of heat storage mediates an anticipatory reduction in exercise intensity during cycling at a fixed rating of perceived exertion. J Physiol 574: 905-915

Tucker R, Rauch LH, Harley YXR, Noakes TD (2004) Impaired exercise performance in the heat is associated with an anticipatory reduction in skeletal muscle recruitment. Pflügers Arch - Eur J Physiol 448: 422-430

Van Ingen Schenau G, Boots P, de Groot G, Snackers R, van Woensel W (1992) The constrained control of force and position in multi-joint movements. Neuroscience 46: 197-207

Vandewalle H, Maton B, Le Bozec S, Guerenbourg G (1991) An electromyographic study of an all-out exercise on a cycle ergometer. Arch Int Physiol Biochim Biophys 99: 89-93

3

Classification of Upper Limb Motions from Around-Shoulder Muscle Activities

Hirokazu Soma, Yuse Horiuchi, Jose Gonzalez and Wenwei Yu
Chiba University
Japan

1. Introduction

In recent years, detecting upper-limb motion intention has attracted growing research attention in order to improve the manipulation of a prosthetic hand. Recording of forearm muscle activity has been used as a signal source to detect wrist and hand motions using different pattern recognition techniques. However, it is difficult to take in consideration body coordinated motions from these signals alone; therefore the movement of the artificial limb can be unnatural, if consider as a part of the whole body coordination, and a dynamical coupling between the user and the prosthesis is impossible. Also, using only forearm muscle activities to drive the artificial limb leaves aside the possibility for higher level amputees to use these systems.

It is well known that most daily-life upper limb activities present a coordination of the shoulder-arm-hand complex. For example, the shoulder, elbow and hand's trajectories are tightly coupled when reaching and grasping an object, or when throwing and catching a ball. It is because of this dependency that research effort had been done to differentiate hand motions using EMG activity of proximal muscles. For example, C. Martelloni et al were able to discriminate different grip types from EMG signals of proximal and distal muscles by statistical means. Also, Xiao Hu et al compared the performance of a Scalar Autoregresive model with a Multivariate AR modeling using EMG data obtained from the bicep, tricep, deltoid, and brachioradialis, successfully classifying different arm movements. Although the results obtained are encouraging, relying only on EMG information is not accurate enough for a robust dynamical control of a prosthetic hand since it is still complex to classify and interpret the information acquired in real time.

In a previous study, we showed the possibility of improving the discrimination rate by using accelerometers, to detect kinematical information from the around-shoulder muscles, along with the EMG signals. In that study we obtained EMG and accelerometer information from only proximal muscles and used an off-line neural network classifier to discriminate different grips and arm positions. Therefore, the objective of this study was to investigate the possibility of associating around-shoulder muscle activity with different grasps and arm positions while reaching for an object using an on-line recognition method. This way we might be able to deduce the user's motion intention and coordinate the prosthetic arm position and movements to his body in a dynamical way.

2. Measurement experiment and analysis

2.1 Experimental setup

2.1.1 Subjects

Three male subjects, all 23 years old, participated in the experiments. They were informed about the experimental procedures and asked to provide their consent. All subjects were healthy with no known history of neurological abnormalities or musculo-skeletal disorders.

2.1.2 Experiment procedure

The subjects were asked to sit comfortably in front of a table. Then, they were asked to move their dominant arm, from an fixed position towards an end-position, and grasp an object (Figure1). Before starting the trial, they had to push a switch button by resting their dominant hand in a natural open flat position. When the trial started they had to extend their arm to reach and grasp an object. Three different object-related grips were used during the experiments, and the object was place in one of five positions five different positions relative to the subject, as denoted in figure 1. The object was placed so as to allow the maximal elbow extension in one of the five directions. Moreover, the height of the chair was regulated for each subject in order to obtain an elbow's angle of 90° (maintaining the trunk erected). Also, the subjects were asked to reach and grasp a total of 20 times for each position and grip, giving a total of 300 (3 objets x 5 position x 20 repetitions) trials. They were able to rest for a few seconds between each trial and were requested not to bend or rotate the trunk in order to prevent translational motions of the shoulder.

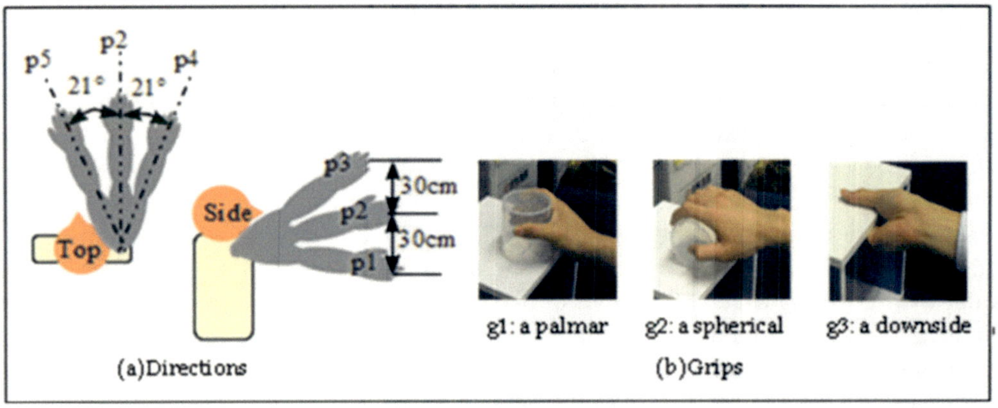

Fig. 1. Experimental setup: Subjects were asked to reach in different positions and grasp with different grips.

2.1.3 Devices

In the experiment, EMG sensor: TYE-1000M, Sikikou Engineering, Japan, was used. The sensor has a band-pass filter with pass frequency band of 10~1000Hz. Muscle activity signals were recorded at a sampling frequency of 400Hz. Generally, the sampling frequency used for EMG recording is of 1 kHz or more, but in order to reduce the processing time and load of the on-line discrimination system, the sampling frequency was decreased. Preliminary experiments showed that this reduction did not significantly affect the recognition. The accelerometer used for measuring the kinematical information from around-shoulder muscles was the MMA7260Q from Freescale Semiconductor Inc. and was sampled at 100Hz.

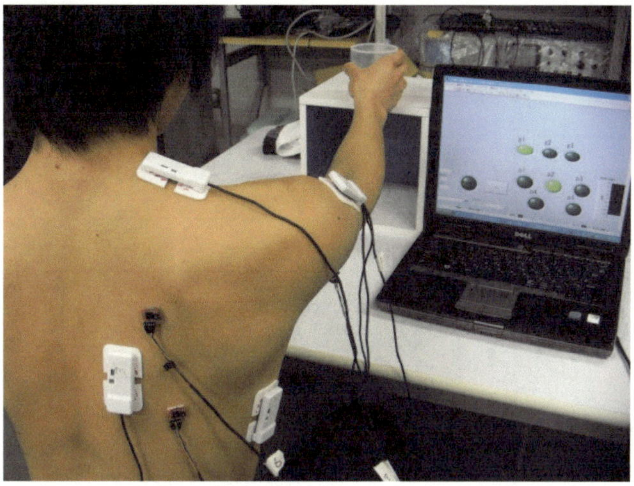

Fig. 2. Experimental setup: Scene of the experiment

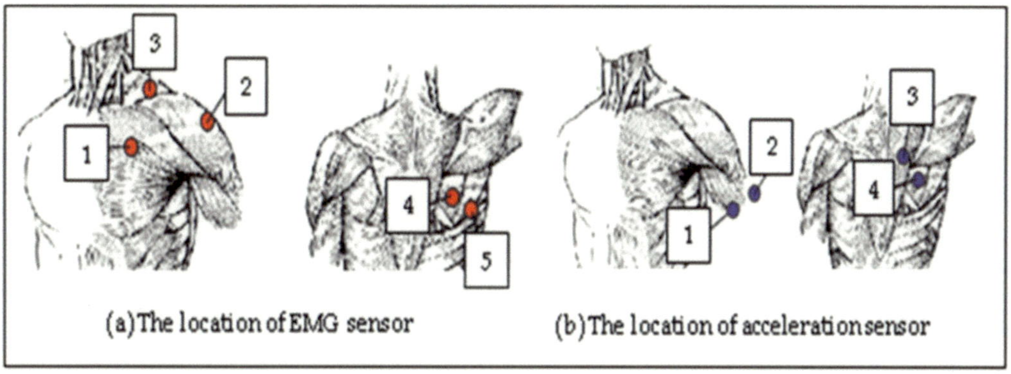

Fig. 3. Location of sensors

In total 5 EMG sensors and 4 accelerometers were placed on the skin surface of the different muscles around the shoulder as shown figure 3. The EMG sensors were placed on top of the following muscles:

1. The clavicular part of pectoralis major muscle.
2. Acromial part of deltoid muscle (central fibers).
3. Descending fibers of trapezius muscle.
4. Ascending fibers of trapezius muscle.
5. Teres major muscle.

The accelerometers were attached to the skin above the following muscles:

1. Short head of biceps brachii muscle.
2. Long head of triceps brachii muscle.
3. Greater rhomboid muscle.
4. Infraspinatus muscle and infraspinous fascia.

2.2 Signal processing and feature extraction

In order to decide a suitable filter for signal processing, a fast Fourier transform was applied to the recorded EMG signals and, as shown in figure 4 (a), the highest power spectrum is located below 150Hz. Accordingly, the EMG signals were filtered with a 150Hz low-pass filter, then a 2Hz high pass filter was applied, and finally, the signal was smoothed by a 50-point moving average window (Fig. 4 (b)).

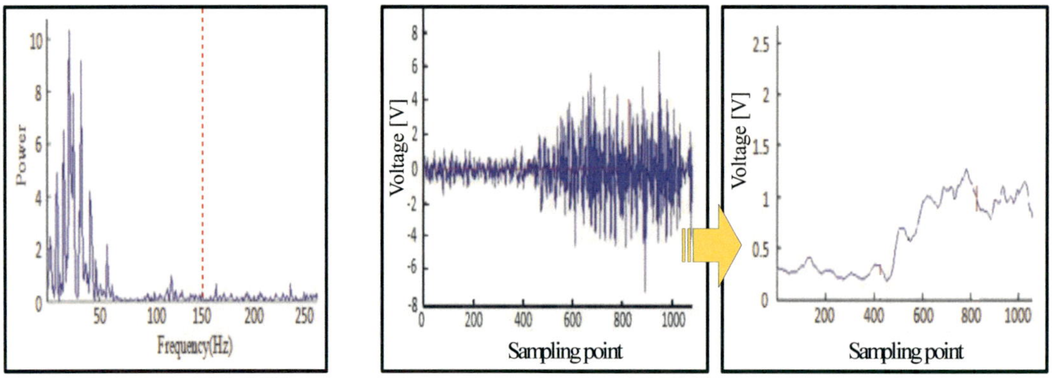

(a) FFT (b) EMG waveform

Fig. 4. EMG signal processing

Fig. 5 shows the original waveform of the acceleration signals (left), to which a 50-point moving average process was applied for smoothing (right of Fig. 5).

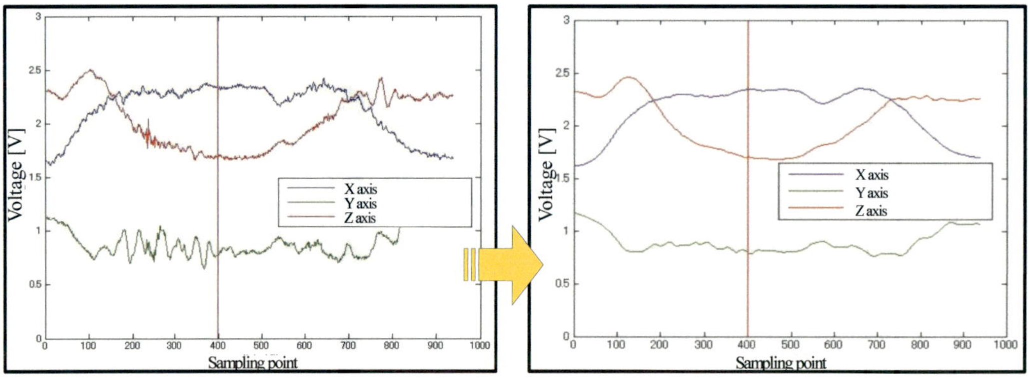

Fig. 5. Acceleration signal processing

3 features were extracted from the data, based on literature of motion recognition from EMG signals, and they were compared in order to investigate their effect. One of the features obtained is the Mean Value (MV) described by equation (1). This value reflects the average amplitude of a biological signal. Another feature is the Subtract Value (SV) described by equation (2), which expresses the amount of change of a biological signal. Also, the Point Value (PV) was obtained as described by equation (3), which observed the temporal amount of EMG of the biological signal. In these equations, T corresponds to the data size used to calculate each feature (200, 400, and 600 points were used in this study). Also, Pi corresponds to the i point of the smoothened EMG and acceleration signals.

$$MV = \frac{1}{T}\sum_{i=0}^{T} P_i \quad (1)$$

$$SV = \sum_{i=1}^{T} |P_i - P_{i-1}| \quad (2)$$

$$PV = P_T - P_0 \quad (3)$$

2.3 Motion discrimination

A back-propagation training based neural network (NN) was used for analysis and classification of the data. It consisted of three layers (input layer, middle layer and output layer). The input layer contained 9 neurons (5 for EMG inputs and 4 for accelerometers), the Middle layer had twice the neuron number as the input layer, and the Output layer had 3 neurons for classifying grips (g1, g2, g3) or 5 neurons to classify positions (p1, p2, p3, p4, p5). The maximal iteration for learning was 2000.

A total of 300 measurements were recorded from each subject. A set of 285 (5 positions x 3 grips x 19 times) measurements were used as the neural network learning data and the remaining 15 measurements (5 positions x 3 grips x 1 times) as the test data, according to the leave-one-out training scheme. After, a different set of 285 measurements was used to train a new neural network and the remaining 15 measurements were used to test it. Following this scheme 20 different neural networks were obtained for each subject. For the off-line analysis the average of the 20 neural networks' discrimination rate was used as the final result. On the other hand, the neural network that showed the best discrimination rate was used as the on-line classifier.

3. Results

In order to analyze the data extracted from the EMG sensors and the accelerometers, an off-line analysis was made. The neural network was tested using different features in order to explore the feasibility of different motion recognition. Thereafter, an on-line discrimination experiment was designed to test and validate whether or not it is possible to classify different arm motion using EMG and acceleration signals from around-shoulder muscles.

3.1 Off-line analysis

For demonstration purposes only the data of one subject is shown in this section, but the results are consistent with the other 2 subjects. Figure 6 shows the results obtained when discriminating the different positions of the arm and figure 7 shows the discrimination rate of the grips used in this study.

It can be observed from the figures that combining the data obtained from the accelerometers and the EMG improves greatly the discrimination rate of the different motions.

3.2 On-line discrimination result

The on-line recognition system used for this experiment consisted of four parts: sampling the signal, processing the signal, extracting signals features, and finally, classifying the signal. A total of 300 trials were performed by each subject (5positions * 3 grips * 20 repetitions).

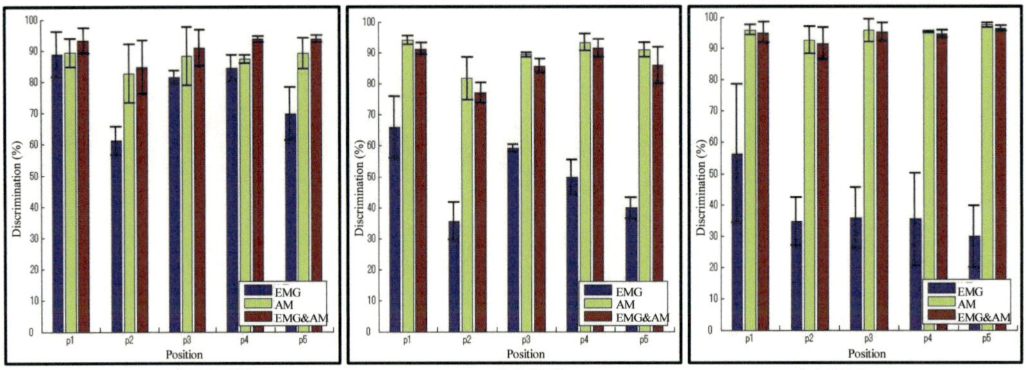

(a) MV (b) SV (c) PV

Fig. 6. The discrimination rate of positions classified by sensor (A.M: accelerometers)

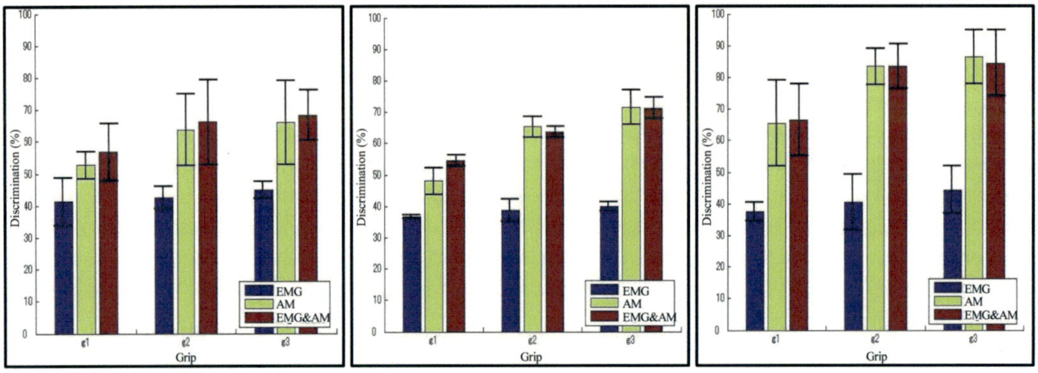

(a) MV (b) SV (c) PV

Fig. 7. The discrimination rate of grips classified by sensor (A.M: accelerometers)

3.2.1 Analysis of discrimination rate

Figure 8 shows a comparison between the discrimination rate of 5 different arm positions and the different data lengths used to calculate each feature (200 points, 400 points, 600 points). Figure 9 shows the same comparison for the discrimination of different grips.

From this results the data length with the highest discrimination rate was selected in order to decide the best feature for each subject, as shown in figure 10 and 11.

Figure 12 shows a comparison of the highest discrimination rate between subjects.

From figure 12, it can be noted that the highest discrimination rates were obtained with different features and data lengths for each subjects. This points out that, by calculating different features, it is possible to assess individual differences in muscle activities, improving the recognition rate for different people.

3.2.2 Analysis of incorrect discrimination

Although good discrimination rates were obtained in the experiment there were times when a position or a grip was wrongly classified. Figure 13 shows how many times an arm position was incorrectly classified as another position. From this data it is possible to determine signal similarities between different arm positions. Additionally, figure 14 show the cases for grip discrimination.

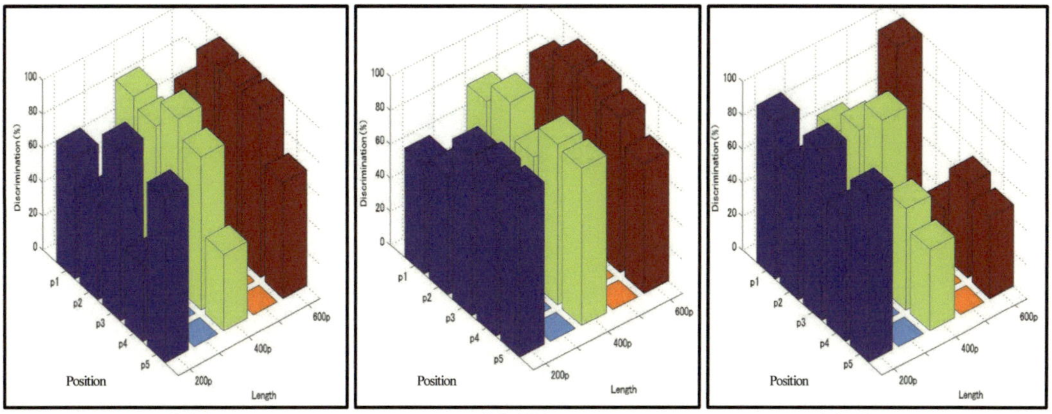

(a) MV (b) SV (c) PV

Fig. 8. The discrimination rate of positions in each data length

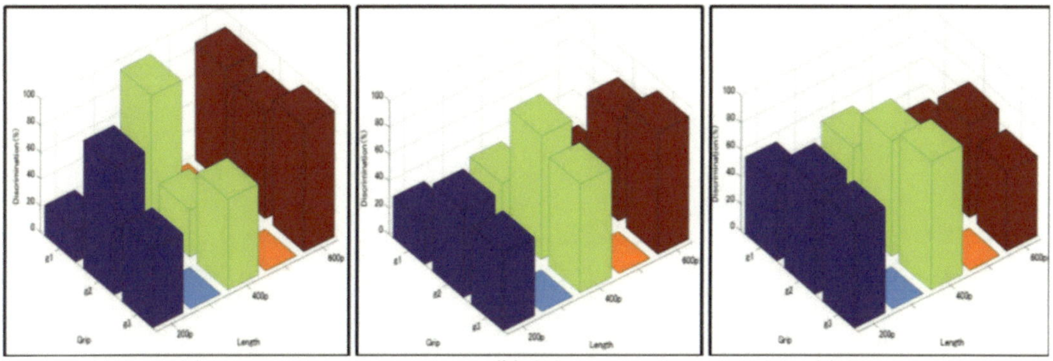

(a) MV (b) SV (c) PV

Fig. 9. The discrimination rate of grips in each data length

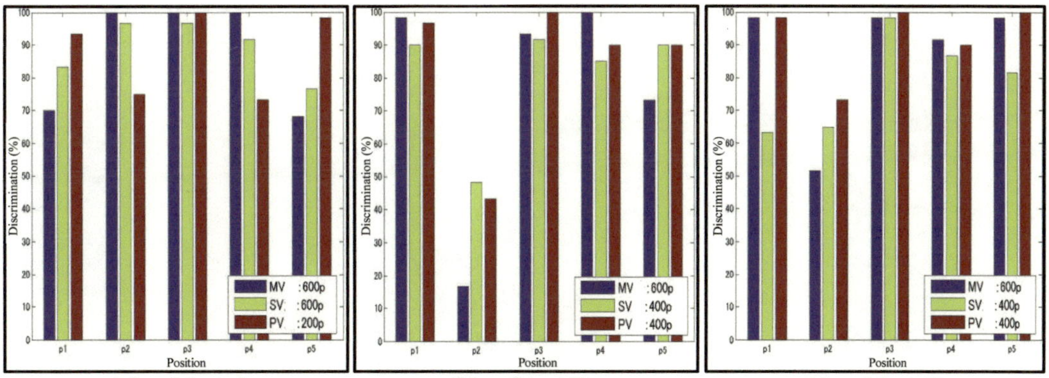

(a) subject A (b) subject B (c) subject C

Fig. 10. The discrimination rate of positions in each subject

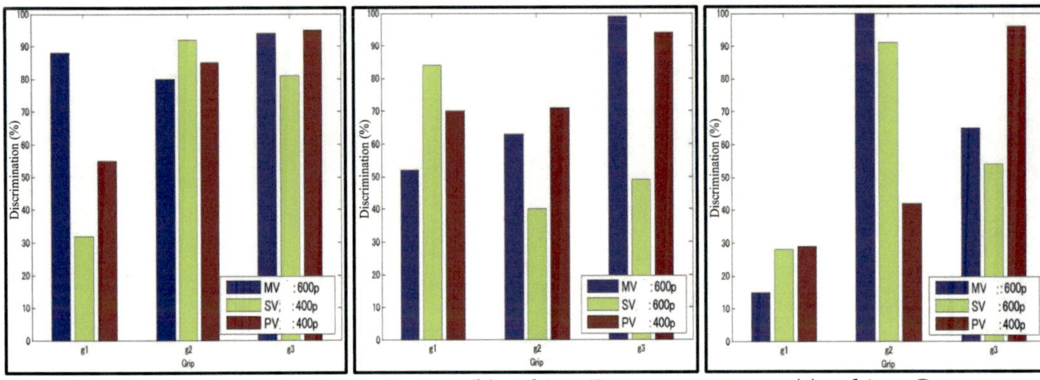

(a) subject A (b) subject B (c) subject C

Fig. 11. The discrimination rate of grips in each subject

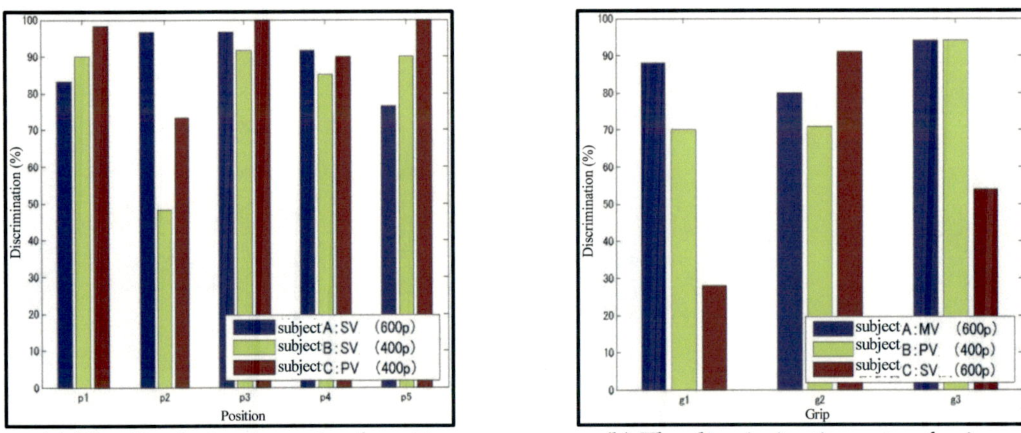

(a) The discrimination rate of positions (b) The discrimination rate of grips

Fig. 12. Comparing the discrimination rate between subjects

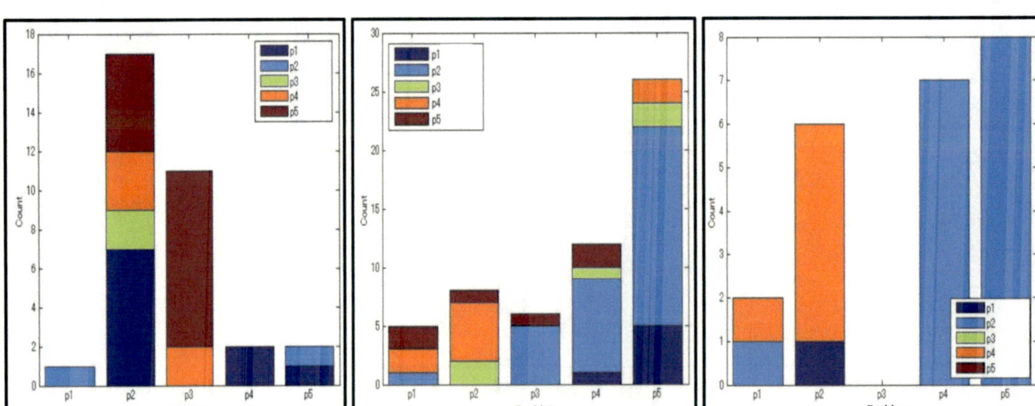

(a) subject A (b) subject B (c) subject C

Fig. 13. Result of incorrect discrimination in positions test

For example in figure 13, for Subject A, p2 was discriminated incorrectly as p1, p4, or p5. Also, for Subject B, p2 had a low discrimination rate, which was discriminated incorrectly as p5 and p4. For Subject C p2 was discriminated incorrectly as p4 and p5, and p4 was discriminated incorrectly as p2. Finally, for all subjects p1 was discriminated incorrectly 36 times, p2 31 times, p3 17 times, p4 21 times, and p5 was 36 times. This results showed that p2 and p5 present difficulties to be recognized.

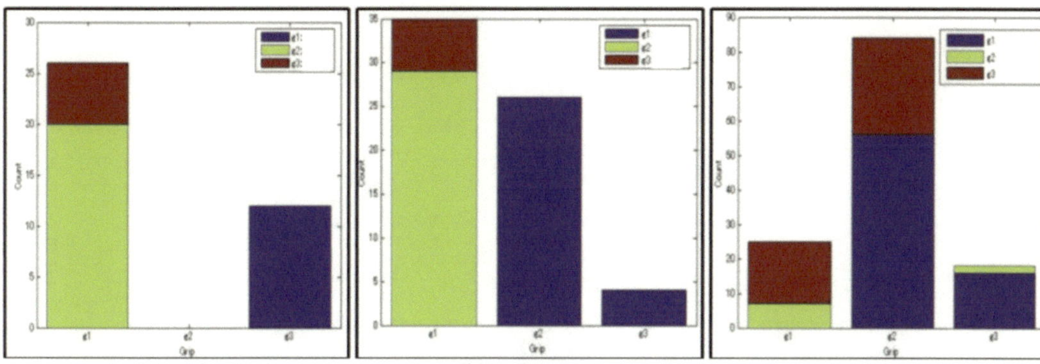

(a) subject A (b) subject B (c) subject C

Fig. 14. Result of incorrect discrimination in grips test

Similarly, figure 14 shows how many times a grip was incorrectly classified as another grip. For Subject A g2 was discriminated incorrectly as g1, and g1 as g3. For Subject B most of the times g1 was mistaken for g2, and for Subject C g1 were discriminated incorrectly as g2. For all subjects g1 was discriminated incorrectly 86 times, g2 110 times, and g3 34 times. This results showed that g1 and g2 were the most difficult grips to be identify.

These mistakes are mainly due to similarities in the recorded muscle activities for each task, but we also explored how the location of the sensors was affecting the discrimination. The contribution of each sensor to the discrimination and the combination of grips and positions with difficult discrimination was investigated using the Tukey-Kramer test. Table 1, 2 and 3 show the result of the analysis of variance for the different positions. In this case the squares with an "O" refers to the data which showed a statistical significant difference between 2 positions (p_i/p_j) and the squares with an "X" refers to the data were there wasn't any significant difference between 2 positions. Also, in the table the sensor that showed more than 7 significant differences between positions are marked with a yellow color. This indicates which location contributed more to the discrimination.

It can be noted from table 1 that, when comparing p2 and p4, only 9 sensors showed a significant difference in their data, and when comparing p2 and p3 only 11 sensors showed a significant difference.

Table 2 shows the results obtained for Subject B. In this case, the comparison between p2 and p3, p2 and p5, p3 and p4 showed a statistical significant difference in only 9 sensors.

Additionally, table 3 shows the results obtained for Subject C. It can be observed that when comparing between p1 and p2, or when comparing between p2 and p4, only 10 sensors showed a significant difference in their data.

This results seems to support the finding showed in figure 13 and p2 is the position most likely to be discriminated incorrectly for all Subjects. Moreover, most of the contribution to the discrimination is mainly due to the accelerometers, and it was difficult to differentiate between position using only the EMG sensors. Also, among all the subjects there wasn't a common EMG sensor that showed more than 7 significant difference between 2 position, which points out how individual differences affect the EMG signals.

	EMG sensor					accelerometer												
						①			②			③			④			
	①	②	③	④	⑤	X	Y	Z	X	Y	Z	X	Y	Z	X	Y	Z	total
p1/p2	○	×	×	×	×	○	○	○	×	○	○	○	○	○	○	○	○	12
p1/p3	○	○	○	○	×	○	○	○	×	○	○	○	×	○	×	○	○	13
p1/p4	○	○	×	○	×	×	○	○	○	○	○	○	○	○	○	○	○	14
p1/p5	○	×	○	○	○	○	○	○	○	○	○	○	×	○	×	○	×	13
p2/p3	○	○	○	○	×	×	○	○	×	×	×	×	○	○	○	×	×	9
p2/p4	×	○	○	○	×	○	○	○	○	○	○	×	×	○	×	○	×	11
p2/p5	○	○	×	○	×	×	○	○	×	○	○	○	○	○	○	○	○	13
p3/p4	○	○	○	○	×	○	○	○	○	○	○	×	○	×	○	○	×	13
p3/p5	○	○	×	×	○	×	○	○	○	○	○	○	×	○	×	○	○	12
p4/p5	○	○	○	○	○	○	×	○	○	○	○	○	○	○	○	○	○	16
total	9	8	6	8	3	6	9	10	6	9	9	7	6	9	6	9	6	

Table 1. The result of the analysis of variance in five positions (Subject A)

	EMG sensor					accelerometer												
						①			②			③			④			
	①	②	③	④	⑤	X	Y	Z	X	Y	Z	X	Y	Z	X	Y	Z	total
p1/p2	×	×	×	○	×	○	○	○	○	○	○	○	○	○	○	○	○	13
p1/p3	○	○	○	○	○	○	○	○	○	○	○	○	○	○	○	○	○	17
p1/p4	×	○	○	×	○	×	○	○	○	○	○	○	○	○	○	○	○	14
p1/p5	×	×	×	○	○	○	○	○	○	○	○	○	×	○	○	○	○	13
p2/p3	○	○	○	×	○	×	○	○	×	○	×	○	×	○	×	×	×	9
p2/p4	×	○	○	×	○	○	○	×	○	○	○	○	×	○	×	×	×	10
p2/p5	×	×	×	○	×	○	×	○	×	×	×	○	○	○	○	○	○	9
p3/p4	×	×	○	×	×	○	○	○	○	○	○	○	×	○	×	×	×	9
p3/p5	×	○	○	○	○	○	○	○	×	×	×	○	○	○	○	×	○	12
p4/p5	×	○	×	○	○	○	○	○	○	○	○	×	○	×	○	×	○	12
total	2	6	6	6	7	8	9	9	7	8	7	9	6	9	7	5	7	

Table 2. The result of the analysis of variance in five positions (Subject B)

	EMG sensor					accelerometer												
						①			②			③			④			
	①	②	③	④	⑤	X	Y	Z	X	Y	Z	X	Y	Z	X	Y	Z	total
p1/p2	×	×	○	×	×	○	○	×	○	○	○	○	○	×	○	×	○	10
p1/p3	×	○	○	○	○	○	○	○	○	○	○	○	○	○	○	○	×	15
p1/p4	×	×	○	○	×	○	○	×	○	○	○	○	○	○	○	○	○	13
p1/p5	×	○	○	○	○	○	○	×	○	○	○	○	○	○	○	○	×	14
p2/p3	×	○	○	×	×	×	○	○	○	○	○	○	○	○	○	○	○	13
p2/p4	×	×	×	○	×	×	○	×	○	○	○	×	○	○	○	○	○	10
p2/p5	○	×	○	○	○	○	○	×	○	○	○	○	×	○	×	○	○	13
p3/p4	×	○	○	○	×	○	○	○	○	○	○	○	×	○	○	○	○	14
p3/p5	×	○	○	○	○	○	○	○	○	○	○	○	○	○	○	○	×	15
p4/p5	×	○	×	○	○	○	○	○	○	×	×	○	○	○	○	○	○	13
total	1	6	8	8	5	8	10	5	10	9	9	9	8	9	9	9	7	

Table 3. The result of the analysis of variance in five positions (Subject C)

	EMG sensor					accelerometer												
						①			②			③			④			
	①	②	③	④	⑤	X	Y	Z	X	Y	Z	X	Y	Z	X	Y	Z	total
g1/g2	×	×	×	○	×	○	×	○	○	○	○	×	×	○	×	×	○	8
g1/g3	×	○	×	×	×	○	○	○	○	○	○	×	×	×	×	×	×	7
g2/g3	×	○	○	×	○	○	×	○	○	○	○	○	×	○	×	×	○	11
total	0	2	1	1	1	3	1	3	3	3	3	1	0	2	0	0	2	

Table 4. The result of the analysis of variance in three grips (Subject A)

Table 4 shows the analysis of variance comparing different grips of Subject A. When comparing g1 and g3 only 7 sensors showed a statistical significant difference. Moreover, the EMG data of sensor 1 didn't showed any statistical difference for any of the comparisons.

Table 5 shows the results obtained from Subject B data. In this case, when comparing g1 and g2, or g1 and g3, only 7 sensors showed a significant difference. The EMG data from sensor 1, 3 and 4 didn't show any significant difference for any of the comparisons.

Finally, table 6 shows the results for Subject C. Comparing the data obtained for g1 and g2 only 6 sensors showed significant differences. The X axis data from the accelerometers 1, 2, 3 and 4 didn't showed any statistical difference in any of the cases.

As an overall, for all subjects, g1 was the most likely grip to be mistaken, which agrees with the result showed in figure 14. Also, the EMG sensor 2 contributed greatly to the discrimination of the grips for all subjects. The information acquired from the Z axis of the accelerometers 1 and 2 also had a great contribution to the discrimination.

	EMG sensor					accelerometer												
						①			②			③			④			
	①	②	③	④	⑤	X	Y	Z	X	Y	Z	X	Y	Z	X	Y	Z	total
g1/g2	×	×	×	×	×	○	×	○	○	×	×	×	○	○	×	○	○	7
g1/g3	×	○	×	×	○	○	○	○	○	×	×	×	×	×	×	×	○	7
g2/g3	×	○	×	×	○	○	○	○	○	○	○	○	○	○	×	○	○	13
total	0	2	0	0	2	3	2	3	3	1	1	1	2	2	0	2	3	

Table 5. The result of the analysis of variance in three grips (Subject B)

	EMG sensor					accelerometer												
						①			②			③			④			
	①	②	③	④	⑤	X	Y	Z	X	Y	Z	X	Y	Z	X	Y	Z	total
g1/g2	○	○	○	○	×	×	×	○	×	×	×	×	×	○	×	×	×	6
g1/g3	○	○	×	×	○	×	○	○	×	○	○	×	×	○	×	×	○	9
g2/g3	○	×	○	×	○	×	○	○	×	○	○	×	×	×	×	○	×	8
total	3	2	2	1	2	0	2	3	0	2	2	0	0	2	0	1	1	

Table 6. The result of the analysis of variance in three grips (Subject C)

In order to verify the effect of the sensors that didn't showed any statistical difference to the discrimination process, we removed the data from these sensors and applied the new data set to the off-line neural network. The sensor data removed was: the EMG sensor 1, the Y axis of accelerometers 3, 4, and the X axis of accelerometer 4 for Subject A; the EMG sensor 1, 3, 4, and the X axis of accelerometers 4 for Subject B; and the X axis of accelerometers 1, 2, 3, 4, and the Y axis of accelerometer 3. Figure 15 shows a comparison between the

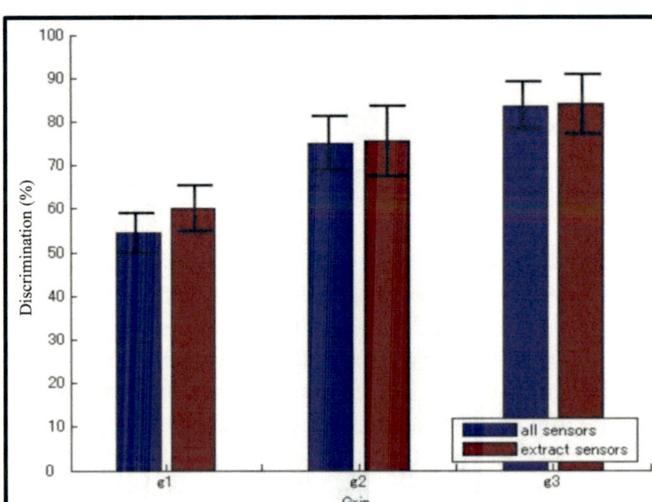

Fig. 15. The result of the discrimination rate of the two cases (all sensors, extract sensors)

discrimination results of using the data from all sensors(17 sensors) and the new data set for each subject (13 sensors for Subject A, 13 sensors for Subject B, and 12 sensors for Subject C). By removing the sensors that didn't have any contribution to the discrimination it is possible to improve the discrimination rate for all grips.

4. Discussion

In order to take full advantage of the many degrees of freedom in current light-weighted dexterous prosthetic hands, research efforts are required to improve the motion intention deduction algorithms available nowadays. The new algorithms have to take into account the whole body dynamics, to aid the amputee to realize natural and intuitive manipulation of the prosthesis. To this date, different data mining methods have been used to extract and predict information from EMG sensors, among which neural networks are the most used method commonly. R. Ashan et al. made a review on the different types of classifiers used until 2009 for EMG extraction for Human Computer Interaction applications. They concluded that the use of neural networks dominates for these applications, but point out the advantages of other methods. Moreover, a statistical approach was used by Hu X et al. in order to model the arm motions. In this case a multivariate analysis of the EMG information approach was used in order to take advantage of the correlation of the EMG activities when making arm movements. The results of these studies show that it is possible to extract arm dynamics information from activities of the proximal muscles. Although these results are encouraging, all of them processed the data off-line, therefore the real time performance of the classifier is not taken into account.

The results of this study shows that it is possible to recognize different arm motion positions and grips in a dynamical way using an on-line classifier. As seen from the results, the discrimination rate for most of the motions was high, but the lowest discrimination rate was observed in reaching position p2, which is reaching an object at the center. In this case, there aren't any distinctive components like in the other motions (for example reaching up or to the sides), making the discrimination very difficult. Also, as expected, the subject variability is very high. This can be due to sensor position or subject's individual muscle strength. Despite this difference, by inspecting different features different positions and grips can be correctly discriminated. Certainly, we need to test more subjects to determine statistically the performance of the system. Another point that has to be taken into account, is that the NN was trained only off-line, which can leave many important features out. This is why currently an on-line training scheme is being developed in order to improve the detection rates, despite of individual differences. Finally, the recognition delay has to be further improved, as for now it is about 1s, which is too slow to use in any real life application.

These preliminary findings are of importance to achieve a dynamical coupling between the person and the machine because, by taking in account the whole body dynamics, it will allow more natural and intuitive manipulation of the robot hand.

5. Conclusion

This study shows that it is possible to distinguish, dynamically, different grips and arm positions from only around-shoulder muscle activities using an online classifier and that the use of EMG and accelerometers improves greatly this discrimination despite individual differences. In near future the recognition delay has to be reduced, and the system has to be tested with real amputees.

6. References

Otsuka, A.; Tsuji, T.; Fulida, O. & Sakawa, M. (2002). Research on Upper Extremity Prosthesis based on Human Motion Analysis-Development of Internally Powered Functional-cosmetic Prosthetic Hand, *Japanese Society of Medical Instrumentation*, Vol.72, No.5

Nishikawa, D.; W, Yu.; Yokoi, H. & Kakazu, Y. (2002). On-Line Supervising Mechanism for Learning Data in SurfaceElectromyogram Motion Classifiers, *System and Computers in Japan 33*, pp.1-11 (1999). On-Line Learning Methods for EMG Prosthetic Hand Controlling, *Institute of Electronics, Information and Communication Engineers*, Vol.No9, pp.1510-1519

Tsukamoto, M.; Kondo, T. & Ito, K. A Prosthetic Hand Control by Non stationary EMG at the beginning of Motion, *The Institute of Electronics, Information and Communication Engineers*

Tsuji, T.; Yoshihiro, T. & Shima, K. (2007). An MMG-based Control Method of Prosthetic Manipulators Using Acceleration Sensors, *Robotics Society of Japan*, Vol.25, No.6

Lacquaniti, F. & Soechting, J. F. (1982). Coordination of arm and wrist motion during a reaching task, *The Journal of Neuroscience*, Vol.2, No.4, pp.399-408

Soechting, J. F. & Flanders, M. (1993). Parallel, interdependent channels for location and orientation in sensorimotor Transformation for reaching and grasping, *Journal of Neurophysiology*, Vol.70, No.2, pp.905-910

Desmurget, M.; Prablanc, C.; Rossetti, U.; Arzi, M.; Paulignam, Y.; Urquizar, C. & Mignot, J. C. (1995). Postural and synergic control for three-dimensional movements of reaching and grasping, *Journal of Neurophysiology*, Vol.74, No.2, pp.905-910

Cothros, N.; Wong, J. D. & Gribble, P. L. (2006). Are there distinct neural representations of object and limb dynamics, *Exp.Brain res*, Vol.173, pp.689-697

Thiel, V. E. & Steenbergen, B. (2001). Shoulder and hand displacements during hitting, reaching and grasping movements in hemiparetic cerebral palsy, *Motor Control*, Vol.5, No.2, pp.166-182

Wilson, F. R. (1998). The Hand: How its use shapes the brain, language and human culture, *Pantheon Books*, New York. ISBN:0679412492

Martellon, C.; Carpaneto, J. & Micera, S. (2008). Classification of Upper arm EMG signals during object-specific grasp. *30th Annual International IEEE EMBS Conference*

Nakamura, R. & Saito, H. (1992). Basic Kinesiology, 4th Ed, *ISHIYAKU publication*

Ahsan, M.; Ibrahimy, M & Khalifa, O. (2009). EMG signal classification for human computer interaction: a review, *Eur J Sci Res*, Vol 33(3), pp.480-501

Hu, X. & Nenov, V. (2004). Multivariate AR modeling of electromyography for the classification of upper arm movements, *Clin Neurophysiol*, Vol115(6), pp1276-87

4

Walking and Jogging: Quantification of Muscle Activity of the Lower Extremities

Begoña Gavilanes-Miranda[1], Juan J. Goiriena De Gandarias[2] and Gonzalo A. Garcia[3]
[1]*Faculty of Physical Activity and Sport Science, University of Basque Country, Vitoria*
[2]*Faculty of Medicine, University of Basque Country, Bilbao*
[3]*Biorobotics Department, Tecnalia, Bilbao*
Spain

1. Introduction

Basmajian (1967) defined locomotion as "the translation of the centre of gravity through space along a path requiring the least expenditure of energy". Taking as reference the centre of gravity (CG) of the body, it has been already established that the trajectory while walking or jogging follows a sinusoidal course (Inman 1968), with two vertical summits per stride (one cycle of locomotion).

During locomotion, the movement of translation of the body is produced by the spatial angular movement of the lower extremities that shows support and non-support phases. The basic unit of measurement in gait analysis is the gait cycle (GC) or stride. The gait cycle is commonly divided into two phases: 1) stance phase, and 2) non-support phase. In walking, in the stance phase there are two periods of double support. In jogging cycle (JC) the phase of non support is composed of two float periods (when both feet are airborne) and between both periods there is one period of swing of the ipsilateral leg.

Walking and jogging present differences at: 1) the velocity pattern, which is higher in jogging, as it implies joint movements of higher amplitude and speed; 2) the duration of cycles and of their respective phases; 3) the kinematics of: a) the peaks of the body CG trajectory (its amplitude and time of appearance), and b) of the joints, as there are wider angular joints displacements and different distribution of arches movements during cycle phases (Novacheck, 1998); 4) the kinetic: a) amplitude, duration, and evolution of the ground reaction force (Mann, 1982), external moments of force, and muscle power (Winter, 1983a and 1983b); b) misalignment of CG between the segments of the leg and of the upper part of the body (head, trunk, and arms); c) inertia; and 5) the mechanisms for saving energy structures (Cavagna & Kaneko, 1977; van Ingen Schenau et al., 1987).

Several studies have compared the muscle activity of the legs during walking and jogging or running. In the works of Mann & Hagy (1980), and Mann (1982), the subjects were trained athletes, and in the work of Ounpuu (1994) they were children. In all the above-mentioned papers the muscle activity was recorded from only one leg, and the muscular activity was qualitatively described rather than quantified. Nilsson et al. (1985) and Gazendam and Hof (2007) quantified the profiles of averaged rectified EMGs at different speeds of locomotion and mode of progression in humans on motor-driven treadmill.

The work here presented was carried out to investigate and to quantify the electromyographic activity (EMG -the weak electric signal produced by contracting muscles) of the lower extremities during walking and jogging and to evaluate the changes produced in jogging. The subjects (who practice regularly physical activities) walked and jogged barefoot at ground level at spontaneous speed. These subjects had a healthy condition, but they were exposed to lesions due to their jogging practice. The aim of the present study was to quantify the changes produced in the EMG signal characteristics (as amplitude and time of occurrence of peak activity) of both legs muscles during jogging compared with walking.

The comparison carried out in this study between the EMG activity of the leg muscles during walking and during jogging can reveal the adaptability of the neuromuscular system against more demanding mechanical needs, and in this way we can learn more about the etiopathology of lesions.

2. Materials and methods

2.1 Subjects

Six male and four female University students who regularly practice jogging (heel-toe style) have participated voluntarily in this study. Five subjects were 19 years old, four of them 20, and one, 30, with an average height of 1.73±0.10m, and a body mass of 64.2±6.0 Kg. The 10 subjects were right lower extremity dominant (determined by the leg they reported to use for shooting a ball). Written informed consent was obtained from all of them. The experimental protocol got the approval of the Scientific Committee of the Basque Institute of Physical Education.

2.2 Instrumentation

The stride phases (support and non-support) were identified by four footswitches (B&L Engineering, Tustin, California) that were taped to each foot sole over the heel, on the heads of the first and fifth metatarsus, and on the tip of the toe. The footswitches (FSs) were activated when the pressure was above 1.5N, producing an on/off output voltage.

For the surface EMG (s-EMG) signals acquisition, circular, three-pole (1.0cm diameter each pole), stainless steel, bipolar surface electrodes (B&L Engineering, Tustin, California) were used. Double differential signals were obtained between each of the outer two active electrodes and a reference central electrode to improve the signal-to-noise ratio and to diminish the cross-talk from adjacent muscles. The centre-to-centre inter-pole distance was 1.5cm. An earth electrode was placed on the wrist. The electrodes had a built-in 320-gain preamplifier, which had an input impedance greater than 20MΩ, minimum common-mode rejection ratio (CMRR) of 95dB (at 50Hz), and a bandwidth from 10Hz to 30KHz (cut-offs at -3dB). The dimensions of the whole body of the electrodes were 5cm x 1.8cm x 0.7cm. An optic-fiber cable transmitted the signals from the connection box, located on the subject, to the acquisition system.

Surface electrodes were chosen for the study of the muscular activity because they offer the following advantages respect to intra-muscular electrodes: they produce no pain neither harm the tissue, they are easier to place, and as already shown by Giroux & Lamontagne (1990), they record statistically similar signals to those obtained with intramuscular wire electrodes. The potential problem of crosstalk was reduced using a double differential technique, which is based on a single amplifier fed with three electrodes (De Luca &

Merletti, 1988; Winter, 1990; Winter et al., 1994). It is already widely accepted that double-differential technique reduces the level of cross-talk (see, *e.g.*, De Luca & Merletti, 1988; and Meinecke et al., 2004). In any case, cross-talk cannot ever be fully cancelled.

In addition, as the subjects were moving during the recordings, surface electrodes gave a more robust signal (free of artifacts) than internal electrodes.

Before performing the recordings, the skin over the target muscles was shaved and then cleaned with alcohol; no gel was used between the skin and the electrodes. Subsequently, the subjects were asked to execute specific movements for each muscle to check the output of the s-EMG electrodes. In order to test the proper functioning of the FSs, the subjects were asked to step on the floor in a way that activated sequentially the FSs. Once the experimental setup was verified, the subjects were asked to walk or jog freely along the laboratory to get used to the electrodes and sensors until they felt comfortable with the equipment and the speeds of consecutive strolls were similar.

Surface EMG was recorded from six target muscles of each leg: rectus femoris (RF), vastus medialis (VM), long head of biceps femoris (BF), semitendinosus (ST), tibialis anterior (TA), and lateral gastrocnemius (LG). Those muscles are the ones normally targeted in the literature, because they are important for the locomotion and because they are superficial and hence easily detectable. In order to obtain a signal with higher amplitude, the electrodes were placed parallel to the fibers direction of each muscle, which was estimated following the work by Wickiewiz et al. (1983). Electrodes were placed on the muscles following the SENIAM recommendations (SENIAM, 1999).

The placement of the electrodes over each target muscle was as follow; RF: at 50% on the line from the anterior iliac spine superior to the superior part of patella; VM: at 80% distal on the line between the anterior iliac spine superior and the joint space of the knee in front of the anterior border of the medial ligament; BF: at 50% on the line between the ischial tuberosity superior and the lateral epicondyle of the tibia; ST: at 50% on the line ischial tuberosity superior and the medial epicondyle of the tibia; TA: at 1/3 proximal on the line between the tip of the fibula and the tip of the medial malleolus; and GL: at 1/3 proximal on the line between the head of the fibula and the heel.

The abovementioned signals (12-channel s-EMG, and two from the FSs status) were registered with a MA-200 (MotionLab Systems, LA, USA) equipped with a Pentium PC endowed with a 16-channel acquisition card CODAS DI 400 PGH (Dataq Instruments, OH, USA) featuring 12 bits of resolution, a gain of x8, a pass-band filter from 10Hz to 1KHz, a CMMR of 40dB, an input impedance above 1MΩ, and a sampling rate of 3 Ksamples/s, as indicated by Merletti (1994).

2.3 Experimental protocol

Individuals were barefoot. Five successive s-EMG recordings were made from each subject while walking and another five recordings while jogging, all of which at spontaneous speed because, as proofed by Kadaba (1989), the s-EMG activity is more reproducible when subjects walk at their spontaneous velocity.

The measurements were carried out in a 10m long laboratory, where the subjects walked at ground level. The average speed (in m/s) was calculated measuring the time required for covering the 10m. There was a one-minute break between each recording. Only the three central cycles of those recordings have been analyzed in order to avoid the acceleration and deceleration effect. All the subjects that participated in the study were athletes, whose ability to start and stop abruptly is quite higher than that of average subjects. Therefore, the effect of acceleration and deceleration is low in this kind of subjects. In any case, the objective of this work was not to study the influence of the locomotion *speed* on the muscular activity, but of the *type* of locomotion, keeping constant the EMG signals acquisition conditions.

2.4 Data analysis
2.4.1 Spatio-temporal parameters

2.4.1.1 Velocity

Average velocity was calculated by measuring with a stopwatch the elapsed time each subject took to cross the 10m length of the laboratory.

2.4.1.2 Temporal components of the locomotion cycle

The signals from the FSs were displayed as a staircase. The time length of support and non-support phases were normalized with respect to the duration of the whole locomotion cycle and expressed as percentages of the respective cycle (gait cycle or jogging cycle), 0% being the beginning of the support phase and 100% the end of the non-support phase.

2.4.2 EMG signal

Surface EMG signals were acquired from six muscles for each leg (RF, VM, BF, ST, TA, and LG). In order to smooth the signal and to reliably determine the s-EMG peak value and its time of occurrence, the raw signals were firstly full-wave rectified and then averaged using a moving window of 50ms length (150 samples), which yielded the linear envelope (LE) corresponding to the s-EMG signal. The LE was used because it closely represents the continuous rises and falls profile of muscular activity as a function of time (Inman et al., 1952).
The intra-subject s-EMG activation profiles were calculated using ensemble averages (EAV) computed as follows: each EAV point was calculated as the average of a 2%-segment of the already averaged s-EMG signal (Winter, 1991) of the 15 selected strides (3 central strides of each stroll x 5 strolls per subject for each locomotion mode).
The s-EMG amplitude normalization of each muscle activity for each subject and for each type of locomotion was performed with respect to the maximum peak of subject's EAV in each type of locomotion (Yang & Winter, 1984). For muscles having two activity peaks, the highest of them was chosen as the normalizing peak and it will be the one referred as "activity peak" hereafter.
The grand ensemble averaged (GEAV) was obtained by averaging the EAV of all the subjects for each kind of locomotion. The electromyographic activity, expressed as GEAV, was analyzed in absolute (GEAV) and normalized (nGEAV) values. Un-normalized values allowed us to appreciate the evolution of the muscle activity when the locomotion changed from walking to jogging (hence increasing the mechanical requirements), while the electrodes remained in the same position.

2.5 Statistical analysis

The mean and the standard deviation (SD) were calculated for the spatio-temporal parameters and for the peak of the lineal envelop (EAV).
The influence of the kind of locomotion on s-EMG peak location and on spatio-temporal parameters (namely, kind of locomotion and percentage of the cycle) was determined applying a t-Student test for independent measurements using *SPSS* statistical package (SPSS Inc., IL, USA), all of them calculated at a significance level of $p < 0.05$.

The coefficient of correlation (CC) between two muscles activity profiles was defined as the ratio between the covariance of those two profiles and its associated standard deviation. The CC cannot exceed 1 in absolute value, and the closer it is to 1, the more similar are the compared profiles. Therefore, the CC provides an index of similarity, and it has been used to measure the similitude of the EMG profile of homologous muscles (those that are the same, but located in different legs).
The inter-subject variability of s-EMG signal was determined by the coefficient of variation (CV –ratio of the standard deviation to the mean) of the average across the 10-subject EAV, which generated an inter-subject EAV and its associated standard deviation.
Locomotion is a complex act that involves the integration of several variables during its learning process; hence, each subject has its own personal way of walking. Therefore, in order to increase our understanding of human locomotion it is necessary to use average values of the muscular activity, so that inter-subject differences can be diminished. Therefore, in this study, the acquired s-EMG signals have been further studied only after the inter-subject reproducibility was assessed, and always from both legs (Inman et al., 1981).

3. Results and discussion

The aim of this study was to analyze: 1) the changes in amplitude on un-normalized electromyographic signal, and 2) the time of appearance of the s-EMG peak from muscles of both legs when the locomotion style changed while the electrodes remained in the same position. All of that after having evaluated and validated the reproducibility of the s-EMG signals. We have quantified the two types of locomotion by using EMG in order to obtain a powerful and objective tool for understanding the origin of lesions that are more frequent in jogging.

3.1 Spatio-temporal parameters

The average speed during walking was 1.33±0.12m/s (mean ± standard deviation), and 2.50 ±0.31m/s in jogging, which implies an average increase of 87%.
Table 1 shows the average time length of each phase in absolute and relative values (respect

Phase	Jogging		Walking	
	average [s]	JC [%]	average [s]	GC [%]
Left leg support	0.26 ±0.02	37.8	0.60 ±0.06	61.0
Left leg non-support	0.45 ±0.03	62.8	0.38 ±0.03	39.0
Right leg support	0.25 ±0.10	35.3	0.59 ±0.07	60.5
Right leg non-support	0.46 ±0.12	64.3	0.38 ±0.04	38.6
Left stride	0.71 ±0.03	100.0	0.99 ±0.08	100.0
Right stride	0.72 ±0.03	100.0	0.97 ±0.09	100.0

Table 1. Comparison of time length of each phase and its corresponding cycle percentage for the jogging cycle (JC) and for the gait cycle (GC). All the values showed significant statistical difference (p<0.05)

to the duration of the whole stride) detected for walking and for jogging. On average, the cycle time for walking was 0.99s for the left leg and 0.97s for the right leg. For jogging, the cycle time decreased to 0.71s and 0.72s respectively. In jogging, the support phase decreased a 50% with respect to the GC and hence, in that short time, a bigger ground reaction force had to be attenuated and bigger and faster displacement of the segments had to be achieved (Mann, 1982). All the above mentioned changes are significant at a certainty level of 95% (p<0.05).

3.2 Reliability of the s-EMG signal

For the muscles studied, the obtained functional patterns for walking and for jogging were similar to those already published (Gazendam & Hof, 2007; Mann & Hagy, 1980; Mann, 1982; and Ounpuu, 1994).
Inter-subject variability was determined by averaging the un-normalized and normalized EAV of the 10 subjects (GEAV). Table 2 shows the CVs calculated from those un-normalized (GEAV) and normalized (nGEAV) grand ensemble averages. A high CV corresponds to a higher inter-subject variability in the s-EMG of the analyzed muscles, and hence of their activity levels (Kadaba, 1989; and Winter & Yack, 1987).

Leg	Muscle	n	Number of observations	CV of GEAV [%]			
				Jogging		Walking	
				uN	N	uN	N
Left Leg	Rectus Femoris	10	50	79	17	41	35
	Vastus Medialis	9	45	49	25	51	34
	Tibialis Anterior	10	50	39	31	30	24
	Biceps Femoris	10	50	67	26	63	37
	Semitendinosus	10	50	56	27	51	25
	Lateral Gastrocnemius	10	50	66	24	47	25
Right Leg	Rectus Femoris	10	50	67	20	51	39
	Vastus Medialis	9	45	34	69	44	59
	Tibialis Anterior	10	50	38	27	31	27
	Biceps Femoris	10	50	61	26	77	28
	Semitendinosus	10	50	59	28	71	25
	Lateral Gastrocnemius	10	50	66	25	55	29

Table 2. Inter-subject (n: number of subjects) coefficients of variation (CV) of un-normalized (uN) and normalized (N) grand ensemble average (GEAV)

In jogging, when the mechanical demand increased, there was a higher inter-subject variability in the LE of the s-EMG of the greater part of the muscles, as showed by the higher values of CV for the un-normalized s-EMG.

The CV of the GEAV obtained from the normalized EAV, was reduced of about 50% in the greater part of the muscles. That CV was in general not too different in both types of locomotion, except for the RF muscle, which showed a higher variability in walking than in jogging, although its muscular activity was smaller in walking. The variability of the EMG has been studied deeper in walking (*e.g.*, Kadaba et al., 1989; and Winter & Yack, 1987) than in jogging (*e.g.*, Karamanidis et al., 2004).

In the present study, the nCV values obtained during walking were smaller than those reported by Kadaba et al. (1989); and by Winter & Yack (1987). The differences found between our CV results and those of the abovementioned studies could be explained by the different computations used in the normalization of the EMG activity: setting the mean value of each subject's EMG over the whole stride period (Winter & Yack, 1987), or smoothing the EMG data using a filter with a low pass cut-off frequency of 12-14Hz (Kadaba et al., 1989).

Other studies normalized the EMG signal of each muscle by the value corresponding to its maximum voluntary contraction (*e.g.*, Arsenault et al., 1986a; and Perry et al., 1993). In the present study we did not use that normalization because it is not always possible to apply it; *e.g.*, in the case of injured subjects and hence it could not be used for the sake of comparison in future works. Instead, we normalized the EMG recordings corresponding to walking and to jogging trials by their respective peak values during locomotion at spontaneous speed because it is a simple and reliable way of obtaining comparable muscular activity profiles (Yang & Winter, 1984) .

In the present work, the nCV of the 10 analyzed subjects were not significantly different (below 35%) in walking and jogging, which points out that there are more similarities than differences in the muscular activity between subjects in both ways of locomotion.

The differences detected on the CV of muscles from a same muscle group can indicate that a muscle has more than one function and a more variable activity, as already pointed out by Winter & Yack (1987).

3.3 Amplitude of myoelectric activity

Figure 1 shows that the muscular activity profiles of five out of the six studied muscles for each leg were similar in walking and in jogging, although there were differences in the sequence of movement arches of hip and knee corresponding to the phases of support and non-support, and also in the direction of the movement arches of the ankle.

The above-mentioned findings support other studies, such as those of Gazendam & Hof (2007); Mann & Hagy (1980); Mann (1982); and Ounpuu (1994).

Figure 1 also shows that there was a similar pattern (nearly identical) between the grand ensemble averages of muscular activity in both legs.

The idea of registering the activity of both legs was to ensure the validity of the assumption made in other works about the symmetry of the activity of both legs.

Table 3 shows the coefficients of correlation (CC) obtained when comparing the GEAVs of homologous muscles (those same muscles in different legs). These findings have provided some support to the assumption of symmetry made in the literature and are on line with the studies de Arseanult et al. (1986b), and by Ounpuu & Winter (1989), who showed the symmetry existing in walking; and by Raibert (1986), who found out that symmetry is desirable because it would simplify control strategies.

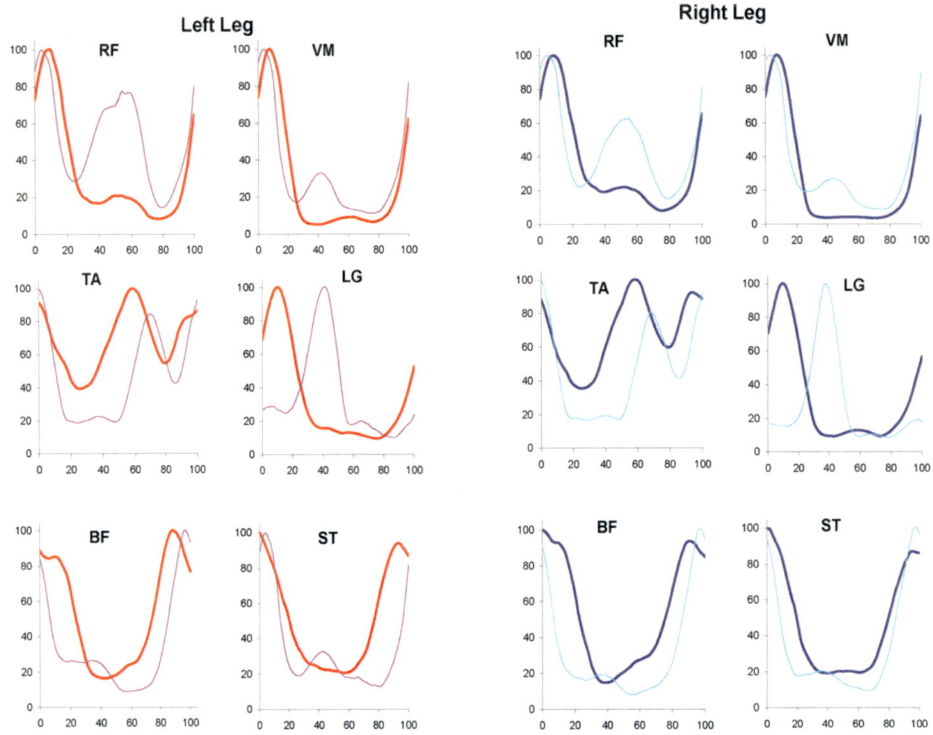

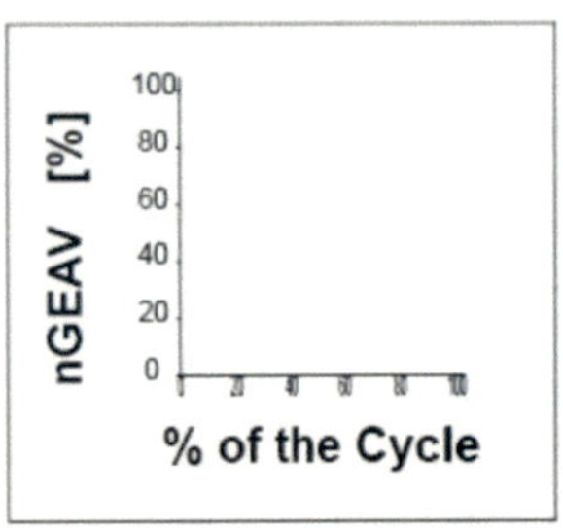

Muscles Acronym	
RF	Rectus Femoris
VM	Vastus Medialis
TA	Tibialis Anterior
LG	Lateral Gastrocnemius
BF	Biceps Femoris
ST	Semitendinosus

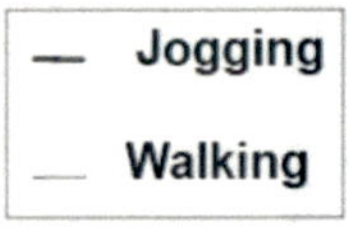

Fig. 1. Normalized grand ensemble average (nGEAV) for left and right leg muscles s-EMG activity. On each graph have been overlapped the activity profile of each muscle in walking (thin line) and in jogging (thick line). It could be appreciated how the peak of each muscle shifted in time in jogging with respect to walking. There was a similar pattern (nearly identical) between the nGEAV of both legs.

Table 4 shows the average of EAV maximum, minimum, and mean amplitudes from ensemble average of all subjects, and their respective standard deviation. Across the different subjects there was a wide range of peak amplitudes as can be seen from the high standard deviation values, which were bigger during jogging. In both types of locomotion, each muscle showed a characteristic level of maximal amplitude. In particular, the peak of the RF was smaller than that of the TA; even though the peak of electrical activity of both muscles was different between subjects. It can be also noted that the TA muscle is always active during jogging, as its minimum values are quite high: 0.39mV and 0.36 mV, which are similar to the average activation levels of TA during walking (0.47mV and 0.51mV). As a matter of fact, 0.39mV and 0.36 mV represent the 40% of its maximal amplitude during jogging cycle.

Muscle	Walking	Jogging
Rectus Femoris	0.96	1.00
Vastus Medialis	0.99	1.00
Tibialis Anterior	1.00	0.96
Biceps Femoris	0.99	0.98
Semitendinosus	0.64	0.99
Lateral Gastrocnemius	0.95	0.99

Table 3. Correlation coefficients between the s-EMG activity grand ensemble averages (GEAV) of homologous muscles

Leg	Muscles	Jogging [mV]						Walking [mV]					
		max	SD	min	SD	mean	SD	max	SD	min	SD	mean	SD
Left Leg	Rectus Femoris	0.52	0.33	0.04	0.02	0.18	0.12	0.16	0.04	0.02	0.01	0.07	0.02
	Vastus Medialis	1.67	0.47	0.07	0.02	0.46	0.13	0.40	0.17	0.04	0.00	0.13	0.05
	Tibialis Anterior	1.50	0.22	0.39	0.19	0.88	0.13	1.01	0.18	0.13	0.04	0.47	0.05
	Biceps Femoris	1.07	0.47	0.12	0.06	0.52	0.19	0.60	0.38	0.04	0.01	0.20	0.09
	Semitendinosus	0.83	0.49	0.11	0.05	0.38	0.18	0.39	0.15	0.04	0.00	0.13	0.05
	Lateral Gastroc.	1.47	0.66	0.12	0.10	0.50	0.25	0.62	0.24	0.05	0.02	0.20	0.07
Right Leg	Rectus Femoris	0.60	0.30	0.04	0.02	0.21	0.09	0.19	0.08	0.02	0.01	0.08	0.03
	Vastus Medialis	1.77	0.37	0.05	0.01	0.46	0.10	0.44	0.19	0.04	0.00	0.14	0.05
	Tibialis Anterior	1.35	0.24	0.36	0.15	0.81	0.17	1.12	0.31	0.16	0.05	0.51	0.10
	Biceps Femoris	1.11	0.62	0.12	0.05	0.52	0.23	0.61	0.43	0.04	0.02	0.19	0.11
	Semitendinosus	1.03	0.66	0.13	0.09	0.46	0.26	0.54	0.40	0.04	0.01	0.18	0.11
	Lateral Gastroc.	1.42	0.59	0.09	0.03	0.47	0.18	0.76	0.34	0.05	0.02	0.21	0.08

Table 4. Walking and jogging: average value of maximal (max), minimal (min), and mean amplitudes from the ensemble average (EAV) of all subjects, and their respective standard deviation (SD)

It is worth noting that, within each mode of locomotion, the amplitude peak was very similar for homologous muscles (see Figure 2). These findings complement the findings of Arsenault et al. (1986b); and Ounpuu & Winter (1989).

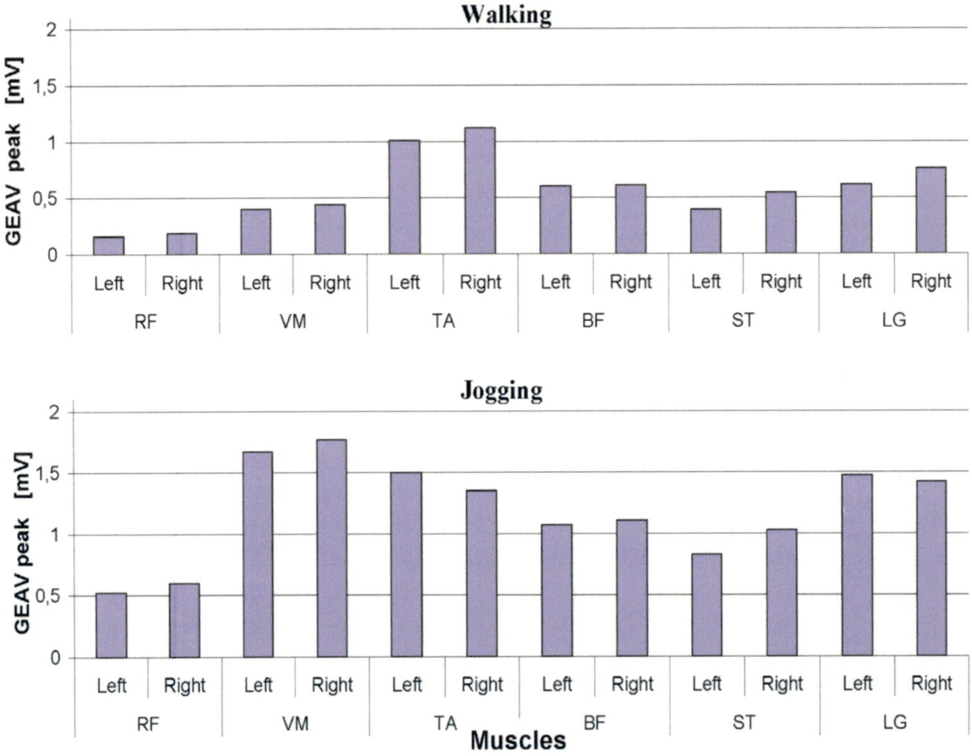

Fig. 2. Peak values of the grand ensemble average (GEAV) for each of the studied muscles for each leg during walking and during jogging. The amplitude peak was very similar for homologous muscles in the two legs for both ways of locomotion.

During jogging, all muscles increased significantly their maximal activity ($p< 0.05$). It can be seen from peak amplitudes that in walking distal muscles were more active than proximal muscles, being TA the muscle showing the biggest peak, and that in jogging it was the proximal muscle VM the most active. The higher sustained level of activity found in the TA agrees with the results of Reber et al. (1993), and indicates that the TA is more susceptible to fatigue and to related injuries.

The electrodes have been left placed on the same locations for each subject while walking than while jogging; therefore, as there was no other changes, the differences observed in the amplitude of the EMG signals of a muscle are due to a different participation of that muscle on the specific type of locomotion.

We have used the absolute (not normalized) signal to precisely quantify the participation of each muscle in each type of locomotion. If the signal was normalized, those changes would have been not detected (as shown in Figure 1), because the bigger EMG signal amplitude obtained while jogging would have been divided by a bigger peak value. However, the use

of the non-normalized values reveals the adaptability of the neuromuscular system against more demanding mechanical needs during jogging.
The recordings of each subject have been averaged because locomotion is a complex act that involves the integration of several variables during its learning process; hence, each subject has its own personal way of walking. Therefore, in order to increase our understanding of human locomotion it is necessary to use average values of the muscular activity, so that inter-subject differences can be diminished, as suggested by Inman et al. (1981).

3.4 Peak amplitude of myoelectric activity and relative increment

In order to find the activity increment during jogging in comparison with walking, the activity peak during jogging was normalized with respect to the peak found during walking.
Table 5 shows the increase of the maximum amplitude expressed in absolute values and in percentage of the maximum amplitude registered during walking. In both legs, the muscles that showed the biggest relative activity increment were the VM and the RF. The minimum relative increase occurred in the TA muscle.
It can be seen that there were different increases of activity of the muscles belonging to the same muscular group. This finding is in line with Gazendam & Hof (2007), who found that the relationship between speed and muscular effort was generally different between muscles of the same group.
The activity peak of muscles belonging to the same group could be very different (RF and VM) or quite similar (BF and ST). In all the cases, the difference in the peak intensity was bigger in jogging (see Table 4), which is in agreement with the results of Gazendam & Hof (2007); and of Montgomery et al. (1994).
The muscles belonging to the same muscular groups RF and VM are innervated by muscular branches of the crural nerve (L2-L4). The BF and ST muscles are innervated by the muscular branches of the sciatic nerve (L4-S2); however, for both legs, the peak and the increase of activity peak between walking and jogging of those muscles belonging to the same group was different. In particular (see Figure 2 and Table 5), the BF showed more activity than the ST in walking, and showed less activity increase in jogging than the ST, even though the BF was more active. The VM showed a higher activity in walking than RF and its activity increased more in jogging than RF. This difference in the activity increment may be due to: 1) their architectural characteristics: mass, muscle fiber length, transversal section area, and pennation angle (Wickiewiz, 1983); 2) the functions they perform in the three-dimensional space; and 3) the amount of joints that they cross. For example, the bigger s-EMG amplitude peak found in the VM in the support phase might be due to its mono-articular and unipennate nature. In addition, this muscle has the roles of: 1) preventing the genu valgum (Perry, 1992), the occurrence of which is more probable in jogging at the beginning of the support phase due to the concomitant dorsal flexion; 2) opposing the flexor action of the LG, which was active and presented, in some subjects, its activity peak at the same time than that of the VM; and 3) controlling the external rotation produced by the activation of the BF. The lesser increment in the peak of RF could be explained by the fact that it is biarticular and bipennate (which facilitates the force production; Gans, 1982). In both walking and jogging, the RF and VM muscles showed the maximum peak at the beginning of the support phase, when there was an extension movement of the hip and a simultaneous flexion of the knee (Mann & Hagy, 1980). If the RF showed high activity during the hip extension, it would oppose that hip movement.

From the mean peak amplitudes it can be seen that, for both legs, during walking the proximal muscles (VM and RF) showed an amplitude peak smaller than that of the distal muscles. When jogging, the proximal muscles showed greater relative increase than the other muscles, which can be due to the importance of the knee for both the movement and the stability. The VM was the muscle showing the bigger peak amplitude; namely, its average peak level was 4 times bigger during jogging (1.67mV and 1.77 mV) than during walking (0.40 mV and 0.44mV).

RF and VM muscles have an important role in the absorption of the mechanical shock resulting from the impact of the heel against the floor. In jogging, the ground reaction force (GRF) is bigger than in walking, and in addition, that shock has to be absorbed in a shorter time, as the contact with the floor passes from being 0,60s to just 0,26s (a reduction to less than a half). Furthermore, the repetition of wrong alignments of the lower limbs can facilitate the production of lesions.

This result complements the studies of Gazendam & Hof (2007); and of Montgomery et al. (1994), and provides support to the results of Taunton et al. (1988) on the prevalence of the patella femoral pain syndrome and of the patellar tendinitis in athletes.

Of the distal muscles, the LG absolute and relative activity during jogging increased more than that of the TA, showing both muscles a similar maximal peak during jogging. Mizrahi et al. (2000b) demonstrated that with the progressing of fatigue in long-distance running, an imbalance in the activities between the ankle plantar and dorsi flexor muscles develops and the muscles that span the tensile surface of the bone becomes less active than those of the opposite side, the result is a decrease in the protection abilities of the muscles.

Leg	Muscle	peak [mV]		Increase [mV]	Increase [%]
		Walking	Jogging		
Left Leg	Rectus Femoris	0.16	0.52	0.37	233
	Vastus Medialis	0.40	1.67	1.27	314
	Tibialis Anterior	1.01	1.50	0.49	49
	Biceps Femoris	0.60	1.07	0.47	79
	Semitendinosus	0.39	0.83	0.44	112
	Lateral Gastrocnemius	0.62	1.47	0.85	137
Right Leg	Rectus Femoris	0.19	0.60	0.41	216
	Vastus Medialis	0.44	1.77	1.33	302
	Tibialis Anterior	1.12	1.35	0.22	20
	Biceps Femoris	0.61	1.11	0.50	81
	Semitendinosus	0.54	1.03	0.49	90
	Lateral Gastrocnemius	0.76	1.42	0.66	86

Table 5. Increase of the s-EMG amplitude peak expressed in absolute values and in percentages respect to the maximum amplitude of the walking cycle

3.5 Appearance time of the activity peak

Figure 1 shows how the peak of each muscle shifted in time in jogging with respect to walking.

Subject	Time of occurrence for the right leg [% of cycle]											
	RF		VM		BF		ST		TA		LG	
	JC	GC	JC	GC	JC	GC	JC	GC	JC	GC	JC	GC
s1	8→12	6	12	N/A	12→14	100	8	4	62	0	8→12	42
s2	8→12	4	10	4	14	0	12	4	94	0	14	40
s3	6→8	46	8	4	84→86	90	0	6	4	0	8→10	38
s4	6→10	4	6→8	4	12	100	94	4	56	0	10	40
s5	8	2	8	2	88	96	2	2	0	0	10	38
s6	8	4	8	4	6	96	4	6	60	N/A	10	32
s7	8	6	8	6	12	100	4→8	4	60	0	12	36
s8	10	42	4	2	0	94	92	2	58	0	6	40
s9	6→10	62	6→8	4	86	98	88	4	56	70	8	36
s10	8	58	2	2	92	98	92	4	4	0	8	44

Subject	Time of occurrence for the left leg [% of cycle]											
	RF		VM		BF		ST		TA		LG	
	JC	GC	JC	GC	JC	GC	JC	GC	JC	GC	JC	GC
s1	16	6	N/A	N/A	90	96	2	96	60	0	10	40
s2	8	4	8	2	16	98	20	98	92	0	10	38
s3	10	56	6	2	14	0	0	98	92	0	8	36
s4	8	6	8	4	14	0	0	0	54	68	12	38
s5	8	2	6→8	0	0	96	2	96	94→98	0	8	34
s6	8	4	8	8	8→10	98	4	98	58→60	0	10	36
s7	12	6	8→10	6	86	98	2	100	58	68	12	36
s8	6	4	6	2	0	96	0	0	56	0	6	34
s9	8	56	8	2	14	36	88	96	58	68	8	36
s10	8	4	6	0	88	98	0	0	60	0	10	36

Table 6. Time of occurrence of the amplitude peak in the ensemble average (EAV) for the muscles of both legs, expressed in percentage of the cycle of walking (GC) and of jogging (JC). (N/A: Not Available)

Table 6 shows, for each subject and for each muscle, the time of EAV peak, which corresponds to the moment of maximum activity of each muscle. In this case, it would be misleading to use the GEAV, as it would yield average values that may actually not appear in any of the real signals. In walking and in jogging the time of appearance of the activity peak of RF, VM, and LG muscles was consistent and always occurred in eccentric contraction; in addition, there was a higher inter-subject variability in the time of occurrence of the IT and TA muscles peak activity.

3.5.1 Rectus femoris

During walking, the peak activity of the RF appeared at different times for each subject; in the majority of the subjects, the peak activity occurred at the loading phase (2-6%GC). In other subjects the peak appeared either at the end of the final stance phase (42%GC), at the pre-swinging phase (58%GC), or at the beginning of the oscillation phase (62%GC).
In jogging, for all the subjects, the peak appeared at the beginning of the support phase (6-12%JC), a bit later than in walking.

3.5.2 Vastus medialis

In walking, the VM muscle of both legs showed its highest activity peak in the loading phase (2-8%GC). In jogging, the peak appeared always at the beginning of stance phase (2-12%JC), but in some subjects it appeared later than in walking. In none of the subjects the peak appeared at the end of the loading phase because the knee extends during the propulsion; while during walking, the knee flexes.

3.5.3 Lateral gastrocnemius

Interestingly, the peak of LG occurred during unipodal support both in walking and in jogging, but in walking at the end and in jogging at the beginning of the unipodal support. The LG peak appeared in eccentric contraction, when it was acting as antagonist (Mann & Hagy, 1980; and Mann, 1982), while dorsal flexion is performed, increasing in this way its efficiency.
In jogging, its activity peak appeared at the same time than that of the VM. This study has confirmed the results of Gazendam et al. (2007), who indicated that in running quadriceps and calf muscles work together in absorbing and generating energy.

3.5.4 Tibialis anterior

The TA muscle presented two peaks. Its maximal amplitude peak in walking, in the greatest part of the subjects, occurred at the beginning of the support phase (0%GC), and -only in a few subjects- in the swinging phase (68-70%GC). In jogging, the peak appeared either at the loading phase (0%JC), in the swing phase (58-62%JC), or in the final flight (92-98%JC).
In any case, the time of appearance of the TA activity peak showed less variability in walking than during jogging. The role of the TA muscle during walking changes depending on the moment in which it becomes active: it acts as antagonist of the plantar flexion if active at the beginning of the support phase, or as agonist of the dorsal flexion if it is active at the beginning of the swinging phase. In jogging, when the TA activity peaked at the very beginning of the loading phase, it facilitated the forward movement of the tibia and hence eased the flexion of the knee. When it peaked in the swing phase and in the final fly, it facilitated the dorsal flexion. Therefore, in jogging, the peak of TA always occurred when it was acting as agonist.

3.5.5 Ischiotibial muscles

The peak of the ischiotibial (ITI) muscles (BF and ST) appeared in the same or in different phases (final non support or initial support). In walking, the maximal amplitude of the BF muscle appeared for nearly all the subjects at the end of the swinging phase (94-100%GC). The peak of the ST occurred in the loading phase (2-6%GC) for the left leg and at the end of the swinging phase (96-100%GC) for the right leg.

The role of the ITI muscles during the swinging phase is to stop the leg in order to ease its standing. Inman (1968) proposed that the deceleration of the oscillating leg by the ITI muscles can contribute even more to the forward movement of the body than the push of the ipsilateral leg.

In jogging, the occurrence of the BF and ST activity peak varied among subjects, appearing indistinctly at the beginning (BF, 0-14%JC; ST, 0-4%JC) or at the end (BF, 86-90%JC; ST, 88-94%JC) of the cycle.

The variability in the time of the peak appearance for the ST and BF muscles supports the theory that forces are optimally distributed between the several muscles that cross a joint (Chao & Rim, 1973; and Crowninshield, 1978).

3.6 Activity pattern of the studied muscles in relation to their mechanical functions during locomotion

The mechanical functions required for the locomotion are: 1) landing impact absorption, 2) dynamic stability, 3) propulsion, and 4) energy conservation (Perry, 1992). The execution of each function depends on a distinct motion pattern.

3.6.1 Landing impact absorption

Muscles amplitude peaks were higher in jogging that in walking and in five or in six (depending on the subject) of the muscles studied for each leg (VM, RF, BF, ST, and LG) the peak occurred mainly in the support phase. These results were as expected because the mechanical requirements for the absorption of the landing impact (the vertical component of the GRF is in the order of 1.5 times each subject's body weight), and the stability requirements (the support during jogging is only on one leg) are bigger in jogging than in walking.

Both in walking and in jogging, the RF and VM muscles showed their peak activity when they were activated eccentrically. The TA muscle controls the plantar flexion in walking, helping to absorb the shock of the landing. As the foot comes in contact with the ground during jogging, dorsiflexion of the ankle takes place. The other mechanism helping to absorb this impact is controlled pronation of foot, which provides flexibility within the foot.

For a deeper study about the influence of the mechanical impact on the lesions, see the works by Mizhrahi et al. (2000a) and (2000b).

3.6.2 Dynamic stability

The stability during walking is improved by the double support, when between two and five (depending on the subject) of the six muscles studied were active and showed their activity peak (TA, VM, and/or RF, and/or BF, and/or ST).

In jogging, the weight is supported when only one leg is on the floor, while the six studied muscle were active. The peak of the VM and of the LG muscles occurred simultaneously; they play an important role in the stabilization of the knee, which is more flexed at the beginning of the support phase in jogging (Man & Hagy, 1980).

The peak of the ITI muscles (flexor muscles of the knee) could also appear at the beginning of the support phase. The co-contraction of VM and BF balances the knee in both sagittal and transversal planes.

In jogging, the support starts with a dorsal flexion (Man & Hagy, 1980); the co-contraction of TA (acting as agonist) and LG (acting as antagonist), facilitates the stability of the foot, which is decreased by the fast changing from supination to pronation (Cavanagh 1987).

Our results, which are in agreement with those of Prilutsky et al. (1998), show that the coordination of the tight muscles does not depend on the type of locomotion, as they are co-activated during both walking and jogging. However, the coordination of the leg muscles is different in walking than in jogging; for example, the TA and LG muscles are co-activated only during jogging.

The co-contraction existing in both ways of locomotion facilitates the movement of the segments, as it has been already established by Falconer & Winter (1985).

3.6.3 Energy conservation, progression, and propulsion

In our study, during jogging, the average speed increment was of 87% respect to walking. In addition, the peak of muscular activity was significantly different (Table 5); but not the peak time, except for the LG (Table 6), the activity of which started earlier in the non-support phase and it was present during the biggest part of the support phase (Figure 1).

It is worth noting that 70% of the energy produced by the muscle is lost as heat (Astrand & Rodhahl, 1980). Furthermore, in jogging the fluctuations of kinetic and gravitational energies are in phase, which produces bigger changes in their sum during stride (McMahon, 1990). In the other hand, in walking the transformation of kinetic energy into potential energy, and vice versa, decreases the work needed to be carried out by the muscles (Eberhart et al., 1954),

The co-contraction of the antagonist muscles (Table 6) plays an important role in the accumulation of elastic energy in the muscles and tendons. During jogging, the wider movements of the joints (Mann 1982) allow active muscles to absorb more energy, which is stored in form of elastic energy. Due to a higher muscular activity (Table 5), there is a bigger amount of elastic energy stored; and, in addition, the speed of the movements facilitates its recovery more efficiently. That energy is released to progress and propel the body up and forward. This result is in line with the study of Cavagna et al. (1964) who established that during jogging tendons elasticity contributes to the 50% of the performed work.

Four out of the six muscles studied are biarticular (RF, BF, ST, and LG) and they perform the energy transfer from one segment to the other (Van Ingen et al., 1987). That is, when a biarticular muscle acts as agonist over one joint and as antagonist over the other joint, the energy accumulated when it operates as antagonist is transferred from the segment to which it operates as antagonist to the segment in which it operates as agonist.

The higher activity showed by the ITI muscles during jogging (Table 4) in the non-support phase (Table 6) decreased the speed of the contralateral leg in the swinging phase and allows the bigger transfer of momentum between the contralateral and ipsilateral legs facilitating the propulsion of the support leg, finding congruent with that of Inman (1968) in walking.

3.7 Injuries in jogging

The comparison carried out in this study between the EMG activity of the leg muscles during walking and during jogging reveals the adaptability of the neuromuscular system against more demanding mechanical needs, and in this way we can learn more about the etiopathogeny of lesions.

An insight on EMG motor-control strategies of individuals without lesions is that the peak activity of the RF, VM, and LG muscles occurs in the eccentric phase. The probability of lesions is higher in eccentric contractions (Lieber, 1992); in addition, as the muscular activity is much higher in jogging, the probability of lesions increases even more. This could be one of the reasons why the musculotendinous lesions are so frequent in runners. Besides, the activity of those muscles occurs when the ITI and TA muscles are highly active; that is, there is a co-contraction of the muscles that cross the hip, knee, and ankle joints. In the case of the knee, the higher activity corresponds to the antagonist muscles. In addition, the higher speed of the movement performed during jogging increases as well the risk of lesions. The continuous activity of the TA at a level greater that 40% of its peak could make it susceptible to fatigue and thus of muscle injury.

Our working hypothesis about the bigger incidence of lesions during jogging is focused on muscular mechanics. However, Mizhrahi et al. (2000a) studied the role of fatigue in the etiology of lesions, and found out that the change due to fatigue exposes the shank to substantially higher impact accelerations, hence increasing the risk of overload injuries. In another study, Mizhrahi et al. (2000b) found that the fatigue-related imbalance in the contraction of the shank muscles develops in parallel to an increase in shank shock acceleration, increasing impact loading. The combination of these two conditions may hamper the loading balance on the tibia and higher risk of stress injury.

In any case, in the conditions in which this study has been carried out (average speeds: walking, 1.33±0.12m/s, and jogging 2.50±0.31m/s; and one-minute break between each recording), fatigue is not probable to appear.

4. Conclusions

The most relevant findings of this work are: (1) In both types of locomotion, each muscle showed a characteristic level of maximal amplitude. (2) In addition, the LE amplitude was very similar for homologous muscles in both legs in walking and in jogging.

Against the more demanding mechanical needs of jogging (when the average velocity increased 87%), the observed adaptations of the neuromuscular system were: 1) significantly bigger activity peak respect to walking of the six studied muscles (the highest peak activity increment was found in VM), which were active also for longer periods of time, even though the support phase was shorter and the non-support phase longer; 2) co-contraction in the three joints of the leg of agonist and antagonist muscles belonging to the same or different segments (*e.g.*, VM and LG); 3) continuous activity of TA; 4) consistent time of appearance of the peak activity during the support phase in the so-called anti-gravitational muscles (RF, VM, and LG), and more variable in the ITI and TA muscles; 5) bigger activity in eccentric contraction of the RF, VM, and LG muscles; and 6) bigger absolute inter-subject variability in the muscle activity for both distal and proximal muscles.

The abovementioned points (1) to (5) could explain the musculotendinous lesions so frequent in runners and provide the basis for the design of specific exercises to prevent those lesions.

5. Future research

As the s-EMG amplitudes obtained from homologous muscles for each subject have been similar, one could be tempted to perform this type of studies on only one leg. However, in this work we have not carried out postural balance studies, which are necessary in order to ensure whether the segment alignment has an influence on muscle activity. That is, it is necessary to

study, for example, lumbar lordosis with weakened abdominal musculature, alignment of the knee, heel, foot, configuration of the forefoot, femoral ante- or retro-version, and symmetry of legs length , as all those factors have an influence on muscle activity.
As future research, the study of the muscular activity and coordination of injured athletes could provide a better insight on the neuromuscular system adaptations during their recovery. The information so gathered could be helpful when designing rehabilitation treatments and for the foreseeing of the probable outcome of a lesion.
In jogging, the frequency of lesions in VM and LG can be due to their higher activity. The analytic training of those muscles could benefit athletes. That analytic training will take into account the contractile and elastic components of the muscles, the intensity of the contraction and of the co-contraction of agonist and antagonist muscles during jogging. The information thus collected from athletes in recovery will bring useful insight into how to avoid lesions.
Long-term studies on several athletes could provide important information about which kind of styles, muscular activation patterns, etc. are more prompt to produce future lesions, so the athletes can train to avoid them.

6. Acknowledgment

Authors thank the volunteers who participated in the experiments carried out for the present work. Thanks also to J. de la Cruz (Department of Applied Economy, University of Basque Country -UPV, Spain), F. Ainz (Department of Physiology, UPV), and to J. Bilbao (Department of Statistics, UPV) for their participation in the analysis of the data; and to S. Rainieri (Food Research Division, AZTI, Spain) for helpful comments on the original manuscript. This study was supported by the Foundation Jesús de Gangoiti Barrera. G.A.G. was supported by an European Marie Curie Post-doctoral Fellowship (ADCOMP project; Contract MEIF CT-2006-025056). The CONSOLIDER INGENIO 2010 program (from the Spanish Ministry of Education) must be acknowledged for supporting partially this work through grant CSD2009-00067.

7. References

Arsenault AB, Winter DA, & Marteniuk RG (1986a). Is there a 'normal' profile of EMG activity in gait? Medical & Biological Engineering & Computing; 1986, 24:337-43.
Arsenault AB, Winter DA, & Marteniuk RG (1986b). Bilaterism of EMG profiles in human locomotion. American Journal of Physical Medicine; 1986, 65(1):1-16.
Astrand PO & Rodhahl K (1980). L'appareil neuromusculaire. In: Précis de Physiologie de l'exercise musculaire. Paris: Masson, 43-96.
Basmajian JV (1967). Human locomotion. In Muscles Alive. Baltimore: The Williams & Wilkins Company, 252-263.
Cavagna GA & Kaneko M. (1977). Mechanical work and efficiency in level walking and jogging. Journal of Physiology; 1977, 268: 467-81.
Cavagna GA, Saibene FP, & Margaria R. (1964). Mechanical work in running. Journal of Applied Physiology; 1964, 19:249-56.
Cavanagh PR (1987). The biomechanics of lower extremity action in distance running. Foot & Ankle; 1987, 7(4):197-217.
Chao EY & Rim K. (1973). Application of optimization principles in determining the applied moments in human leg joint during gait. Journal of Biomechanics; 1973, 6:497-510.

Crowninshiel RD (1978). Use of optimization techniques to predict muscle force. Journal of Biomechanics Engineering; 1978, 100:88-92.

De Luca CJ & Merletti R. (1988). Surface myoelectric signal cross-talk among muscles of the leg. Electromyography and Clinical Neurophysiology; 1988, 69:568-75.

Eberhart HD, Inman VT, & Bresler B. (1954). In: The principal elements in human locomotion. P Klopstig and P Wilson editors. New York, Hafner: 437-71.

Falconer K & Winter DA (1985). Quantitative assessment of co-contraction at the ankle joint in walking. Electromyography and Clinical Neurophysiology; 1985, 25:135-49.

Gans C. (1982). Fiber architecture and muscle function. Exercise and Sports Sciences Reviews; 1982, 10:160-207.

Gazendam M. & Hof L. (2007). Averaged EMG profiles in jogging and running at different speeds. Gait & Posture, 2007;(25):604-14.

Giroux B. & Lamontagne M. (1990). Comparisons between surface electrodes and intramuscular wire electrodes in isometric and dynamic conditions. Electromyography and Clinical Neurophysiology 1990;30:397-405.

Ingen Schenau GJ Van, Bobbert J, & Rozendal RH (1987). The unique action of biarticular muscles in complex movements. Journal of Anatomy 1987;155:1-5.

Inman VT (1968). Conservation of energy in ambulation. In Bull Procc Res BPR 1968;10(9):26-35.

Inman VT, Ralston HJ, Saunders JB, Feinstein B., & Wright EW Jr (1952). Relation of human electromyogram to muscular tension. Electroencephalography and Clinical Neurophysiology 1952;4:187-94.

Inman VT, Ralston HJ, Saunders JB, & Frank T (1981). Human walking. Williams and Wilkins Baltimor , London. Page 2.

Kadaba MP, Ramakrishnan HK, Wootten ME, Gainey J, Gorton G , & Cochran GVB (1989). Repeatibility of kinematic, kinetic and electromyographic data in normal adult gait. Journal of Orthopaedic Research 1989;7:849-60.

Karamanidis K., Arampatzis A., & Brüggemann GP (2004). Reproducibility of electromyography and ground reaction force during various running techniques. Gait & Posture, April-2004,19(2):115-23.

Lieber RL (1992), Skeletal muscle response to injury. In John P Butler, Editor. Skeletal muscle structure and function. Baltimore: Williams & Wilkins, 1992: 260-292.

Mann RA & Hagy J. (1980). Biomechanics of walking, running and sprinting. The American Journal of Sports Medicine. 1980;8(5):345-50.

Mann RA (1982). Biomechanics of running. In: Mack RP editor. American Academy of Orthopaedics Surgeons. Symposium on the foot and leg in running sports. St Louis: Mosby: 1-29.

McMahon TA (199). Spring-like properties of muscles and reflexes in running. In Winters JM, Woo S LY, editors. Multiple muscle systems. Biomechanical and movement organization. New York: Springer-Verlag: 578-90.

Meinecke L., Disselhorst-Klug C., & Rau G. (2004): Crosstalk and Coactivation in Bipolar Surface EMG Data: A New Methodology for Detection, Discrimination and Quantification; in the 25th Congress of the International Society of Electrophysiological Kinesiology (ISEK), Boston, Massachusetts, June 2004, p. 87.

Merletti R. (1994). Surface electromyography: possibilities and limitations. Journal of Rehabilitation Sciences 1994; 7(3):24-35.

Mizrahi J., Verbitsky O., Isakov E., & Daily D. (2000a). Effect of fatigue on leg kinematics and shank shock in long distance running. Human Mvmnt. Science, 19(2): 139-151.

Mizrahi J., Verbitsky O., & Isakov E. (2000b). Fatigue-related loading imbalance on the shank in running: a possible factor in stress fractures. Annals Biomed. Eng., 28:463-469.

Montgomery WH, Marilyn P., & Perry J. (1994). Electromyographic analysis of hip and knee musculature during running. The American Journal of Sports Medicine. 1994;22(2):272-78.

Nilsson J., Thorstensson A., & Halbertsma J. (1985); Changes in leg movements and muscle activity with speed of locomotion and mode of progression in humans? Acta Physiol Scand; 1985. 123(4):457-75.

Novacheck TF (1998). The biomechanics of running. Gait & Posture 1998;7:77-95.

Ounpuu S. (1994) The biomechanics of walking and jogging. Clinics in Sports Medicine 1994;13(4):843-63.

Ounpuu S. & Winter D. (1989). Bilateral electromyographical analysis of the lower limbs during walking in normal adults. Electroencephalography and Clinical Neurophysiology 1989;72:429-38.

Perry J. (1992). Basic functions. In Gait analysis: normal and pathological function. Thorofare, NJ: Slack.

Perry J., Bontrager EL, Bogey RA, Gronley JK, & Barnes LA (1993). The Rancho EMG analyzer: a computerized system for gait analysis. Journal of Biomechanics Engineering 1993;15:487-97.

Prilutsky BL, Gregor RJ, & Ryan MM (1998). Coordination of two-joint rectus femoris and hamstrings during the swing phase of human walking and running. Experimental Brain Research 1998;120:479-89.

Raibert MH (1986). Symmetry in running. Science 1986, 231:1292-94.

Reber L., Perry J., & Pink M. (1993). Muscular control of the anke in running. The American Journal of Sports Medicine. 1993;21(6):805-10.

SENIAM (1999). European recommendations for surface electromyography,1999.

Taunton E., Mckenzie DC, & Clement DB (1988). The role of biomechanics in the epidemiology of injury. Sports Medicine 1988; 6: 107-120.

Wickiewiz TL, Roland R., Perry L., Powell BS, & Edgerton R. (1983). Muscle architecture of the human lower limb. Clinical Ortopaedics and Related Research 1983;179:275-83.

Winter DA (1983a). Biomechanical motor patterns in normal walking. Journal of Motor Behaviour. 1983;15:(4)302-30.

Winter DA (1983b). Moments of force and mechanical power in jogging. Journal of Biomechanics 1983;16:(1)91-97.

Winter DA & Yack HJ (1987). EMG profiles during normal human walking: stride-to-stride and inter-subject variability. Electroencephalography and Clinical Neurophysiology 1987; 67:402-11.

Winter DA (1990). Biomechanical and motor control of human movement, 2nd edn. New York:Wyley, 1990.

Winter DA, Fugelvand AJ, & Archer SE (1994). Crosstalk in surface electromyography: theoretical and practical estimates. Journal of Electromyography and Kynesiology 1994;4:15-26.

Winter DA (1991). Electromyogram recording, processing, and normalization: procedures and considerations. Journal of Human Muscle Performance 1991;1(2):5-15.

Yang JF & Winter DA (1984). Electromyographic amplitude normalization methods: improving their sensitivity as diagnostic tools in gait analysis. Archives Physical Medical Rehabilitation 1984;65:517-21.

Part 2

EMG Processing and Noise Reduction

5

EMG Signal Noise Removal Using Neural Netwoks

Vijay R. Mankar
Head of Department, Govt. Polytechnic, Amravati
India

1. Introduction

The bioelectric potentials associated with muscle activity constitute the Electromyogram, abbreviated as EMG. These potentials may be measured at the surface of the body near a muscle of interest or directly from the muscle by penetrating the skin with needle electrodes. Since most EMG measurements are intended to obtain an indication of the amount of activity of a given muscle, or group of muscles, rather than that of an individual muscle fiber, the pattern is usually a summation of the individual action potentials from the fibers constituting the muscle or muscles being measured. EMG electrodes pick up potentials from all muscles within the range of the electrodes, hence potentials from nearby large muscles may interfere with attempts to measure the EMG from smaller muscles, even though the electrodes are placed directly over the small muscles. Where this is a problem, needle electrodes inserted directly into the muscle are required. [Bronzino, J.D. (ed), 1995]
The action potential of a given muscle (or nerve fiber) has a fixed magnitude, regardless of the intensity of the stimulus that generates the response. Thus, in a muscle, the intensity with which the muscle acts does not increase the net height of the action potential pulse but does increase the rate with which each muscle fiber fires and the number of fibers that are activated at any given time. The amplitude of the measured EMG waveform is the instantaneous sum of all the action potentials generated at any given time. Because these action potentials occur in both positive and negative polarities at a given pair of electrodes, they sometimes add and sometimes cancel. Thus, the EMG waveform appears very much like a random-noise waveform, with the energy of the signal a function of the amount of muscle activity and electrode placement. Typical EMG waveforms are shown in Figure 1.

2. EMG measurements

Although action potentials from individual muscle fibers can be recorded under special conditions, it is the electrical activity of the entire muscle that is of primary interest. In this case, the signal is a summation of all the action potentials within the range of the electrodes, each weighted by its distance from the electrodes. Since the overall strength of muscular contraction depends on the number of fibers energized and the time of contraction, there is a correlation between the overall amount of EMG activity for the whole muscle and the strength of muscular contraction. In fact, under certain conditions of isometric contraction, the voltage-time integral of the EMG signal has a linear relationship to the isometric

voluntary tension in a muscle. There are also characteristic EMG patterns associated with special conditions, such as fatigue and tremor.
The EMG potentials from a muscle or group of muscles produce a noiselike waveform that varies in amplitude with the amount of muscular activity. Peak amplitudes vary from 25 µV to about 5 mV, depending on the location of the measuring electrodes with respect to the muscle and the activity of the muscle. A frequency response from about 5 Hz to well over 15000 Hz is required for faithful reproduction. [Childers, D.G., J.G. Webster, 1988]

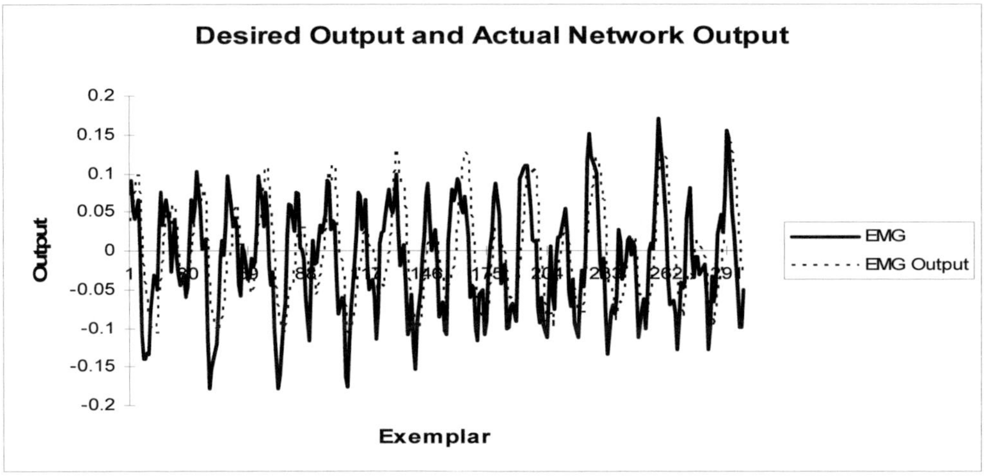

Fig. 1. Typical electomygram waveform showing EMG signal and EMG output signal.

The amplifier for EMG measurements, like that for ECG and EEG, must have high gain, high input impedance and a differential input with good common-mode rejection. However, the EMG amplifier must accommodate the higher frequency band. In many commercial electromyographs, the upper-frequency response can be varied by use of switchable lowpass filters. [Cromwell, L.,et al., 1980, John G. Webster, 2001] Unlike ECG or EEG equipment, the typical electromyograph has an oscilloscope readout instead of a graphic pen recorder. The reason is the higher frequency response required. Sometimes a storage cathode-ray tube is provided for retention of data, or an oscilloscope camera is used to obtain a permanent visual record of data from the oscilloscope screen.
The EMG signal can be quantified in several ways. The simplest method is measurement of the amplitude alone. In this case, the maximum amplitude achieved for a given type of muscle activity is recorded. Unfortunately the amplitude is only a rough indication of the amount of muscle activity and is dependent on the location of the measuring electrodes with respect to the muscle. Surface, needle, and fine-wire electrodes are all used for different types of EMG measurement. Surface electrodes are generally used where gross indication are suitable, but where localized measurement of specific muscles is required, needle or wire electrodes that penetrate the skin and contact the muscle to be measured are needed. As in neuronal firing measurements, both unipolar and bipolar measurements of EMG are used. [Brush, L.C., Cohen, B.J., 1995]
Another method of quantifying EMG is a count of the number of spikes or, in some cases, zero crossings, that occur over a given time interval. A modification of this method is a count of the number of times a given amplitude threshold is exceeded. Although these

counts vary with the amount of muscle activity, they do not provide an accurate means of quantification, for the measured waveform is a summation of a large number of action potentials that cannot be distinguished individually.

The most meaningful method of quantifying the EMG utilizes the time integral of the EMG waveform. With this technique, the integrated value of the EMG over a given time interval, such as 0.1 second, is measured and recorded or plotted. As indicated above, this time integral has a linear relationship to the tension of a muscle under certain conditions of isometric contraction, as well as a relationship to the activity of a muscle under isotonic contraction. As with the amplitude measurement, the integrated EMG is greatly affected by electrode placement, but with a given electrode location, these values provide a good indication of muscle activity.[Tompkins, W. J., 1999, Cromwell L. et al., 2004]

In another technique that is sometimes used in research, the EMG signal is rectified and filtered to produce a voltage that follows the envelope or contour of the EMG. This envelop, which is related to the activity of the muscle, has a much lower frequency content and can be recorded on a pen recorder, frequently in conjunction with some measurement of the movement of a limb or the force of the muscle activity.

3. Sources of errors

Errors can occur in a multitude of ways. These errors need to be considered, although may not be always present simultaneously:

- Errors due to tolerance of electronic components.
- Mechanical errors in meter movements.
- Component errors due to drift or temperature variation.
- Errors due to poor frequency response.
- In certain types of instruments, errors due to change in atmospheric pressure or temperature.
- Reading errors due to parallax, inadequate illumination, or excessively wide ink traces on a pen recording.

Two additional sources of error should not be overlooked. The first concerns correct instrument zeroing. Another source of error is the effect of the instrument on the parameter to be measured, and vice versa. This is especially true in measurements in living organisms. These errors lead to the noise in a system.

All semiconductor junctions generate noise, which limits the detection of small signals. Op Amps have transistor input junctions, which generate both noise-voltage sources and noise-current sources as indicated in Figure 2. For low source impedance, only the noise voltage v_n is important; it is large compared with the i_nR drop caused by the current noise i_n. The noise is random, but the amplitude varies with frequency. For example, at low frequencies the noise power density varies as 1/f (flicker noise), so a large amount of noise is present at low frequencies. At the midfrequencies, the noise is lower and can be specified in rms units of $V.Hz^{-1/2}$. In addition, some silicon planar-diffused bipolar integrated-circuit op amps exhibit bursts of noise. [Geddes, L.A., L.E. Baker, 1989] The noise currents flow through the external equivalent resistances so that total rms noise voltage is

$$v_t = \{[v_n^2 + (i_nR_1)^2 + (i_nR_2)^2 + 4kTR_1 + 4kTR_2]BW\}^{1/2}$$

where R_1 and R_2 = equivalent source resistances

v_n = mean value of the rms noise voltage, in V.Hz$^{-1/2}$, across the frequency range of interest,
BW = noise bandwidth, Hz.
i_n = mean value of the rms noise current, in A Hz$^{-1/2}$, across the frequency range of interest,
k = Boltzmann's constant, T = temperature, K,

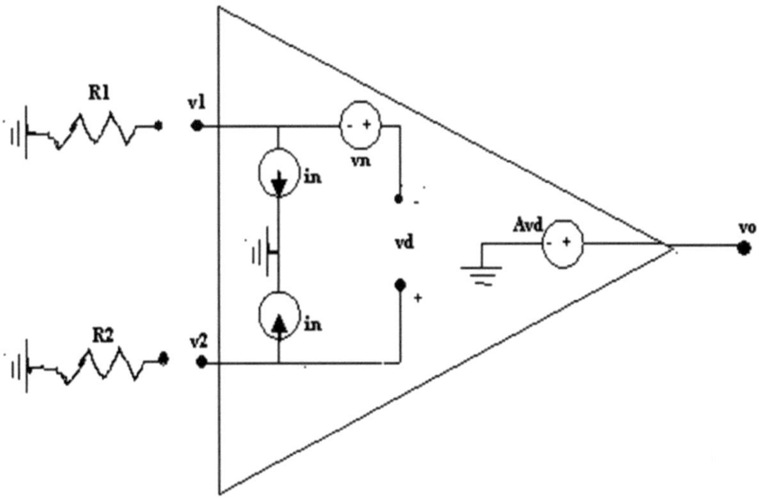

Fig. 2. Noise sources in an Op Amp

Signal enhancement in noisy environment is a challenge problem since decades. Noise is added to a signal under measurement almost in an uncontrolled manner. Signal-processing systems pick-up"unwanted" noise signal alongwith desired signal. These noise signals result in performance degradation of those systems. Noise classification can be used to reduce the effect of environmental noises on signal processing tasks. NN's are proposed as alternative optimization techniques to handle problems in signal processing. Prior a neural network maps each input feature vector into output vector, it must have first learnt the classes of feature vectors through a process that partitions a set of feature vectors. This is called discrimination or classification, which involve machines learning.

4. Importance of neural networks

A Neural Network is a massively parallel distributed processor made of simple processing element having natural propensity for storing experimental knowledge and making it available for use. It has the ability to acquire the knowledge from its environment through a learning process and to store acquired knowledge through inter-neuron connection strengths (synaptic weights). The procedure used to perform the learning process is called a learning algorithm, the function of which is to modify the synaptic weights of the network in an orderly fashion to attain a desirable design objective.

The use of neural network offers the useful properties and capabilities like nonlinearity, input/output mapping, adaptivity, evidential response, contextual information, fault tolerance, VLSI implementability, uniformity of analysis and design and neurobiological analogy. Neural networks, because of their massively parallel nature, can perform computation at a very high rate. Neural networks can adapt to a change in the data and learn the characteristics of input signals due to their adaptive nature. Neural networks can also perform functional approximation and signal filtering operation because of their nonlinear nature. Hence, neural networks are widely used for problem solving in engineering that are difficult for conventional computers or human beings [Haykin, S, 1986].

Neural networks are composed of simple elements operating in parallel. These elements are inspired by biological nervous systems. As in nature, the network function is determined largely by the connections between elements. A neural network can be trained to perform a particular function by adjusting the values of the connections (weights) between elements. Commonly neural networks are adjusted, or trained, so that a particular input leads to a specific target output. Such a situation is shown below.

The network is adjusted, based on a comparison of the output and the target, until the network output matches the target. Typically many such input/target pairs are used, in this supervised learning, to train a network as shown in figure 3.

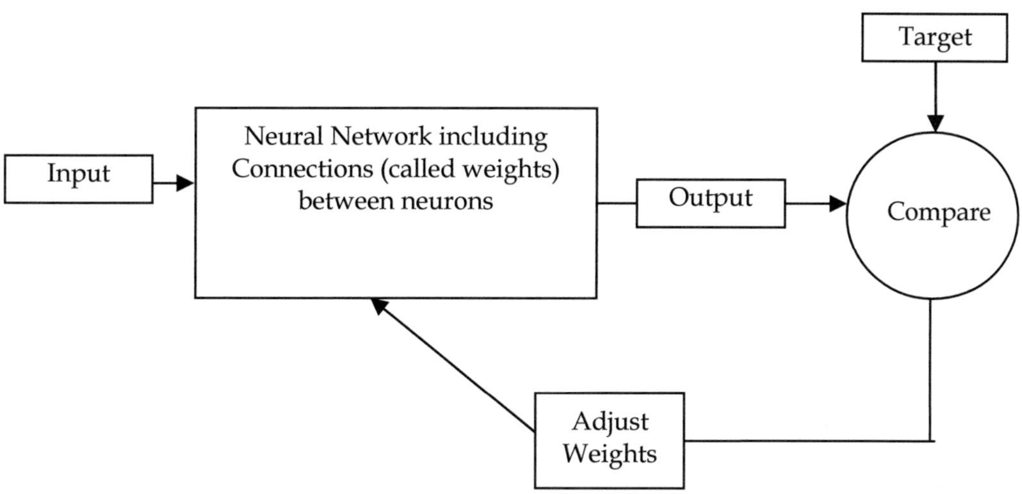

Fig. 3. Neural Network in Supervised Learning Mode.

Batch training of a network proceeds by making weight and bias changes based on an entire set (batch) of input vectors. Incremental training changes the weights and biases of a network as needed after presentation of each individual input vector. Incremental training is sometimes referred to as "on line" or "adaptive" training. Neural networks have been trained to perform complex functions in various fields of application including pattern recognition, identification, classification, speech, vision, control systems and signal processing.

The supervised training methods are commonly used, but other networks can be obtained from unsupervised training techniques or from direct design methods. Unsupervised networks can be used, for instance, to identify groups of data. Certain kinds of linear networks and Hopfield networks are designed directly. In summary, there are a variety of kinds of design and learning techniques that enrich the choices that a user can make. The field of neural networks has a history of some five decades but has found solid applications only in the past fifteen years, and the field is still developing rapidly. Neural network will be a useful tool for industry, education and research, a tool that will help users find what works and what doesn't, and a tool that will help develop and extend the field of neural networks.

5. Neural network approach

There are numerous real life situations where the exactness of the measurements is required. In Biomedical applications, due to complicated situations, the measurements are noisy. Neural Networks can be used to obtain reasonably good accuracy in removal of noise or elegantly filtering out the desired signals. At a high level, the filtering problem is a special class of function approximation problem in which the function values are represented using time series. A time series is a sequence of values measured over time in the discrete or continuous time units. Literature survey revealed that the Neural Networks can also be effectively used for solving the nonlinear multivariable regression problem. [Xue, Q.Z., et. al., 1992, Richard D. de Veaux, et. al., 1998] Also, there is a wide scope for an exact neural network with the performance indices approaching to their ideal values, i.e. MSE = 0, and correlation coefficient r = 1 [J.C. Principe, et. al. , 2000].

Signal filtering from present observations is a basic signal processing operation by use of filters. Conventional parametric approaches to this problem involve mathematical modeling of the signal characteristics, which is then used to accomplish the filtering. In a general case, this is relatively a complex task containing many steps for instance model hypothesis, identification and estimation of model parameters and their verification. However, using a Neural Network, the modeling phase can be bypassed and nonlinear and nonparametric signal filtering can be performed. As the thresholds of all neurons are set to zeros, unknown variables for one step ahead filtering are only the connection weights between the output neurons and the jth neuron in the second layer, which can be trained by available sample set [Widrow, B, et al., 1975].

In the last decade, NN, have given rise to high expectations for model free statistical estimation from a finite number of sample. The goal of predictive learning is to estimate or learn an unknown functional mapping between the input variables and the output variables, from the training set of known input output samples. The mapping is typically implemented as a computational procedure in software. Once the mapping is obtained from the training data, it can be used for predicting the output value, given only the values of the input variables [Khandpur R.S., 2001]. In the research work referred, the several techniques for noise removal from biomedical signals like EMG, [Abdelhafid Zeghbib, et. al.,2007, Umut Gundogdu, et. al., 2006] EEG, [Mercedes Cabrerizo, et. al.,2007, David Coufal, 2005], and ECG [Mahesh S. Chavan, et. al.,2006, Hafizah Husain, Lai Len Fatt, 2007] using signal processing techniques [Chunshien Li, 2006, M.Areziki, et. al.,2007,] and neural networks have been presented.

5.1 Recurrent networks

Recurrent networks are the proper neural network to be selected when identifying a nonlinear dynamical process. Such networks are attractive with their capabilities to perform highly nonlinear dynamic mapping and their ability to store information for later use. Moreover, they can deal with time-varying input or output through their own natural

temporal operation. There are two types of recurrent neural networks: fully recurrent neural networks and partially recurrent neural networks. Many learning algorithms have been developed. Partially recurrent networks are back-propagation networks with proper feedback links. It allows the network to remember cues from the recent past. In these architectures, the nodes receiving feedback signals are context units. According to the kind of feedback links, two major models of partially recurrent networks are encountered as described below.[Ezin C. Eugène, 2008]
Fully Recurrent Networks feed back the hidden layer to itself. Partially recurrent networks start with a fully recurrent net and add a feedforward connection that bypasses the recurrency, effectively treating the recurrent part as a state memory. These recurrent networks can have an infinite memory depth and thus find relationships through time as well as through the instantaneous input space. Most real-world data contains information in its time structure. Recurrent networks are the state of the art in nonlinear time series prediction, system identification, and temporal pattern classification.

5.2 Jordan network

This network model is realized in adding recurrent links from the network's output to a set of context units Ci, of a context layer and from the context units to themselves. Context units copy the activations of output node from the previous time step through the feedback links with unit weights. Their activations are governed by the differential equation

$$C'i(t) = - \alpha Ci(t) + yi(t)$$

where the yi's are the activations of the output nodes and α is the strength of the self-connections.
Despite the use of the Jordan sequential network to recognize and distinguish different input sequences with sequences of increasing length, this model of network encounters difficulties in discriminating on the basis of the first cues presented.

5.3 Multilayer perceptron approach

Multilayer Perceptrons (MLPs) are layered feedforward networks typically trained with static backpropagation. These networks have found their ways into countless applications requiring static pattern classification. Their main advantage is that they are easy to use, and that they can approximate any input/output map. The key disadvantages are that they train slowly, and require lots of training data (typically three times more training samples than network weights). The multilayer perceptron (MLP) is one of the most widely implemented neural network topologies. For static pattern classification, the MLP with two hidden layers is a universal pattern classifier. In other words, the discriminant functions can take any shape, as required by the input data clusters. When the weights are properly normalized and the output classes are normalized to 0/1, the MLP achieves the performance, which is optimal from a classification point of view. In terms of mapping abilities, the MLP is believed to be capable of approximating arbitrary functions,which is important in the study of nonlinear dynamics, and other function mapping problems.
MLPs are normally trained with the backpropagation algorithm. The LMS learning algorithm proposed by Widrow can not be extended to hidden PEs, since the desired signal is not known. The backpropagation rule propagates the errors through the network and

allows adaptation of the hidden PEs. Two important characteristics of the multilayer perceptron are its nonlinear processing elements (PEs) which have a nonlinearity that must be smooth and their massive interconnectivity i.e. any element of a given layer feeds all the elements of the next layer. The multilayer perceptron is trained with error correction learning, which means that the desired response for the system must be known.

Jordan (1986) described the first MLP architecture with recurrent connections for sequence generation. The input layer has two parts: plan units representing external input and the identity of the sequence and state units that receive one-to-one projections from the output layer, forming decay trace STM. After a sequence is stored into the network by back propagation training, it can be generated by an external input representing the identity of the sequence. This input activates the first component of the sequence in the output layer. This component feeds back to the input layer and, together with the external input, activates the second component, and so on. A particular component of a sequence is generated by the part of the sequence prior to the component, earlier components having lesser roles due to exponential decay. Elman (1990) later modified Jordan's architecture by having the hidden layer connect to a part of the input layer, called the context layer. The context layer simply duplicates the activation of the hidden layer in the previous time step. Elman used this architecture to learn a set of individual sequences satisfying a syntactic description, and found that the network exhibits a kind of syntax recognition. This result suggests a way of learning high-level structures, such as natural language grammar.

5.4 Elman neural network

Elman Neural Network (ENN) is a type of partial recurrent neural network, which consists of two-layer back propagation networks with an additional feedback connection from the output of the hidden layer to its input layer. The advantage of this feedback path is that it allows ENN to recognize and generate temporal patterns and spatial patterns. This means that after training, interrelations between the current input and internal states are processed to produce the output and to represent the relevant past information in the internal states. As a result, the ENN has been widely used in various fields from a temporal version of the Exclusive-OR function to the discovery of syntactic or semantic categories in natural language data. However, since ENN often uses back propagation (BP) to deal with the various signals, it has proved to be suffering from a sub-optimal solution problem. At the same time, for the ENN, it is less able to find the most appropriate weights for hidden neurons and often get into the sub-optimal areas because the error gradient is approximated. [Yves St-Amant, et al., 1998]

In the Elman neural network, after the hidden units are calculated, their values are used to compute the output of the network and are also all are stored as "extra inputs" (called context unit) to be used when the next time the network is operated. Thus, the recurrent contexts provide a weighted sum of the previous values of the hidden units as input to the hidden units. The activations are copied from hidden layer to context layer on a one for one basis, with fixed weight of 1.0 (w=1.0). The forward connection weight is trained between hidden units and context units as well as other weights. [Edward A. Clancy, 1995] Both the Jordan and Elman networks have fixed feedback parameters and there is no recurrence in the input-output path. These networks can be trained approximately with straight Back propagation. Elman's context layer receives input from the hidden layer, while Jordan's context layer receives input from the output as shown in figure 4.

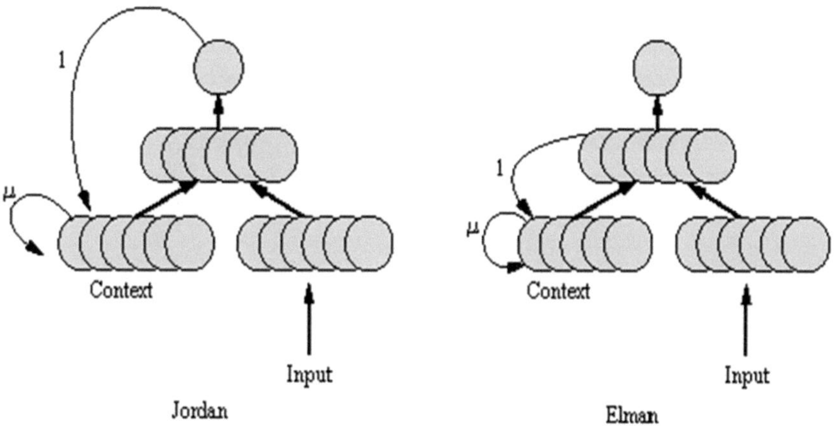

Fig. 4. Jordan and Elman network.

5.5 Generalized feedforward networks

Generalized feedforward networks are a generalization of the MLPs such that connections can jump over one or more layers. In theory, a MLP can solve any problem that a generalized feedfoward network can solve. In practice, however, generalized feedforward networks often solve the problem much more efficiently. A classic example of this is the two spiral problem. Without describing the problem, it suffices to say that a standard MLP requires hundreds of times more training epochs than the generalized feedforward network containing the same number of processing elements.

5.6 Modular feedforward Networks

Modular Feedforward Networks are a special class of MLP. These networks process their input using several parallel MLPs, and then recombine the results. This tends to create some structure within the topology, which will foster specialization of function in each sub-module. In contrast to the MLP, modular networks do not have full interconnectivity between their layers. Therefore, a smaller number of weights are required for the same size network (i.e. the same number of PEs). This tends to speed up training times and reduce the number of required training exemplars. There are many ways to segment a MLP into modules. It is unclear how to best design the modular topology based on the data. There are no guarantees that each module is specializing its training on a unique portion of the data.

5.7 Principal Component Analysis Networks (PCAs)

Principal Component Analysis Networks (PCAs) combine unsupervised and supervised learning in the same topology. Principal component analysis is an unsupervised linear procedure that finds a set of uncorrelated features, principal components, from the input. A MLP is supervised to perform the nonlinear classification from these components. The fundamental problem in pattern recognition is to define data features that are important for the classification (feature extraction). One wishes to transform the input samples into a new space (the feature space) where the information about the samples is retained, but the dimensionality is reduced. This will make the classification job much easier. Principal component analysis (PCA) is such a technique. PCA finds an orthogonal set of directions in the input space and provides a way of finding the projections into these directions in an ordered fashion. The first principal component is the one that has the largest projection. The orthogonal directions are called the eigenvectors of the correlation matrix of the input vector, and the projections the corresponding eigenvalues. Since PCA orders the projections, the dimensionality can be reduced by truncating the projections to a given order. The reconstruction error is equal to the sum of the projections (eigenvalues) left out. The features in the projection space become the eigenvalues. This projection space is linear. PCA is normally done by analytically solving an eigenvalue problem of the input correlation function. Also, PCA can be accomplished by a single layer linear neural network trained with a modified Hebbian learning rule.

5.8 Radial Basis Function (RBF) Networks

Radial Basis Function (RBF) Networks are nonlinear hybrid networks typically containing a single hidden layer of processing elements (PEs). This layer uses gaussian transfer functions, rather than the standard sigmoidal functions employed by MLPs. The centers and widths of the gaussians are set by unsupervised learning rules, and supervised learning is applied to the output layer. These networks tend to learn much faster than MLPs. If a generalized regression (GRNN) / probabilistic (PNN) net is chosen, all the weights of the network can be calculated analytically. In this case, the number of cluster centers is by definition equal to the number of exemplars, and they are all set to the same variance. This type of RBF is used only when the number of exemplars is so small (<100) or so dispersed that clustering is ill-defined. Radial basis functions networks have a very strong mathematical foundation rooted in regularization theory for solving ill-conditioned problems. The RBF networks can be constructed as shown in figure 5. Every input component (ρ) is brought to a layer of hidden nodes. Each node in the hidden layer is a ρ multivariate Gaussian function,

$$G(x;x_i) = exp\left[\frac{-1}{2\sigma_i^2}\sum_{k=1}^{p}(x_k - x_{ik})^2\right]$$

of mean x_i (each data point) and variance σ_i. These functions are called radial basis functions. Finally, linearly weight the output of the hidden nodes to obtain

$$F_{(x)} = \sum_{i=1} w_i\left(G(x;x_i)\right)$$

But, it may lead to a very large hidden layer (number of samples of training set).

This solution can be approximated by reducing the number of PEs in the hidden layer, but cleverly position them over the input space regions, i.e. where more input samples are available. This requires the estimation of the positions of each radial basis function and its variance (width), as well as computes the linear weights.

Self-Organizing Feature Maps (SOFMs) transform the input of arbitrary dimension into a one or two dimensional discrete map subject to a topological (neighborhood preserving) constraint. The feature maps are computed using Kohonen unsupervised learning. The output of the SOFM can be used as input to a supervised classification neural network such as the MLP. This network's key advantage is the clustering produced by the SOFM which reduces the input space into representative features using a self-organizing process. Hence, the underlying structure of the input space is kept, while the dimensionality of the space is reduced. These nets are one layer nets with linear PEs but use a competitive learning rule. In such nets there is one and only one winning PE for every input pattern (i.e. the PE whose weights are closest to the input pattern). In competitive nets, only the weights of the winning node get updated. Kohonen proposed a slight modification of this principle with tremendous implications. Instead of updating only the winning PE, in SOFM nets the neighboring PE weights are also updated with a smaller step size. This means that in the learning process (topological) neighborhood relationships are created in which the spatial locations correspond to features of the input data. These data points that are similar in input space can be mapped to small neighborhoods in Kohonen's SOFM layer.

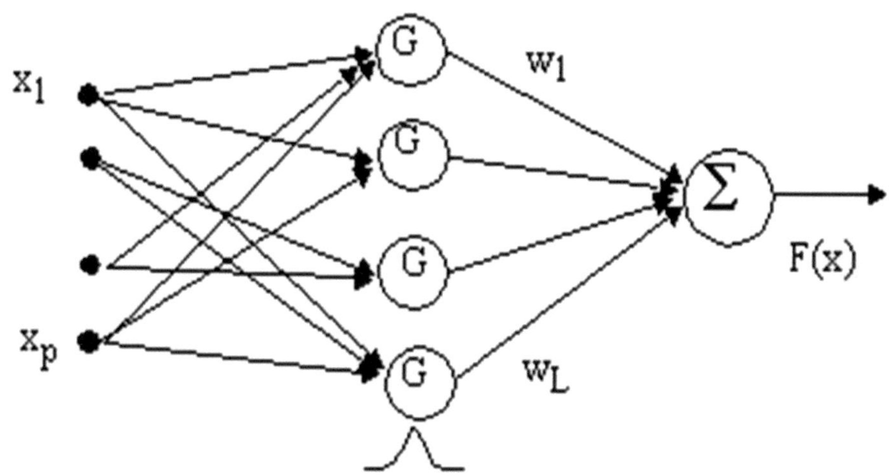

Fig. 5. Radial Basis Function (RBF) Network

6. Performance measures

6.1 MSE (Mean Square Error)

The formula for the mean square error is

$$MSE = \sum_{j=0}^{p}\sum_{i=0}^{n}\left(d_{ij} - y_{ij}\right)^2 / NP$$

where P = number of output processing elements, N= number of exemplars in the data set, y_{ij} = network output for exemplar i at processing element j, d_{ij} = desired output for exemplar i at processing element j.

Learning of a neural network is a stochastic process that depends not only on the learning parameters, but also on the initial conditions. Thus, if it is required to compare network convergence time or final value of the MSE after a number of iterations, it is necessary to run each network several times with random initial conditions and pick the best.

6.2 r (Correlation coefficient)

The size of the mean square error (MSE) can be used to determine how well the network output fits the desired output, but it doesn't necessarily reflect whether the two sets of data move in the same direction. For instance, by simply scaling the network output, the MSE can be changed without changing the directionality of the data. The correlation coefficient (r) solves this problem. By definition, the correlation coefficient between a network output x and a desired output d is:

$$r = \frac{\frac{\sum_i (x_1 - \bar{x})(d_1 - \bar{d})}{N}}{\sqrt{\frac{\sum_i (d_1 - \bar{d})^2}{N}} \sqrt{\frac{\sum_i (x_1 - \bar{x})^2}{N}}}$$

The Numerator is the covariance of the two variables and the denominator is the product of the corresponding standard deviation. The correlation coefficient is confined to the range [-1,1]. When r = 1, there is a perfect positive linear correlation between x and d, that is, they co-vary, which means that they vary by the same amount. When r = -1, there is a perfectly linear negative correlation between x and d, that is, they vary in opposite ways. When r = 0, there is no correlation between x and d, that is, the variables are uncorrelated. Intermediate values reveal partial correlations, e.g. r = 0.9, which states that the fit of the linear model to the data is reasonably good.
Correlation Coefficient, r tells how much of the variance of d is captured by a linear regression on the independent variable x, and hence r is a very effective quantifier of the modeling result. It has the greatest advantage with respect to the MSE as it is automatically normalized, while the MSE is not. But, r is blind to the differences in means as it is a ratio of variances, i.e. as long as the desired data and input co-vary, r will be small, in spite of the fact that they may be far apart in actual value. Hence, both parameters(r and MSE) are required when testing the results of regression.

6.3 The N/P ratio

It describes the complexity of a neural network and is given by
N/P = Total Training Samples / Number of connection weights.

6.4 Time elapsed per epoch per exemplar (t)

It helps to calculate the speed of a network and is given by
t = Time elapsed for n samples / (n samples x total training samples)

7. Database descriptions

The EMG signal appears like a random-noise waveform, with the energy of a signal, a function of amount of the muscle activity and electrode placement. The waveform was obtained at a sweep speed of 10 milliseconds per cm; amplitude of 1 mV per cm. The data related to EMG noise signal was obtained from standard data sources available. (Veterans Administration Hospital, Portland) The EMG signal under consideration had three sample patterns, 408, 890 and 1500 samples. Out of total samples, 50% samples constitute the training set, 20% samples are used for cross-validation and 30% samples are chosen for testing set. The training set is used to train the neural network. During the learning, the weights and biases are updated dynamically using the back propagation algorithm. The validation set is used to determine the performance of the neural network on patterns that are not trained during learning. Its major goal is to avoid the over training during the learning phase. The testing set is used to check the overall performance of the network. The input PE and output PE were chosen to be one, as it is a single input (i.e. noisy EMG input) and a single output (i.e. desired or filtered EMG output), SISO system. The neural network defined has the other parameters like context unit (time) = 0.8, transfer function = Tanhaxon, learning rule = momentum. Termination criterion for experimentation is minimum MSE in both training and cross-validation stages with maximum epochs = 1000 and learning rate is fixed to 0.01. MSE criterion is limited to 1%.

The noisy EMG and desired EMG signals are inputted to Neural Networks and desired signal is expected with mean square error limited to 1%. The MLP, General Feed Forward, Modular Neural Network, Jordan/ Elman Network, RBF Neural Network, and Recurrent Network neural networks have been tried for optimal performance and it is found that the Neural Networks are optimally performing. The performance measures like MSE and Correlation Coefficient (r) are specified in the table 8. [Strum R. D., 2000, Andrzej Izworski, et al., 2004]

8. Simulation

The results are obtained on Neuro Solutions platform and accordingly, simulations are carried out on noisy EMG input and desired EMG signal. The noisy EMG input was inputted to different neural networks with number of hidden layers varying from 2 to 4. The neural networks with input, hidden and output layer with varying parameters like processing elements, transfer function, learning rule, step size and momentum were tested with maximum epoch value, 1000.

After training the Neural Networks on a noisy input and desired output data values with different sample patterns and under different (training, cross-validation and testing samples swapped) conditions, the expected results were obtained with minimum MSE and maximum correlation coefficient around the estimated values as shown below. The other parameters like processing element per hidden layer, transfer function, learning rule were also varied. The results for optimum parameters for SISO system under consideration are given in following tables.

a) GEN. FF. NN, (05, 05, 07), 60% TR, 15% CV, 25% Test SP

Figure 6 depicts the variation of average of minimum MSE for 5 runs vs. number of PEs in the second hidden layer It is observed that for five processing elements in the second hidden layer, the MSE on CV attained its minimum value. When the PE's are increased beyond 5, the MSE on CV was seen to increase. Therefore, 5 PE's are chosen for second hidden layer.

Figure 7 depicts the variation of average Training MSE vs. number of Epochs. Five different runs with new random initialization of connection weights of NN's are shown below. It is observed that for each run (training cycle), average MSE decreases as number of epochs increases. It is worthwhile to notice that this trend of decrease in MSE is consistent for 5 runs.

Figure 8 shows the variation of desired output and actual NN output vs. number of exemplars. The covariance between the desired output and the actual NN output is indicated by the correlation coefficient, r = 0.636240018.

The neural network was trained five times and the best performance with respect to MSE of training was observed during the 1st run at the end of 1000 epochs. Similarly, the best Cross-Validation performance was noticed during the 4th run at the end of 12 epochs, as depicted in the following table 1.

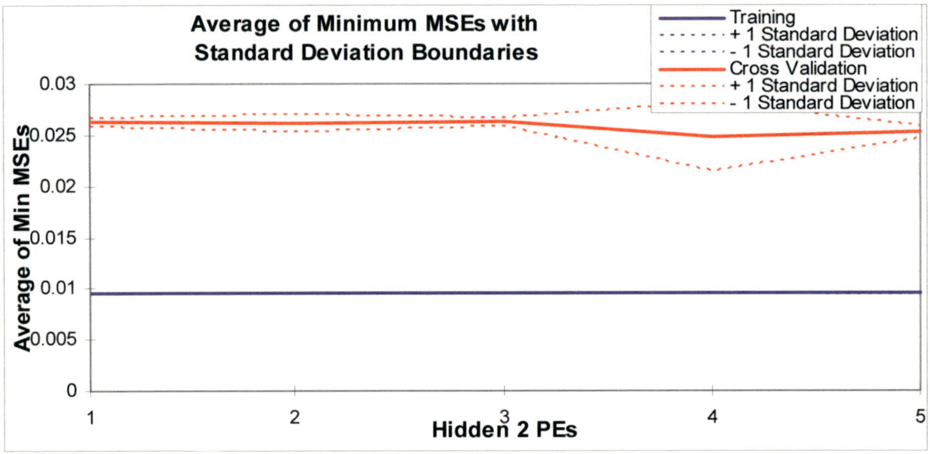

Fig. 6.

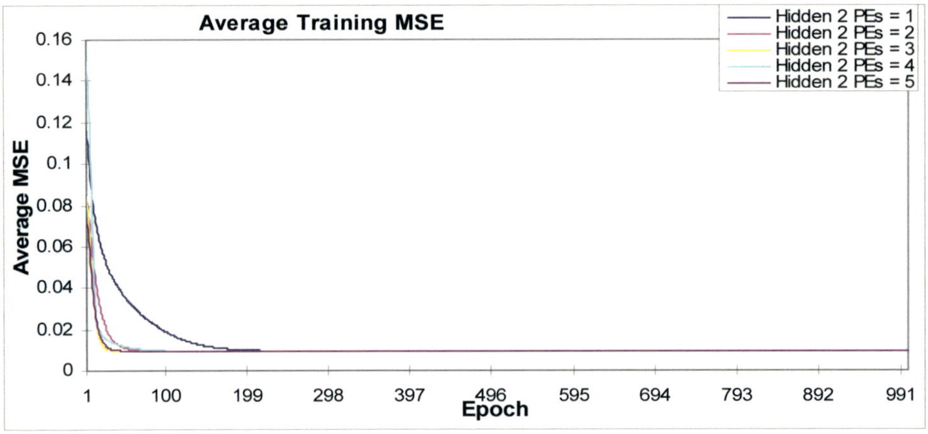

Fig. 7.

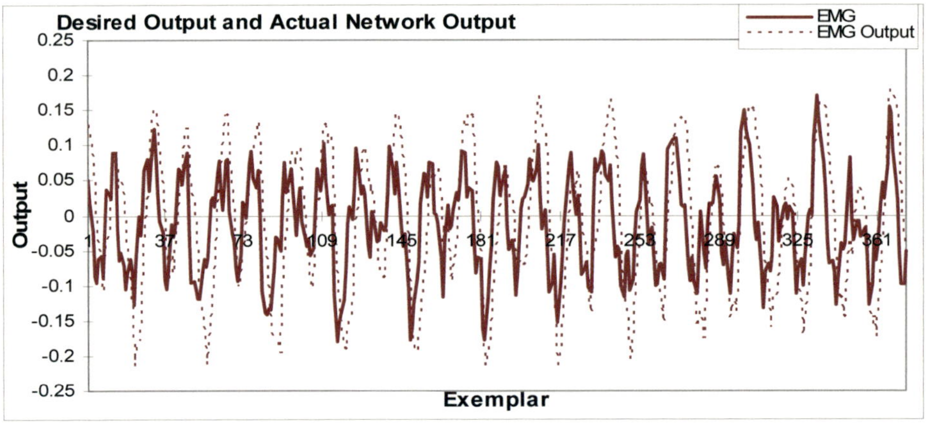

Fig. 8.

Best Networks	Training	Cross Validation
Hidden 2 PEs	5	4
Run #	1	4
Epoch #	1000	12
Minimum MSE	0.009501057	0.018979003
Final MSE	0.009501057	0.018979003

Table 1.

Different performance measures are listed in the following table 2.

Performance	EMG
MSE	0.004679485
NMSE	1.318501294
MAE	0.068195457
Min Abs Error	5.04679E-05
Max Abs Error	0.176143173
r	0.636240018

Table 2.

b) JORDAN / ELMAN NN, (08, 04, 02), 50% TR, 20% CV, 30% Test SP

Figure 9 depicts the variation of average of minimum MSE for 5 runs vs. number of PEs in the second hidden layer It is observed that for four processing elements in the second hidden layer, the MSE on CV attained its minimum value. When the PE's are increased beyond 4, the MSE on CV was seen to increase. Therefore, 4 PE's are chosen for second hidden layer.

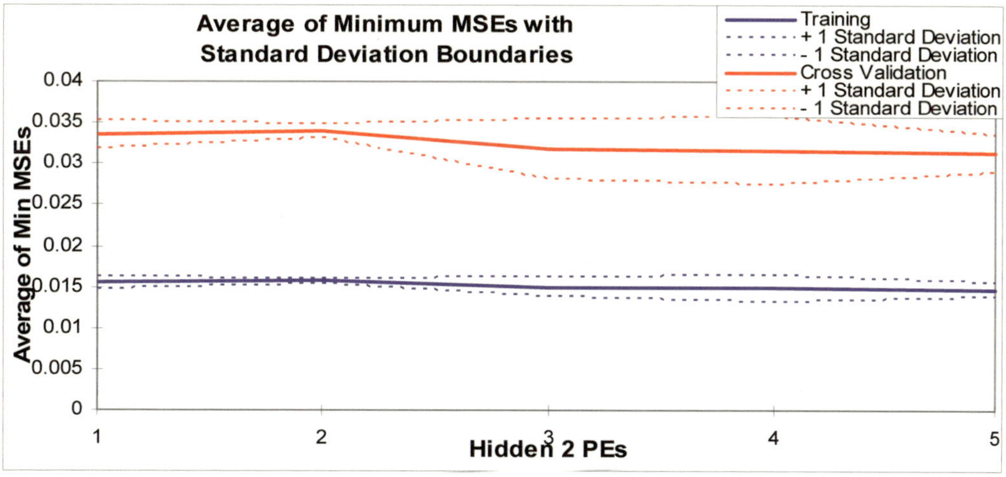

Different performance measures are listed in the following table 3.

Performance	EMG
MSE	0.015119372
NMSE	0.812867701
MAE	0.103271719
Min Abs Error	9.59247E-05
Max Abs Error	0.42812628
r	0.805945071

Figure 10 depicts the variation of average Training MSE vs. number of Epochs. Five different runs with new random initialization of connection weights of NN's are shown below. It is observed that for each run (training cycle), average MSE decreases as number of epochs increases. It is worthwhile to notice that this trend of decrease in MSE is consistent for 5 runs.

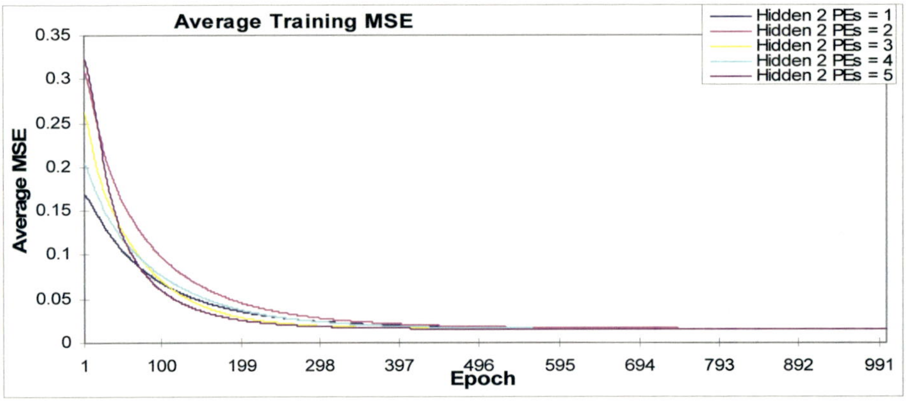

Figure 11 shows the variation of desired output and actual NN output vs. number of exemplars. The covariance between the desired output and the actual NN output is indicated by the correlation coefficient, r= 0.805945071

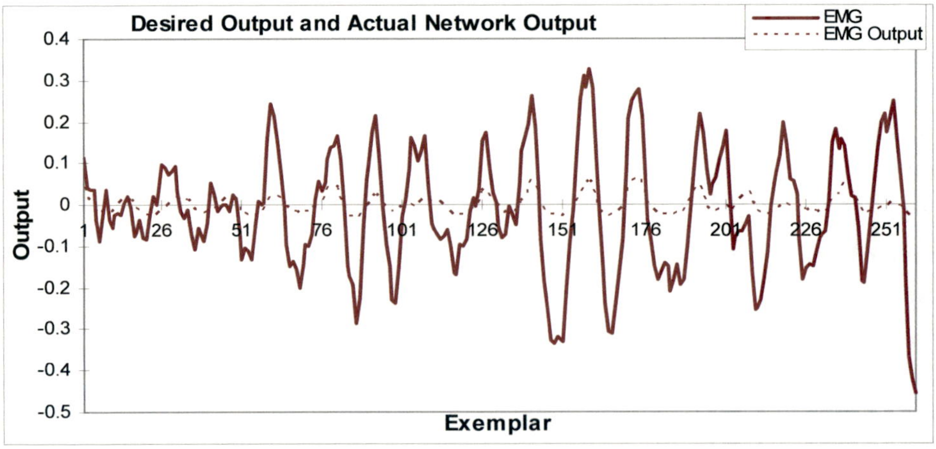

The neural network was trained five times and the best performance with respect to MSE of training was observed during the 2nd run at the end of 1000 epochs. Similarly, the best Cross-Validation performance was noticed during the 2nd run at the end of 1000 epochs, as depicted in the following table 4.

Best Networks	Training	Cross Validation
Hidden 2 PEs	4	4
Run #	2	2
Epoch #	1000	1000
Minimum MSE	0.009983631	0.021040779
Final MSE	0.009983631	0.021040779

c) GEN. FF NN, (04, 02), 50% TR, 20% CV, 30% Test SP

Figure 12 depicts the variation of average of minimum MSE for 5 runs vs. number of PEs in the first hidden layer. It is observed that for four processing elements in the first hidden layer, the MSE on CV attained its minimum value. When PEs are increased beyond 4, the MSE on CV was seen to increase. Therefore, 4 PEs are chosen for first hidden layer.

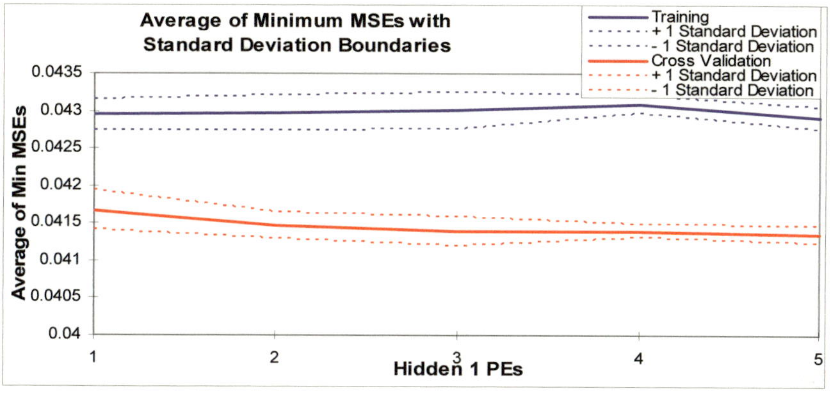

Figure 13 depicts the variation of average Training MSE vs. number of Epochs. Five different runs with new random initialization of connection weights of NNs are shown below. It is observed that for each run (training cycle), average MSE decreases as number of epochs increases. It is worthwhile to notice that this trend of decrease in MSE is consistent for all the five runs.

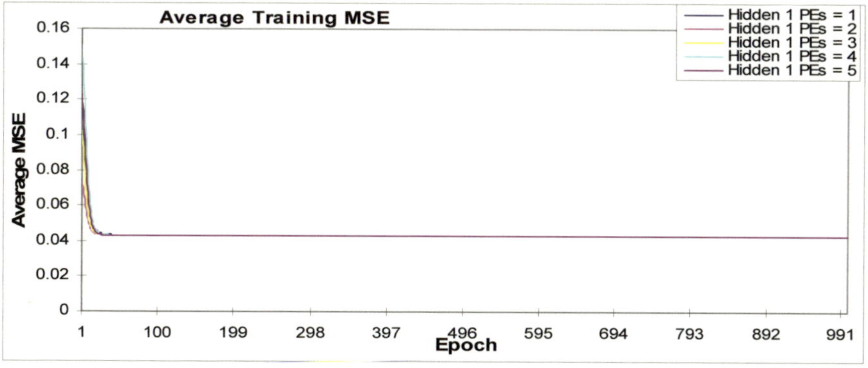

Figure 14 shows the variation of desired output and actual NN output vs. number of exemplars. The covariance between the desired output and the actual NN output is indicated by the correlation coefficient, r= 0.662274425.

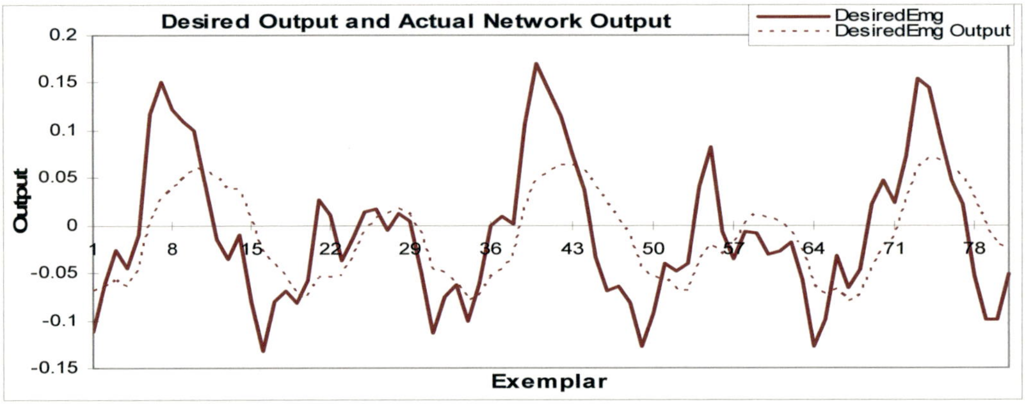

Different performance measures are listed in the following table 5.

Performance	DesiredEmg
MSE	0.003100258
NMSE	0.566522078
MAE	0.04580669
Min Abs Error	0.001058364
Max Abs Error	0.123692824
r	0.662274425

The neural network was trained five times and the best performance with respect to MSE of training was observed during the 1st run at the end of 1000 epochs. Similarly, the best Cross-Validation performance was noticed during the 2nd run at the end of 23 epochs, as depicted in the following table 6.

Best Networks	Training	Cross Validation
Hidden 1 PEs	3	5
Run #	1	2
Epoch #	1000	23
Minimum MSE	0.04264781	0.041166622
Final MSE	0.04264781	0.041874009

The optimum results experiment-wise are presented in table 7 in consolidated form.

Expt. No.	Type of ANN	Hidden Layer Variation H1H2H3	Correlation Coefficient r	MSE			N/P	t (μ sec)
				Training	Cross validation	Testing		
01	Gen.NN	05,05,07	0.636240018	0.009501057	0.018979003	0.004679485	12.5	6.2
02	Jor/Elmn	08,04,02	0.805945071	0.009983631	0.021040779	0.015119372	9.782	6.5
03	Gen.NN	04,02	0.662274425	0.04264781	0.041874009	0.003100258	14.5	57.7

9. Conclusion

EMG signal is a very important biomedical signal associated with muscle activity, giving useful information about nerve system in order to detect abnormal muscle electrical activities that occur in many diseasesand conditions like muscular dystrophy, inflammation of muscles, pinched nerves, peripheral nerve damages, amyotrophic lateral sclerosis, disc herniation, myasthenia gravis, and others. The detection and measurement of low frequency and lower magnitude EMG signals is noise-prone. Removal of noise from an EMG signal using various Neural Networks has been studied. It is demonstrated that Jordan/Elman Neural Network and Generalized Feed Forward Neural Network elegantly reduce the noise from the EMG signal.

One of the simplest methods is to observe the better performing network, how the MSE, which is the square difference between the network's output and the desired response, changes over training iterations. The goal of the stop criterion is to maximize the network's generalization. If the training is successful and the network's topology is correct, the network will apply its 'past experience' to the unseen data and will produce a good solution. If this is the case, then the network will be able to generalize based on the training set. It is observed that the networks presented in Table 7 are exhibiting better MSE values in the training, cross-validation and testing phase, which are distinctly designed. The MSE values are found to be in the desired range i. e. nearly equal to 0.01 in all the phases. The networks are not memorizing the training patterns, nor rattling in the local minima. These networks can be considered to provide good generalization.

The difference between the noisy EMG signal and the desired EMG signal is computed as a performance measure (MSE) and is found to be in the expected range approaching to 0.01. The minimum MSE criterion is found satisfactory (0.0099-0.01) in trained Jordan/Elman Neural Network and found to perform better during testing phase (0.01) as it is evident from all similar graphs as in Figure 9.

The correlation coefficient 'r' is a very effective quantifier of the modeling results, which describes the covariance between the desired output and the actual neural network's output. As can be seen from Table 7, the generalized neural network is found to have maximum correlation coefficient 'r' value, under several varying test conditions. The generalized neural network is found to effectively utilize the knowledge embedded in the input data and the desired response as compared to MLP, Modular Neural Network, Jordan/ Elman Network, RBF Neural Network, Time Lag Recurrent Network and Recurrent Neural Network. The 'r' is nearly close to 1 in most of the experiments, indicating a better linear correlation between the desired output and the actual neural network's output. Only the result of three Neural Networks have been presented here.

Also, the correlation coefficient (r) is found to be in the desired range (0.805945071 at sr. no. 2 Table 7), so that the network output and the desired output co-varies, i.e. varying by the same amount as depicted in figure 11.

As can be seen from the Table 7, the number of hidden layers used in the topology is either 2 or 3. This indicates that a simple neural network configurations can be very conveniently used to better generalize the input/ output mapping, in accordance with the theory of generalization, which correlates the number of PEs in the hidden layer, number of hidden layers with the mapping ability of the neural networks. N/P ratio describes the complexity of the neural network. The obtained values (9.782 to 14.5) of the ratio N/P shows that the neural network so designed is simpler to design and is capable of good generalization, with a better ability to learn from training exemplars. The neural networks presented in Table 7. are found to have smaller number of degrees of freedom achieving the desired performance and hence the networks can be said to be optimal.

Also, moderately smaller values of N/P shows that the Jordan/ Elman Neural Network so designed is simpler to design and is capable of generalization.

The time elapsed per epoch per exemplar (t) helps to calculate the speed of a network. Time t describes the training time elapsed per epoch per exemplar. Smaller values of t make it evident that the designed neural network requires less training time and hence, is faster.

Thus, from above, it can be concluded that Neural Networks can be designed to perform better as far as the overall performance is concerned. The designed neural networks have right combination of PEs and hidden layers to solve the given problem with acceptable training times and performance. Other neural networks are also performing optimally and are situation dependent. Accordingly, an optimal network needs to be selected for a particular application.

10. References

Bronzino, J.D. (ed), "The Biomedical Engineering Handbook", Boca Raton, FL: CRC Press, 1995

Brush, L.C. et al.," The guide to Biomedical Standards ",20th ed. Bera, CA: Quest publishing Co., 1995.

Cohen, B.J.," Medical Terminology: An Illustrated Guide", 2nd ed. Philadelphia: Lippincott, 1995.

Cromwell, L., F. J. Webell, and E.A. Pfeiffer."Biomedical Instrumentaion and Measurements", 2nd ed. Englewood Cliffs. NJ: Prentice-Hall, 1980.

John G. Webster (Ed.), "Medical Instrumentation : Application and Design", 3rd ed., John Wiley and Sons, Inc. 2001

Tompkins, W. J. (ed.) "Biomedical Digital Signal Processing" PHI, ND, 1999.

Cromwell L., Weibell F. J., Pfeiffer E.A. "Biomedical Instrumentation and Measurements", PHI, N.D., 2004

Ezin C. Eugène, " Discriminating Noisy Sentences with Partially Recurrent Neural Networks", www.cari-info.org/actes 2006/ 59.pdf, 30.06.2008.

Xue, Q.Z., Hu, Y. H. and Tompkins, W.J. 1992." Neural-Network-based Adaptive Matched Filtering for QRS Detection", IEEE Trans. Biomed Engg., BMN-39(4): 317-29.

Richard D. de Veaux, Jennifer Schumi, Jason Schweinsberg. Lyle H. Ungar, "Prediction Intervals for Neural Networks via Nonlinear Regression", Technometrics, Vol. 40, No. 4, pp. 273-282, Nov. 1998.

J.C. Principe, N.R. Euliano and W.C. Lefebvre, "Neural and Adaptive Systems", New York, USA: John Wiley and Sons, Inc. 2000.

Haykin, S "Adaptive Filter theory", Englewood Cliffs, NJ: Prentice Hall, 1986.

Widrow, B, Glover, J.R., John M., et al "Adaptive Noise Canceling Principles and Applications", Proc. IEEE, 63(12): 1692-1716, 1975.

Khandpur R.S. "Handbook of Biomedical Instrumentation" , Tata McGraw-Hill, N.D., 2001.

Abdelhafid Zeghbib, et. al., "Sampling Frequency and Pass-Band Frequency Effects on Neuromuscular Signals (EMG) Recognition", Proc. of 6th WSEAS Intl. Conf. on Signal Processing, Robotics and Automation, Corfu Island, Greece, Feb.16-19, 2007, pp 107-114.

Umut Gundogdu, et. al., "Investigation of Muscle Fatigue Using Temporal and Spectral Moments", Proc. of 5th WSEAS Intl. Conf. on Signal Processing, Istanbul, Turkey, May 27-29, 2006, pp10-14.

Mercedes Cabrerizo, et. al., "EEG Analysis using Neural Networks for Seizure Detection", Proc. of 6th WSEAS Intl. Conf. on Signal Processing, Robotics and Automation, Corfu Island, Greece, Feb.16-19, 2007, pp 121-126.

David Coufal, "Classification of EEG Signals by Radial Neuro-Fuzzy System", Proc. of 4th WSEAS Intl. Conf. on Computational Intelligence, Man-Machine Systems and Cybernetics, Miami, Florida, USA, Nov. 17-19,2005, pp 224-232.

Mahesh S. Chavan, et. al., "Use of Kaiser Window For ECG Processing", Proc. of 5th WSEAS Intl. Conf. on Signal Processing, Robotics and Automation, Madrid, Spain, Feb.15-17, 2006, pp285-289.

Hafizah Husain, Lai Len Fatt, "Efficient ECG Signal Classification Using Sparsely Connected Radial Basis Function Neural Network", 6th WSEAS Intl. Conf. on Circuits, Systems, Electronics, Control and Signal Processing, Cairo, Egypt, Dec. 29-31, 2007, pp 412-416.

M.Areziki, et. al., "Analysis of Fast Recursive Least Squares Algorithms for Adaptive Filtering", Proc. of 11th WSEAS Intl. Conf. on Systems, Agios Nikolaos, Crete Island, Greece, Jul.23-25, 2007, pp 474-481.

Chunshien Li, "Adaptive Noise Cancellation with Computational-Intelligence-based Approach", Proc. of 5th WSEAS Intl. Conf. on Signal Processing, Istanbul, Turkey, May 27-29, 2006, pp93-98.

Edward A. Clancy, Neville Hogan, "Multiple Site Electromyograph Amplitude Estimation", IEEE Trans. on Biomedical Engineering, Vol. 42, No. 2, Feb.1995, pp 203-211.

Yves St-Amant, Denis Rancourt, Edward A. Clancy, "Influence of Smoothing Window Length on Electromyogram Amplitude Estimates", IEEE Trans. on Biomedical Engineering, Vol. 45, No. 6, June 1998, pp 795-800.

Lin Wang, Thomas S. Buchanan, "Prediction of Joint Moments using a Neural Network Model of Muscle Activations from EMG Signals", IEEE Trans. on Neural Systems and Rehabilitation Engineering, Vol. 10, No. 1, Mar. 2002, pp 30-37.

Andrew Hamilton-Wright, Daniel W. Stashuk, "Physiologically Based Simulation of Clinical EMG Signals", IEEE Trans. on Biomedical Engineering, Vol. 52, No. 2, Feb. 2005, pp 171-183.

ZhiQiang Zhang, Zheng Tang and Catherine Vairappan, "A Novel Learning Method for Elman Neural Network Using Local Search", Neural Information Processing - Letters and Reviews Vol. 11, No. 8, pp 181- 188, August 2007.

Geddes, L.A., and L.E. Baker, "Principles of Applied Biomedical Instrumentation", 3rd ed. New York: Wiley, 1989.

Strum R. D., Kirk D.E., "Contemporary Linear Systems Using Matlab", Thomson Learning, 2000.

Childers, D.G., J.G. Webster (ed.), "Evoked potentials", Encyclopedia of Medical Devices and Instrumentation. New York: Wiley, 1988, pp. 1245-1254.

Andrzej Izworski, Piotr Bamia, "Interpretation of the Biomedical Signals using RBF- type Neural Networks", WSEAS trans on Circuits and systems, Issue 9, Vol.3, Nov 2004, pp 1799-1803.

Electromyography Pattern-Recognition-Based Control of Powered Multifunctional Upper-Limb Prostheses

Guanglin Li
Key Lab of Health Informatics of Chinese Academy of Sciences (CAS)
Shenzhen Institutes of Advanced Technology, CAS
P. R. China

1. Introduction

The human history has been accompanied by accidental trauma, war, and congenital anomalies. Consequently, amputation and deformity have been dealt with, one way or another, throughout the ages. More than one million individuals in the United States today are living with limb amputations (Adams et al., 1999), in which there are approximately 100,000 patients with an upper limb amputation. The wars in Iraq and Afghanistan have added to this number. According to the survey results of the Second China National Sample Survey on Disables (SCNSSD 2006) led by the National Statistics Bureau in 2006, approximately 8% of physical disables, or 2.26 million people, live with limb amputations in China alone. Natural disasters and accidents have been making this number increase. The massive earthquakes that occurred in May 2008, Sichuan Province, China, recently increased about 20 thousand of new limb amputees. Expectations for control of upper limb prostheses have always been high because of the standard established by able-bodied dexterity.

Most commercially available upper limb prostheses are either body-powered or electrical motor powered. The body-powered prostheses are operated by certain movements of the amputees' body through a system of cables, harnesses, and sometimes, manual control. In order to operate a body-powered prosthesis, the upper limb amputees have to possess significant strength and control over various body parts, including the shoulders, chest, and residual limb which must have sufficient residual limb length, musculature, and range of motion. Exaggerated movements of the body are captured by harness systems and are transferred through cables to operate the hand, wrist, or elbow movements of a prosthesis. With some advantages such as low cost, high reliability, and some kinesthetic feedback provided by the harness system, body-powered prostheses are still widely accepted by the upper limb amputees worldwide, especially in some developing countries. However, with this inappropriate control approach, body-powered upper limb prostheses are limited in utility, frustratingly slow to operate, awkward to maintain, and can operate only one joint at a time.

Myoelectric signals detected with electrodes placed on the skin surface overlying the muscles, well-known as electromyography (EMG), have been used in control of motorized upper-limb prostheses for several decades (Kay & Newman, 1975; Parker & Scott, 1986). The myoelectric control approach was proposed in the 1940s, but the myoelectric prostheses could not be viably made into clinical applications in that day due to the technical limitations. With the advances of technologies, especially electronic technologies, a significant progress has been made in the development of myoelectric prosthesis control during the 1960s. The first commercialized myoelectric prosthesis, a powered hand, was developed in the USSR (Kobrinski et al., 1960) in 1960, and later more myoelectric prostheses had been developed one after the other in different countries. A multifunctional myoelectric hand was developed in Japan (Kato et al., 1969), in 1969, and the first myoelectric elbow prosthesis was developed in the United States (Lyman et al., 1976), in 1970s. The three-state myoelectric controller was developed for the control of a three function device with a single muscle (Dorcas & Scott, 1966) in Canada. However, before several major commercial companies such as Otto Bock and Viennatone invested in the field, the production of powered myoelectric prostheses was pretty small. Beginning in the 1970s, the powered upper-limb myoelectric prostheses were clinically and routinely fitted to upper-limb amputees. Currently, most commercially available motorized upper-limb prostheses are controlled by using EMG signals from the residual muscles of an amputated arm. Commercial electronic prostheses and prosthetic components are sold by several companies, including Liberating Technologies, Inc, Otto Bock, Shanghai Kesheng Prostheses Co, and Touch Bionics.

The control strategies of upper-limb myoelectric prostheses use surface electromyogram (EMG) amplitude to control the prosthetic devices in either on/off or proportional mode. The EMG signals are recorded from one or two electrodes and processed by band-pass filtering, rectifying, and low-pass filtering to get the envelope amplitude of EMG signals, as shown in Fig. 1. Threshold of EMG signal amplitude is then applied to determine the minimum level of contraction necessary to initiate a movement. In the on/off control mode, the speed of prosthetic movements is constant. When two electrodes are used to control one degree of freedom (DOF), it is possible to use proportional control, in which the speed of movement is proportional to the amplitude of the myoelectric signal.

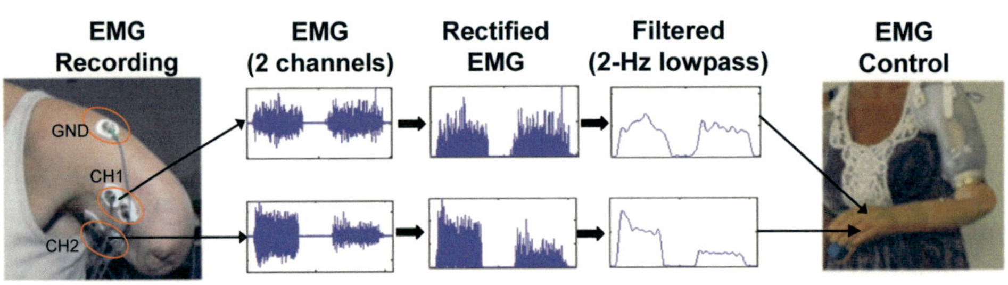

Fig. 1. Schematic diagram of conventional two-site EMG prosthesis control system

Most commercially available upper-limb myoelectric prostheses use a pair of muscles (usually an agonist/antagonist pair) to control one degree of freedom: one EMG signal from a flexor muscle and one from an extensor muscle, as shown in Fig. 1. Each of two movements in a joint DOF is assigned to a separate control muscle, such as hand opening to biceps and hand closing to triceps. When the EMG amplitude from one control muscle (such as biceps) is greater than a given threshold (T1 for biceps muscle), the associated prosthetic movement (hand opening) is selected and performed by an electric motor, as shown in Fig. 2. The logical circuitry in the controller of a myoelectric prosthesis allows only one of the DOF movements to be active at a time.

This control mode allows choosing the physiologically appropriate control muscles associated to the movement functions for an intuitive control of a prosthesis, but requires two control muscles for each prosthetic DOF. The control approach works fairly well if only one joint DOF is required such as for a transradial amputee, where two remaining forearm muscles (flexor and extensor) are used to control a powered hand DOF (hand opening/closing). If wrist rotation is desired, the users must activate an external switch or co-contract the two forearm muscles to shift from hand mode to wrist rotation mode. The same forearm flexion and extension EMG signals are then used to control the wrist rotator.

For higher level amputees, given a limited number of muscles available after amputation, it is difficult to control multiple DOF using this conventional control mechanism (Hudgins, 1993; Sears, 1992). For example, for a transhumeral amputee, the remaining arm muscles only have parts of biceps and triceps which can serve as EMG signal sites to control prosthetic movements. When all the three joint DOFs of elbow, wrist, and hand are required, the user must trigger a "mode switch" such as making a co-contraction of the agonist/antagonist muscle pair to sequentially select which of these joints is desired to be actuated. Obviously, switching to different modes is slow and cumbersome. Moreover, using a same agonist/antagonist pair to control different joint DOFs is non-intuitive and very difficult for users to learn the contraction/co-contraction of these muscles, because the applicable residual muscles may not be physiologically associated with the joint DOFs (such as using the residual biceps and triceps muscles to control hand opening and closing).

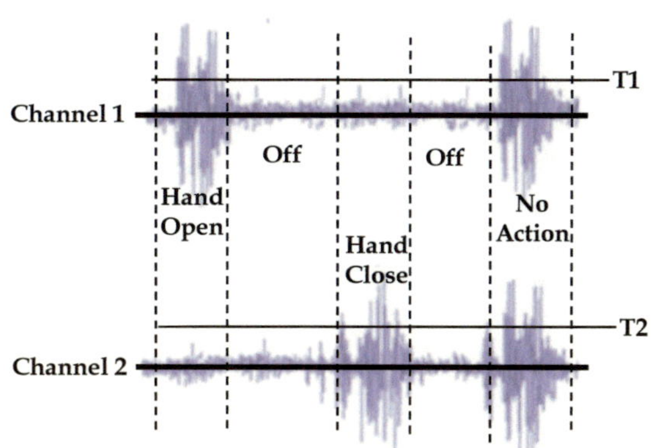

Fig. 2. Two-channel EMG amplitudes based prosthesis control

An alternative strategy is one-site EMG prosthetic control approach that has been used in a three-state myoelectric control system (Dorcas & Scott, 1966). In this control approach, the amplitude range of the one-site EMG signals that are generated from a relaxed muscle state to the full contraction is divided into three segments, as depicted in Fig. 3. Each segment has an associated amplitude threshold and corresponds to a specific prosthetic movement function (S1 for no movement, S2 for hand closing, and S3 for hand opening). In order to perform a specific movement function, the user must try to produce a constant muscle contraction to keep the EMG amplitude in the range of the associated segment. Theoretically, this approach can control a number of prosthetic functions. However, the number of functions that an amputee can control with acceptable accuracy is limited to two per control muscle (Vodovnik, 1967). In addition, like the two-site EMG control approach, using this method to control a prosthetic function also is non-intuitive and very hard for users to learn the contraction procedures of muscles.

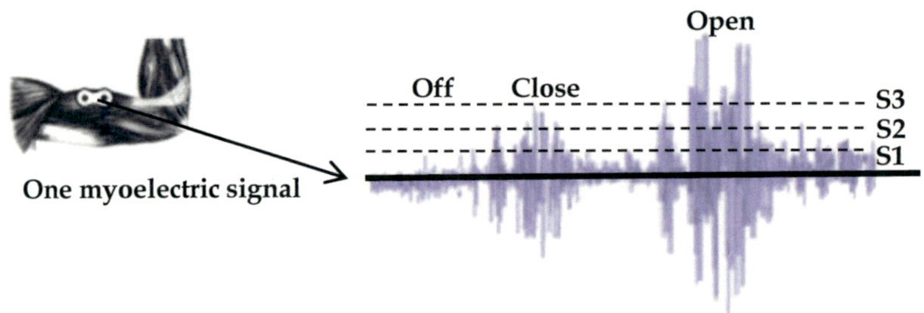

Fig. 3. One-channel EMG amplitude based prosthesis control

A promising alternative to myoelectric control is to measure the actual muscle movement, since this method is impervious to external variables, yet captures the individual movement of the muscles. It is very difficult, however, to capture this movement. Zheng et al. (Zheng et al., 2005) have attempted to measure muscle movement using sonomyography. Although the technique has provided impressive results, it is not currently feasible to implement the required instrumentation in a form factor suitable for integration in a prosthesis. Miniature muscle tunnel cineoplasties (Marquardt, 1987; Beasley, 1966), in which the tendons of muscles are connected to external cables, offer a more accurate measurement of tendon excursion. However, it has not seen much clinical interest in the world due to the invasive nature of this method.

Electrically powered upper-limb myoelectric prostheses have several advantages over body-powered prostheses. The user of a myoelectric prosthesis is freed of cables and harnesses that are required in body-powered and mechanical switch control. The myoelectric signal is noninvasively recorded on the skin surface of the residual arm and the muscle activity required to generate prosthesis control signals is relatively small. However, with the limitations of currently available myoelectric prostheses discussed above, it is estimated that only 50% of patients with an upper limb amputation use a myoelectric prosthesis. These disabled people have always been expecting high performance artificial upper-limb systems to restore the motion functions involved in their lost arms.

Recently, a significant progress of the advanced physical prostheses or components with a number of degrees of freedom has been made worldwide. Several multifunctional hands and wrists are under development or even in clinical trial. Touch Bionics has released a prosthetic hand with individually driven fingers and thumb. The Otto Bock Michelangelo Hand, the Southampton Hand (Kyberd & Chappell, 1994; Kyberd et al., 2001) and Cyberhand (Carrozza et al., 2002; 2004; 2006) have been in development in Europe for many years. However, without a new control approach that allows the user to operate a multifunctional myoelectric prosthesis intuitively and easily, these newly developed prostheses or components could not be practically usable and clinically viable.

A significant improvement over the conventional control method of current myoelectric prostheses is the use of EMG pattern recognition based control strategy (Hudgins et al., 1993; Saridis & Gootee, 1982; Kang et al., 1995; Park & Lee, 1998; Englehart et al., 1999; Englehart & Hudgins, 2003; Chan & Englehart, 2005; Ajiboye & Weir, 2005; Sebelius et al.,

2005; Hargrove et al., 2007; Momen et al., 2007). This new control approach is grounded on the assumption that EMG patterns contain rich information about the intended movements involved in a residual limb. Using a pattern classification technique, the distinguishing characteristics of EMG patterns can be used to identify a variety of different intended movements. Once a pattern has been classified, a command is sent to a prosthesis controller to implement the movement, as shown in Fig. 4. With this new control method the user elicits the contraction corresponding to the DOF that they want to control, and the classifier chooses the appropriate class of motion. As a result, the user has intuitive control and rapid selection of each function, as the intended movement matches the prosthesis function. This control approach may allow users to more easily operate their myoelectric prostheses with multiple degrees of freedom.

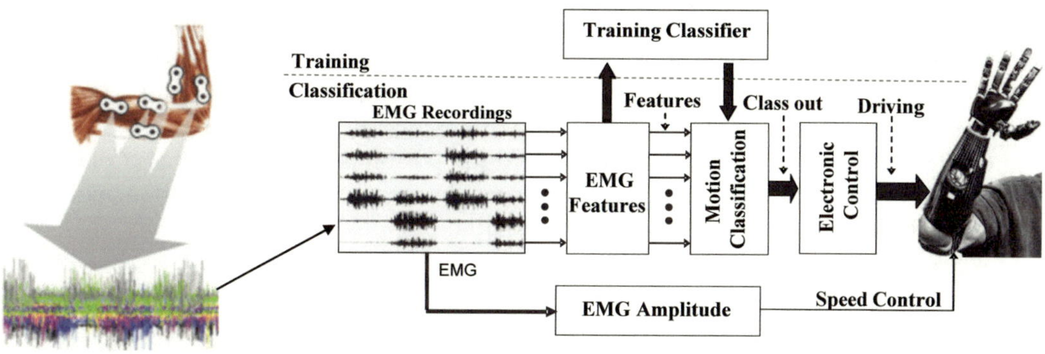

Fig. 4. Schematic diagram of EMG pattern-recognition-based prosthesis control system

In the next sections of this chapter, some important issues related to this new control strategy of multifunctional myoelectric prostheses, such as EMG signal processing and analysis and the performance of pattern recognition algorithms, will be introduced. Then, a newly proposed and developed neural-machine interface technology called Target Muscle Reinnervation (TMR) will be briefly described. TMR technology has the ability to provide additional myoelectric sources for improvement of control performance of a multifunctional prosthesis. Finally, the quantification of control performance of multifunctional myoelectric prostheses will be discussed and the real-time control performance in manipulating a virtual-reality arm and a powered physical transradial prosthesis by upper-limb amputees will be quantized and analyzed.

2. Pattern-recognition-based control approach

As explained in the previous section, current myoelectric control strategies use information from the EMG based on an estimate of the amplitude or the levels of EMG change for controlling a single device in a prosthetic limb, such as a hand, an elbow, or a wrist. These control methods have been commercially available and clinically viable to meet the need of upper-limb amputees for a powered prosthesis. However, the conventional control mode is not able to reliably control multiple functions, as required in high-level limb deficiencies. So a new control strategy is needed to deal with this difficult problem in control of a multifunctional myoelectric prosthesis. This section describes the newly proposed control strategy, EMG pattern-recognition-based control approach, which promises to deliver multifunction control of a myoelectric prosthesis. Although a full-fledged practical

implementation is still awaited, many previous studies conducted to investigate the performance of this new control technology have shown its capabilities of developing the next generation of multifunction and microprocessor-driven myoelectric prosthetic systems.
In general, an EMG pattern-recognition-based prosthetic control approach involves performing EMG measurement (to capture more and reliable myoelectric signals), feature extraction (to retain the most important discriminating information from the EMG), classification (to predict one of a subset of intended movements), and multifunctional prosthesis control (to implement the prosthetic operation of the predicted class of movement), as illustrated in Fig. 4. The details of each stage of a pattern recognition based control strategy are discussed in the following sections.

2.1 Multi-channel EMG acquisition

EMG signal measurement: In EMG pattern-recognition-based control of a multifunctional prosthesis, multi-channel myoelectric recordings are needed to capture enough myoelectric pattern information for the accurate classification of multiple classes of intentional movements. This raises two primary concerns in practice: number of myoelectric channels and configuration of electrode placement (electrode positions). The number and placement of electrodes would mainly depend on how many classes of movements are demanded in a multi-functional prosthesis and how many residual muscles of an amputee are applicable for myoelectric control. It is obvious that the more the classes of movements are involved in a prosthesis, the more the myoelectric electrodes are required to get more myoelectric signals. Using more myoelectric electrodes may increase the number of myoelectric signals captured, but it simultaneously adds more complexity, weight, and cost to a prosthesis. For the amputees with different upper-limb amputation levels, the motion classes that they demand and their remaining arm muscles available for myoelectric control are highly variable. Thus an appropriate analysis must be performed to determine the number and placement configuration of myoelectric electrodes required to control multifunctional upper-limb prostheses, accordingly.
Pattern recognition has been used in different laboratories worldwide for development of transradial prosthesis control because the forearm contains the residual wrist muscles, allowing wrist function to be readily controlled, and some residual hand muscles, for limited multifunction hand control. For myoelectric transradial prostheses, the EMG signals are measured from residual muscles with a number of bipolar electrodes (8-16) which are generally placed on the circumference of the remaining forearm. In a recent study (Li et al., 2010), 12 self-adhesive bipolar electrodes were used to record EMG signals, in which 8 of the 12 electrodes were uniformly placed around the proximal portion of the forearm and the other 4 electrodes were positioned on the distal end. A large circular electrode was placed on the elbow of the amputated arm as a ground.
The primary motion classes that may be highly required by a transradial amputee are wrist flexion/extension, wrist rotation (pronation/supination), and hand open/close. The preliminary analysis that was recently performed (Li et al., 2010) shows that for the six basic motion classes, using six optimally selected electrodes could produce an average classification accuracy of around 92%. In addition, this study also showed that for different transradial amputees, the locations of the optimal electrode placement are variable. This study used a straightforward, exhaustive search algorithm to determine the optimal electrodes based on the 12-channel EMG recordings for each subject.

EMG signal conditioning and acquisition: EMG signals captured with surface electrodes are commonly filtered by a band-pass filter to improve signal quality. Properly choosing the frequency band for the band-pass filter would be of importance for improving the control performance of a myoelectric prosthesis. At the higher frequency side of signal spectrum, a low-pass filter is used to attenuate the unwanted high-frequency components in EMG signals and avoid aliasing signal distortion. Generally, the cut-off frequency of a low-pass filter is determined by the requirement of the Nyquist sampling theory, which should be equal or less than half of signal sampling rate. At the lower frequency side of signal spectrum, the cut-off frequency of a high-pass filter is determined by the need to remove slow variations in the signals caused by the motion artifacts such as electrode shift and cable movement. Almost all the previous studies of EMG pattern recognition based prosthesis controls adopted a high-pass cut-off frequency ranging from 5 Hz to 20 Hz. The lower frequency components of EMG spectrum mainly contain the information on the firing rates of active motor units, which may be important for some EMG studies. However, these components may not make a significant contribution to the movement classification in EMG-based movement analysis. It is known that the cable motion artifacts typically have a frequency range of 1-50 Hz and the power density of electrode motion artifacts is up to 20 Hz. Thus a high-pass filter of 5-20 Hz could not effectively attenuate the motion artifacts, which may impair control accuracy and stability of a myoelectric prosthesis. Therefore, a higher high-pass cut-off frequency will be expected to significantly reduce more motion artifacts in the captured EMG signals; this may enhance the control accuracy and stability of a myoelectric prosthesis. The results from our recent study (Li et al., 2011) showed that the accuracy for the classification of a number of classes of arm movements could not benefit much from acquiring more low frequency components of EMG signals. Including 20-100 Hz frequency band components of EMG signals only slightly increased the classification accuracy in both of able-bodied subjects (about 0.25%) and amputees (about 1.6%). This suggests that a higher high-pass cut-off frequency such as 50Hz-60Hz can be used to remove or reduce more low-frequency motion artefacts from EMG recordings for improving the control stability of a multifunctional myoelectric prosthesis.

With the exception of a few cases, the major power (about 95%) of surface EMG signals is accounted for by harmonics up to 400-500Hz (Clancy et al., 2002) and most of the EMG components with a frequency of more than 500 Hz are contributed by electrode and equipment noise or environmental interference. Thus, the widely used sampling rate in surface EMG studies (Clancy et al., 2002; Ives & Wigglesworth, 2003) is around 1,000 Hz. This sampling rate was also adopted in most studies of EMG pattern recognition prosthesis control (Ajiboye & Weir, 2005; Sebelius et al., 2005; Hargrove et al., 2007; Li et al., 2010). It is obvious that using a high sampling rate may involve more high-frequency contents in myoelectric signals captured with surface electrodes, but it simultaneously adds more processing and computational complexity to the controller of a prosthesis. With the limited computation capability of a microprocessor-based prosthetic controller embedded into the socket of a prosthesis, it would be desired in EMG signal acquisition to use a low sampling rate without compromising much with prosthesis control performance. Our recent investigations (Li et al., 2011) showed that using a 500-Hz sampling rate, the average classification accuracy for the subjects with upper-limb amputation only dropped around 2.0% in comparison of a 1-kHz sampling rate. Compared to a 1-kHz sampling rate, using a 500-Hz sampling rate can save about 50% storing memory and reduce 50% data processing time with a slight accuracy sacrifice; this will greatly simplify the design and implementation of a microprocessor-based prosthetic controller. In addition, fast data processing speed may allow us to use more sophisticated pattern recognition algorithms and additional control strategies such as prosthetic adaptive control and majority vote in decision making to further improve the control performance of multifunctional myoelectric prostheses.

2.2 EMG feature extraction

An EMG pattern associated to a limb movement is described with the features extracted from EMG recordings. The choice of a feature set has a significant influence on the performance of the EMG pattern classifier. Commercially available myoelectric controllers only use the smoothed amplitude myoelectric signals as their feature. With the need of providing more information about the EMG patterns in each channel, multivariate features sets have been proposed and used in EMG pattern-recognition-based control of multifunctional prostheses. The most intuitive features are based on time-domain statistics such as mean absolute value, mean absolute value slope, variance of the EMG signals, zero crossing, slope sign changes (Hudgins et al., 1993), which need less computational resources in comparison to frequency-domain features and time-frequency features such as autocorrelation coefficients, spectral measures, short-time Fourier transform, wavelet transform, and wavelet packet transform. Because of their relative ease of implementation and high performance, the time-domain features have been widely used in most previous studies.

EMG pattern recognition is performed on windowed EMG data. EMG recordings from all recording channels are segmented into a series of analysis windows either with or without a time overlap, as shown in Fig.5. The window length is usually 100-250 ms. Overlapping analysis windows are used to maximally utilize the continuous stream of data and to produce a decision stream that is as dense as possible, with regard to the available computing capacity (Englehart and Hudgins, 2003). For overlapping window analysis, the operational delay in real-time control due to data buffering would be the duration of the overlapping (e.g., 50 ms) instead of the length of the window (e.g., 150 ms). The EMG features are extracted from each analysis window as a representation of EMG signal pattern. For each analysis window, a feature set is extracted on each of all the recording channels, producing an L-dimensional feature vector (corresponding to the L features). After concatenating the feature sets of all the channels, the entire EMG feature matrix ($L \times C \times W$, where L, C, and W are the number of features, the number of channels, and the number of analysis windows, respectively) from the training set is provided to a classifier for training.

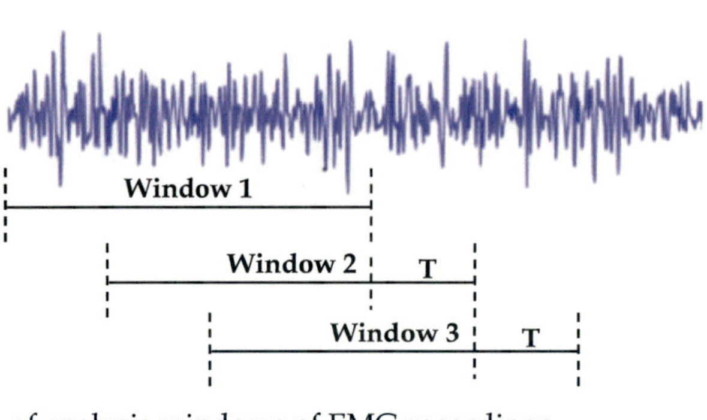

Fig. 5. Segmentation of analysis windows of EMG recordings

2.3 EMG pattern recognition classifier

The goal of a pattern recognition based classifier is to discriminate the intended movements from the EMG recordings as accurately as possible. Many classification techniques have been investigated, including linear discriminate analysis (Hargrove et al., 2007; Li et al., 2010), Bayesian statistical methods (Huang et al., 2005), artificial neural networks, and fuzzy logic (Ajiboye & Weir, 2005). All report similar classification accuracies (92-98% accuracy), and there is no statistical difference across a subject pool [38], provided the classifiers are properly tuned and use a good set of features. The linear discriminant analysis (LDA) classifier (Tou and Gonzalez, 1974) has been widely used in previous studies for classification of different movements. More complex and potentially more powerful classifiers may be constructed, but it has been shown in previous work (Hargrove et al., 2007) that the LDA classifier does not compromise classification accuracy. Compared with other classifiers, the LDA classifier is much simpler to implement and much faster to train.

It is worth noting that many previous studies have used able-bodied subjects to assess the feasibility and performance of pattern-recognition algorithms using EMG signals from forearm muscles. Using various pattern classification techniques, such as linear discriminant analysis (LDA), artificial neural networks, and fuzzy logic, high accuracies (>93%) for classification of six to ten wrist and hand movements were consistently achieved in many previous studies. This suggests that a variety of pattern-recognition algorithms can be used to predict the able-bodied subject's actual hand or arm movements with high accuracies. Use of able-bodied subjects is reasonable with the simple goal of comparing classification accuracy of different pattern recognition algorithms in discriminating EMG patterns. However, the limb amputees are the final users of a myoelectric prosthesis. In some of these previous studies for able-bodied subjects, electrodes were placed on the proximal portion of forearm to mimic the case of people with transradial amputations. However, unlike the able-bodied subjects who could do a hand or arm movement physically, limb amputees perform an intended movement using their phantom hand or arm. Limited works have been done in subjects with a limb amputation. A recent study involved six subjects with transradial amputations (five transradial amputees and one congenital below-elbow failure of formation) and used 8 electrodes placed on the residual forearm for EMG recordings (Sebelius et al, 2005). This study showed a low average accuracy (approximately 70%) for classification of 10 arm classes (wrist flexion/extension plus 8 hand grasps) with an artificial neural network - based classifier. Another study (Li et al., 2010) that was conducted on five unilateral transradial amputees also found high pattern recognition accuracies (around 94%) on the intact limbs—in which EMG data was collected from both forearm and intrinsic hand muscles—and significantly lower accuracies (around 79%) on the amputated limb. It is obvious that the classification accuracy achieved with an amputated arm is significantly lower than that with an intact arm. Thus this suggests that the performance assessment of a classifier in identifying a number of movements for control of a multifunctional myoelectric prosthesis should use the people with limb amputations.

2.4 Evaluation of classification performance

Historically, investigators quantified the EMG pattern recognition performance with the simple goal of comparing the classification accuracy of different pattern recognition algorithms. In general, the EMG recordings from performing a movement are divided into two parts. One part of EMG data is used as the training data set and another part serves as the testing data set. For a subject, a specific classifier is built using the training EMG data set. Then the performance of a trained classifier in identifying a movement is evaluated using the testing data set and measured by the classification accuracy, which is defined as

$$\frac{\text{Number correctly classified samples}}{\text{Total number of testing samples}} x 100\% \tag{1}$$

The classification accuracies in identifying all the classes of movements are averaged to calculate the overall classification accuracy for a subject.

2.5 Multifunctional prosthesis control

For multifunctional prosthesis control, a classifier is offline trained by having the user to perform repetitions of a number of motion classes that will be involved in the prosthesis. Then in the real-time application, the trained classifier sequentially determines which motion class the user is employing based on a set of EMG features. The duration of making a decision of the classifier would be the time increment of an overlapping analysis window. When a motion class is recognized, a motor control command is sent to the prosthesis controller for completion of the motion. The classification is repeated at overlapping intervals to provide continuous control of a myoelectric prosthesis.

3. Neural-machine interface for improvement of control performance

3.1 A paradox

As discussed above, EMG pattern recognition based control strategy seems highly promising in developing the novel myoelectric prosthetic systems that may allow users to more easily and intuitively operate their prostheses with multiple degrees of freedom. The usability and performance of the pattern recognition approach in control of a multifunctional myoelectric prosthesis are premised on whether the users have enough residual muscles as sources of myoelectric control signals. This premise may be true for people with a below-elbow amputation. Their remaining forearm contains the residual wrist muscles, allowing wrist function to be readily controlled, and some residual hand muscles for control of hand movements (Fig. 6(a)). Since their elbow joint is intact, there is no need to restore the movements associated with elbow. High accuracies are consistently achieved in different studies using different processing techniques, for six classes of basic wrist and hand movements, as illustrated in Fig. 7. Thus the clinical implementation of a pattern recognition control system with wrist movements and one hand grasp looks promising for people with transradial amputations, based on the results of these previous studied. However, this premise is hardly true for people with an above-elbow or shoulder disarticulation amputation. In a transhumeral amputee only portion of biceps and triceps muscles remains (Fig. 6(b)), which would provide enough myoelectric signals for control of elbow function, but there are no remaining muscles for control of wrist and hand functions. For a person with whole shoulder disarticulation amputations, there is no any arm muscle remained as control signal (Fig. 6(c)), whereas they have a need to restore whole arm joint functions (shoulder, elbow, wrist, and hand). The less the arm muscles remain after amputations, the more the arm joint functions need to be restored in a prosthesis. It is quite a paradox.

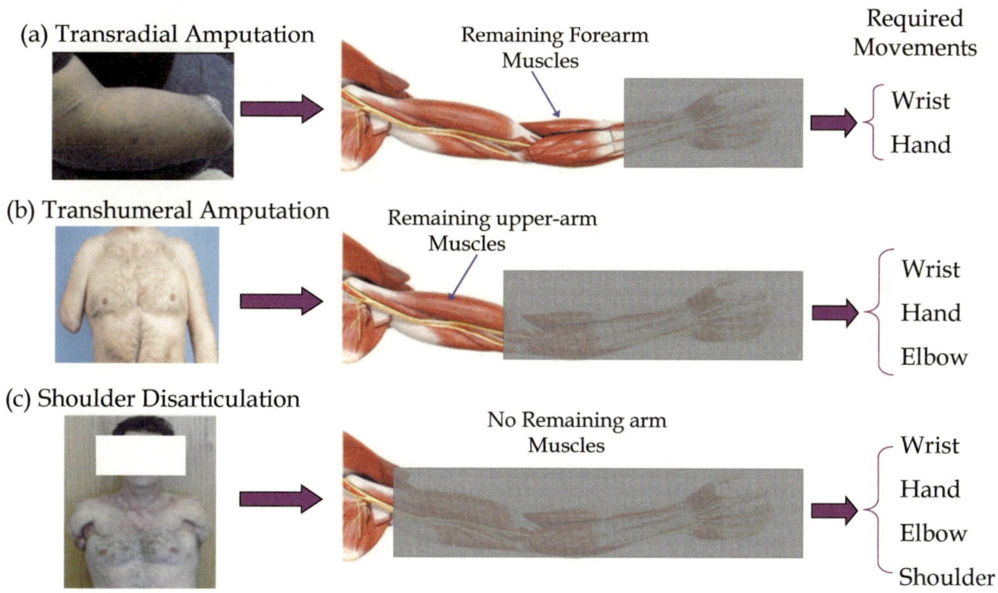

Fig. 6. Different level upper-limb amputations.

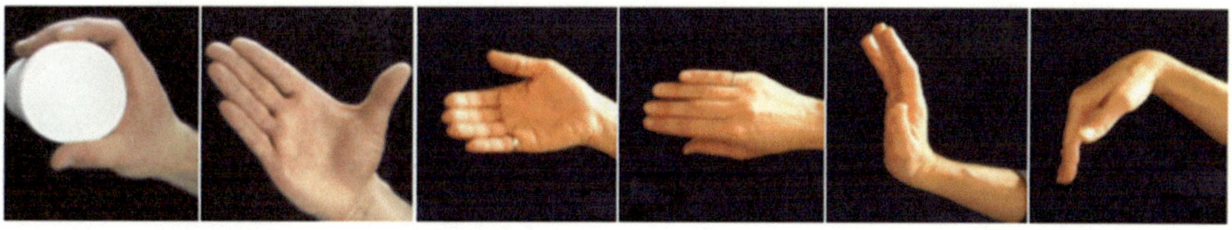

Fig. 7. Six basic wrist and hand movements.

3.2 Neural prostheses

It is obvious for people with high-level arm amputations that additional control information associated to arm movements is needed to see the realization of myoeletric prostheses with multiple degrees of freedom. An exciting concept called neuroelectric control has received considerable attention. Three so-called neural-machine interface techniques emerged and have been investigated for control of neural prostheses. They are brain-computer interface (BCI), peripheral never interface (PNI), and targeted muscle reinnervation (TMR), as shown in Fig. 8.

With BCI or PNI prosthetic control, neural sensors need to be directly connected to either the cortex or the residual nerves to capture the neural signals associated with arm movements as control signals of artificial neuroprostheses (DeLuca, 1978; Hoffer & Loeb, 1980; Edell, 1986; Hochberg et al., 2006). Although this concept offers the hope of improved control there are several inherent problems such as the mechanical sensitivity of nervous tissue, the permanence of sensor array fixation, and the fibrosis of sensor recording tips. In addition, the neural signal is very small, difficult to record and ease to be contaminated by various interference and noise in surrounding environment. An inherent challenge in the neural interface is that only a relatively small number of motor nerve fascicles may be sampled (with respect to all fascicles within a nerve bundle), making it difficult to construct a complete representation of motor intent. Motor nerves also atrophy when they are not connected to muscle, which could compound these problems. A further difficulty arises in transmitting the signals out of the body. This requires either chronic percutaneous wires (which tend to become infected) or complex transmitter-receiver systems. Finally, the durability of the implanted hardware is a critical issue. With these limitations of the BCI and PNI technologies, the works of many years have not yet resulted in any usable system of multifunctional neuroprosthesis. Prosthetic control systems are required to function for a long time (from several years to decades). The TMR technology may be considered as using muscle as a biological amplifier of the neural signal to circumvent many of the problems of BCI or PNI control and makes additional control signals accessible without implanted hardware into body.

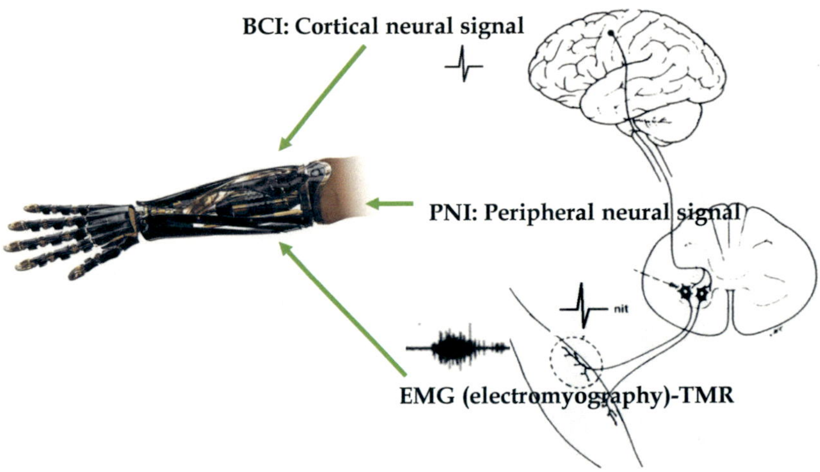

Fig. 8. Three emerging neural-machine interface techniques for control of neuroprostheses.

3.3 Target muscle reinnervation

EMG pattern recognition based prosthesis control strategy is not applicable for people with above-elbow amputations because few muscles remain in their residual arm from which to extract myoelectric control signals. To address this challenge, a new neural machine interfacing (NMI) technology called targeted muscle reinnervation (TMR) have been recently proposed and developed at Rehabilitation Institute of Chicago (RIC), which has the ability to improve control performance of multifunctional myoelectric upper-limb prostheses (Kuiken et al., 2009; Zhou et al., 2007). Neural information that controlled the limb prior to amputation remains in the residual peripheral nerves. TMR uses the residual nerves from an amputated limb and transfers them onto alternative muscle groups that are not biomechanically functional since they are no longer attached to the missing arm. During the nerve transfer procedure, target muscles are denervated so that they can be reinnervated by the residual arm nerves that previously traveled to the arm prior to amputation. The reinnervated muscles then serve as biological amplifiers of the amputated nerve motor commands (Kuiken, 2003). During the surgery subcutaneous tissue is removed so that surface EMG signals are optimized for power and focal recording. Fig. 9 schematically shows the TMR technique in a person with shoulder disarticulations. TMR thus provides physiologically appropriate EMG control signals that are related to previous functions of the lost arm. Successful TMR allows voluntary motor control signals that used to activate muscles in the amputated limb to activate these newly reinnervated muscles.

TMR technique has been successfully performed in some dozens of people with transhumeral and higher upper-limb amputations worldwide. The relevant studies showed that TMR can provide a rich source of additional control data that are physiologically related to the missing limb. The high classification accuracy was consistent within subjects, demonstrating good repeatability. It was also high between subjects who had had different surgical procedures and had different remaining posttraumatic anatomy and geometry of their target muscle, demonstrating that the surgical concept can be applied to a broad array of injury levels (Zhou et al, 2007).

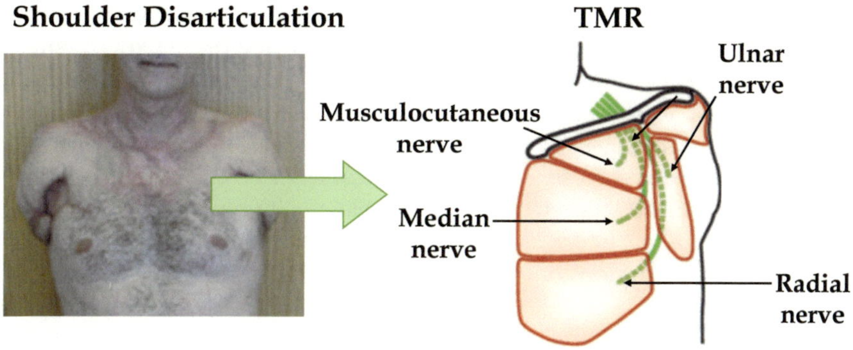

Fig. 9. Schematic diagram of TMR technique (Kuiken et al., 2009)

4. Quantification of real-time control performance

It is a challenge to evaluate the real-time control performance of EMG pattern recognition based prostheses, especially in the case that there are no multifunctional prosthetic systems available. Note that almost all of the previous studies used classification accuracy to evaluate the performance of pattern recognition algorithms. Classification accuracy is the ability of the algorithm to appropriately recognize the desired movements during each time window (usually 100-200 ms) while the subject holds different movements for several seconds. This accuracy is calculated by post-processing EMG recordings and is not a true measure of real-time function of a myoelectric prosthesis. Thus, in order to know whether the residual muscles following amputation can provide stable EMG information for accurate real-time control of multifunctional prostheses, the real-time performance metrics are required to examine the clinical robustness and accuracy of pattern recognition control.

4.1 Virtual prosthesis control

The controllable degrees of freedom are limited by the mechanical degrees of freedom available in the prosthesis. Currently, physical myoelectric prostheses with multiple degrees of motion freedom are not available yet, resulting in a challenge in quantitatively evaluating the real-time control performance. To deal with this challenge, the virtual reality (VR) based platforms have been developed for the purposes of development and performance quantification of multifunctional myoelectric prosthesis control system (Li et al, 2010; Kuiken et al., 2009). These VR platforms are designed to create an efficient, flexible, and user-friendly environment for prosthetic control algorithm development in the laboratory, application in a clinical setting, and eventual use in an embedded system. The major function modules of this platform include multi-electrode EMG recording (up to 16 channels), classifier training and testing in offline, virtual and physical prosthesis control in real time, real-time motion testing for quantification of control performance. Using this platform, we can choose an arbitrary number of motion classes (up to 22 upper-limb movements) as the targets of a virtual prosthesis. This platform has served as an important research platform to perform many lines of research works at RIC group and others.

A pilot work (Lock et al., 2005) has shown that offline classification accuracy across different classifiers has only a weak correlation with real-time performance in an objective task. This indicates that real-time performance metrics are required to examine the clinical robustness of various pattern recognition techniques and improvements. Towards this end, RIC has developed a protocol in which subjects must control a virtual arm. Experiments with the virtual prosthesis are performed immediately following classifier training. Subjects are instructed to follow visual prompts for each movement. A virtual arm which responded to the class decisions allows subjects to observe the real-time results of their movement commands. Subjects are asked to sequentially perform a series of motions and to maintain each muscle contraction until the virtual arm completed the movement. Dynamic data in performing each movement are recorded and used to quantitatively evaluate the speed and consistency of pattern recognition control in real time.

4.2 Real-time performance metrics

To assess important control parameters and gain insight into the feasibility of clinically implementing EMG pattern recognition based controllers for upper limb amputees, the three real-time performance metrics have been first proposed and used by the research group at RIC (Li et al., 2010). These metrics could also be used for comparing conventional myoelectric control and any new neural-machine-control systems that may evolve in the future. The three performance metrics are:

Motion-Completion Rate (MCR) is defined as the percentage of successfully completed motions. This metric is a measure of performance reliability. A motion trial will be considered completed if it is successfully performed through the full range of motion within the designated time limit. If the target movement is not completed within the time limit, the movement will be considered a failure.

Motion-Completion Time (MCT) is defined as the time taken to successfully complete a movement through the full range of motion. This metric is a measure of speed of use. MCT is measured as the time from the onset of movement to the completion of the intended movement.

Motion-Selection Time (MST) is defined as the time taken to correctly select a target movement. This quantity represents how quickly motor command information (here represented with myoelectric signals) could be translated into the correct motion predictions. MST is measured as the time from the onset of movement to the first correct prediction of the movement. The onset of movement was identified as the time of the last "no movement" classification; this corresponded to approximately a 5% increase in the mean absolute value of the baseline EMG signals.

4.3 Real-time performance in amputees

Recently, several studies have been conducted to use these real-time performance metrics for quantification of real-time control performance in amputees. The real-time performance metrics was first used by the RIC's group to quantify the control performance of virtual prosthesis control in five TMR patients with transhumeral or shoulder disarticulation amputations. Ten classes of different elbow, wrist, and hand movements were included in the study (Kuiken et al., 2009). According to this study, the mean motion selection and motion completion times for hand grasp patterns were 0.38 seconds and 1.54 seconds, respectively. These patients successfully completed a mean of 96.3% of elbow and wrist movements and 86.9% of hand movements within 5 seconds, compared with 100% and 96.7% completed by controls. These results suggest that reinnervated muscles can produce sufficient EMG information for real-time control of advanced artificial arms.

Later, another study was done by the RIC's group in five people with unilateral transradial amputees (Li et al., 2010). Same metrics were used to quantify the real-time performance of virtual prosthesis control in these amputees. Based on the results of this study, the wrist movements could be selected and completed quickly with both the amputated and intact limbs, with no difference between arms. Similarly, the motion-completion rates for wrist movements with both arms were close to 100%. When hand grasps were successfully performed in 5 s or less with the amputated arm, they were selected and completed just as quickly as with the intact arm, but fewer hand grasps were successfully performed with the amputated limb. From these findings, it appears that motion-completion rate was the most telling performance metric. It is obvious that a high completion rate will be needed for adequate prosthesis function and to prevent user frustration.

Note that Quantifying operation of a virtual arm allows measurement of some useful metrics in the laboratory. However, the ultimate goal is for amputees to operate more dexterous prosthetic arms. Controlling a real prosthesis introduces many practical challenges, such as stability of EMG signal recording, interference from muscles controlling remaining joints, and the effects of tissue loading and arm dynamics.

5. Summary

The limb muscle cells can be activated by an intentional limb movement to generate myoelectric signals which are able to be recorded using electrodes. The surface recordings of myoelectric signals are effective and important input signals in control of prostheses for people with limb amputations. EMG pattern-recognition-based control systems of myoelectric prostheses rely on the myoelectric signal to convey information regarding intent from the user to the prosthesis controller. The previous efforts have showed that using a pattern classification technique, an intentional movement can be predicted with the distinguishable characteristics of EMG patterns; this new method allows users to intuitively operate their myoelectric prostheses with multiple degrees of freedom.

Many encouraging progresses have been made in EMG pattern-recognition-based control of multifunctional prostheses. However, currently there is no any multifunctional myoelectric prosthesis system available for clinical use. The primary limitation may be lack of reliability and stability of current pattern recognition control, which have substantially hindered this technique from getting clinical applications. Further research and development need to be conducted before field trials can be performed. Improving EMG signal recording repeatability and stability are required to minimize or eliminate daily classifier training.

Work is ongoing to develop more robust surface EMG recording systems and prosthetic interfaces. Adaptive pattern-recognition algorithms also may improve the stability of control. Various existing hierarchical control schemes may be more robust for some patients; customization of control hierarchy is an accepted practice in modern prosthetics. These early trials of TMR technique demonstrate its feasibility and realization in control of complex multifunction myoelectric prostheses.

6. Acknowledgment

The author would like to thank Dr. Todd Kuiken's team at Neural Engineering Center for Artificial Limbs, Rehabilitation Institute of Chicago, USA, for supports. This work was supported in part by the Shenzhen Governmental Basic Research Grand #JC200903160393A and JC201005270295A the National Natural Science Foundation of China under Grant #60971076, Hong Kong Innovation and Technology Fund (ITF) #GHP/031/08, and the Shenzhen Engineering Laboratory of Motion Function Rehabilitation Technology.

7. References

Adams, P. F.; Hendershot, G. E. & M. A. Marano, M. A. (1999). Current Estimates from the National Health Interview Survey, 1996. Vol.10 (200), *National Center for Health Statistics.*

Ajiboye, AB. & Weir, RF. (2005). A heuristic fuzzy logic approach to EMG pattern recognition for multifunctional prosthesis control, *IEEE Trans. Neural Sys. Rehab. Eng.*, vol. 13, pp. 280-291.

Beasley, R. W. (1966). The tendon exteriorization cineplasty, *Inter-Clin Info Bull*, Vol. 5, pp. 6-8.

Carrozza, M.C.; Massa, B.; Micera, S.; Lazzarini, R.; Zecca, M. & Dario, P. (2002). The development of a novel prosthetic hand - Ongoing research and preliminary results, *IEEE/ASME Transactions on Mechatronics*, Vol. 7, pp. 108-114.

Carrozza, M.C.; Suppo, C.; Sebastiani,F.; Massa, B.; Vecchi, F.; Lazzarini, R.; Cutkosky, M.R. & Dario, P. (2004). The SPRING hand: Development of a self-adaptive prosthesis for restoring natural grasping, *Autonomous Robots*, Vol. 16, pp. 125-141.

Carrozza, M.C.; Cappiello, G.; Micera, S.; Edin, B.B.; Beccai, L. & Cipriani, C. (2006). Design of a cybernetic hand for perception and action, *Biological Cybernetics*, Vol. 95, pp. 629-644.

Chan, AD. & Englehart, K. (2005). Continuous myoelectric control for powered prostheses using hidden Markov models, *IEEE Trans. Biomed. Eng.*, vol. 52, pp. 121-124.

Clancy, E. A.; Morin, EL. & Merletti, R. (2002). Sampling, noise-reduction and amplitude estimation issues in surface electromyography, *J. Electromyogr. Kinesiol.*, Vol. 12, pp.1-16.

DeLuca, CJ. (1978). Control of Upper-Limb Prostheses - Case for Neuroelectric Control, *J. Med. Eng. Technol.*, vol. 2, pp. 57-61.

Dorcas, D. S. & Scott, R. N. (1966). A three-state myoelectric control, *Med. Biol. Eng.*, Vol. 4, pp. 367-372.

Edell, DJ. (1986). A Peripheral-Nerve Information Transducer for Amputees - Long-Term Multichannel Recordings from Rabbit Peripheral-Nerves, *IEEE Trans. Biomed. Eng.*, vol. 33, pp. 203-214.

Englehart, K.; Hudgins, B.; Parker, PA. & Stevenson, M. (1999). Classification of the myoelectric signal using time-frequency based representations, *Med. Eng. Phys.*, Vol. 21, pp. 431-38.

Englehart, K. & Hudgins, B. (2003). A robust, real-time control scheme for multifunction myoelectric control, *IEEE Trans. Biomed. Eng.*, Vol. 50, pp. 848-54.

Hargrove, L.; Englehart, K. & Hudgins, B. (2007). A comparison of surface and intramuscular myoelectric signal classification, *IEEE Trans. Biomed. Eng*, vol. 54, pp. 847-853.

Hochberg, LR.; Serruya, MD.; Friehs, GM.; Mukand,JA.; Saleh, M.; Caplan,AH.; Branner,A.; Chen, D.; Penn,RD. & Donoghue,JP. (2006). Neuronal ensemble control of prosthetic devices by a human with tetraplegia, *Nature*， vol. 442, pp. 164-171.

Hoffer, JA. & Loeb, GE. (1980). Implantable Electrical and Mechanical Interfaces with Nerve and Muscle, *Ann. Biomed. Eng.*, vol. 8, pp. 351-360.

Huang, YH.; Englehart, K.; Hudgins, B. & Chan, AD. (2005). A Gaussian mixture model based classification scheme for myoelectric control of powered upper limb prostheses, *IEEE Trans. Biomed. Eng.*, vol. 52, pp. 1801-1811.

Hudgins, B. S.; Parker, P. A. & Scott, R. N. (1993). A new strategy for multi-functional myoelectric control, *IEEE Trans. Biomed. Eng.*, Vol. 40(1), pp. 82-94.

Ives, J. C. & Wigglesworth, JK. (2003). Sampling rate effects on surface EMG timing and amplitude measures, *Clin. Biomech.*, Vo. 18,pp. 543 - 552.

Kang, W.J.; Shiu, J.R.; Cheng, C.K.; Lai, J.S.; Tsao, H.W & Kuo, T.S. (1995). The application of cepstral coefficients and maximum likelihood method in EMG pattern recognition, *IEEE Trans. Biomed. Eng.*, Vol. 42, pp. 777-85.

Kato, I., et al. (1969). Multifunctional myoelectric hand prosthesis with pressure sensory feedback system—WASEDA Hand-4P, *Proc 3rd Int Symp External Control of Human Extremities*, Dubrovnik, Yugoslavia, pp. 155-170.

Kay, H. & Newman, J. (1975). Relative incidence of new amputations. *Orthotics and Prosthetics*, Vol. 29, pp. 3-16.

Kobrinski, A. E., et al. (1960). Problems of bioelectric control, in J. F. Coles, ed., Automatic and remote control, Proc 1st IFAC Int Conf, Vol. 2, Butterworths, London.

Kuiken, T.; Li, G.; Lock, B.; Lipschutz, R.; Miller, L.; Stubblefield, K. & Englehart, K. (2009). Targeted muscle reinnervation for real-time myoelectric control of multifunction artificial arms, *JAMA.*, vol. 301, pp. 619-628.

Kuiken, T. (2003). Consideration of nerve-muscle grafts to improve the control of artificial arms, *Journal of Technology and Disability*, vol. 15, pp. 105-111.

Kyberd, P.J. & Chappell, P.H. (1994). The Southampton Hand - an Intelligent Myoelectric Prosthesis, *Journal of Rehabilitation Research and Development*, Vol. 31, pp. 326-334.

Kyberd, P.J.; Light, C.; Chappell, P.H.; Nightingale, J.M.; Whatley, D. & Evans, M. (2001). The design of anthropomorphic prosthetic hands: A study of the Southampton Hand, Robotica, Vol. 19, pp. 593-600.

Li, G.; Schultz, AE. & Kuiken, TA. (2010). Quantifying pattern recognition based myoelectric control of multifunctional transradial prostheses, *IEEE Trans. Neural Syst. Rehabil. Eng.*, Vol. 18, pp. 185-192.

Li, G.; Li, Y.; Yu, L. & Geng, Y. (2011). Conditioning and sampling issues of EMG signals in motion recognition of multifunction myoelectric prostheses, *Ann. Biomed. Eng.*, vol. 39(6), pp.1779-1787.

Lock, B.; Englehart, K. & Hudgins, B. (2005). Real-Time Myoelectric Control in a Virtual Environment to Relate Usability vs. Accuracy, *presented at MyoElectric Controls Symposium,* New Brunswick, Fredericton.

Lyman, J. H.; A. Freedy, A. & Prior, R. (1976). Fundamental and applied research related to the design and development of upper-limb externally powered prostheses, *Bull Prosthet Res.*, Vol. 13, pp.184-195.

Marquardt, E. (1987). Come-back of the pectoral cineplasty, *J Assoc Child Prosthet Orthot Clin,* Vol. 22, pp. 32.

Momen, K.; Krishnan, S. & Chau, T. (2007). Real-time classification of forearm electromyographic signals corresponding to user-selected intentional movements for multifunction prosthesis control, *IEEE Trans. Neural Sys. Rehab. Eng.*, vol. 15, pp. 535-542.

Park, S.H. & Lee, S.P. (1998). EMG pattern recognition based on artificial intelligence techniques, *IEEE Trans. Rehab. Eng.,* Vol. 6, pp. 400-405.

Parker, P.A. & Scott, R.N. (1986). Myoelectric control of prostheses. *Crit. Rev. Biomed. Eng.*, Vol. 13, pp. 283-310.

Saridis, G.N. & Gootee, T.P. (1982). EMG pattern analysis and classification for a prosthetic arm, *IEEE Trans. Biomed. Eng.,* Vol. 29, pp. 403-12.

Sears, H. H. (1992). Trends in upper-extremity prosthetic development, *In: Atlas of Limb Prosthetics,* edited by J. H. Bowker, and J. W. Michael. St. Louis: Mosby.

Sebelius, FC.; Rosen, BN. & Lundborg, GN. (2005). Refined myoelectric control in below-elbow amputees using artificial neural networks and a data glove, *J. Hand Surg. Am.*, vol. 30, pp. 780-789.

Vodovnik, L.; Kreifeldt, J.; Caldwell, R.; Green, L.; Silgalis, E. & Craig, P. (1967). Some topics on myoelectric control of orthotic/prosthetic systems, *Rep EDC 4-67-17,* Case Western Reserve University, Cleveland, OH.

Y. Zheng, Y.; Chan, M.M.F.; Shi, J.; Chen, X. & Huang, Q.H. (2005). Sonomyography: Monitoring morphological changes of forearm muscles in actions with the feasibility for the control of powered prosthesis, *Med. Eng. Phys.,* Vol.28(5), pp. 405-415.

Zhou, P.; Lowery, M.; Englehart, K.; Huang, H.; Li, G.; Hargrove, L.; Dewald, J. & Kuiken, T. (2007). Decoding a new neural-machine interface for control of artificial limbs, *J. Neurophysiol.*, vol. 98, pp. 2974-2982.

Part 3

Force Estimation

7

Pinching Effort Evaluation Based on Tendon Force Estimation

Atsutoshi Ikeda, Yuichi Kurita and Tsukasa Ogasawara
Nara Institute of Science and Technology
Japan

1. Introduction

The quantitative evaluation of product usability is important for product design. Most products, e.g. digital cameras, remote controls, and cellphones, have holding and operation parts where the hands are placed. The pinching effort which is the feeling when an user picks up and controls a product is important for product usability. Demands for product design that considers the pinching effort have increased. However, quantitative evaluation of sensibility is difficult. A questionnaire survey using a semantic differential method is commonly used for the subjective evaluation of the usability. In recent years, quantitative evaluation methods have been proposed based on physical data that are measurable by sensors. Radhakrishnan & Nagaravindra (1993) analyzed the force distribution during grasping a tube. Kong & Freivalds (2003) measured the maximum pulling force, the surface EMG (electromyogram), and the contact force, when pulling seven different meat hooks. They also developed a biomechanical hand model to estimate the tendon force. These research methods addressed the quantitative evaluation of a power grasp using the whole hand (palm and fingers).

On the other hand, some research methods in biomechanics have proposed an accurate musculoskeletal model of the human hand and fingers; An et al. (1979) established a three-dimensional normative hand model based on X-ray image analysis. Brook et al. (1995) introduced a dynamic index finger model using a set of moment arm coefficients and elongation equations. Sueda et al. (2008) developed a method for generating motions of tendons and muscles for hand animation. Holzbaur et al. (2005) developed a biomechanical model of the upper extremity, Flanagan et al. (2006) discussed control strategies of the human fingertips, Valero-Cuevas (2005) proposed a detailed model of the human finger, including neuro-musculo-skeletal interactions. Also, in robotics, there have been a lot of research methods related to skin and muscle modeling. For example, Nakamura et al. (2005) proposed a computation method of somatosensory information from motion-capture data. Tada & Pai (2008) developed a simple finger shell model that is efficient to quickly simulate the finger surface deformation. However, these research methods were not applied to the quantitative evaluation of product usability.

A goal of this research is to design an evaluation system of product usability using a simulation in conjunction with multiple sensors, such as contact sensors, pressure sensors, and force sensors. Fig. 1 shows the concept of the evaluation system, which is designed to correlate the obtained sensor data with the human sensory information. Ikeda et al. (2008) has

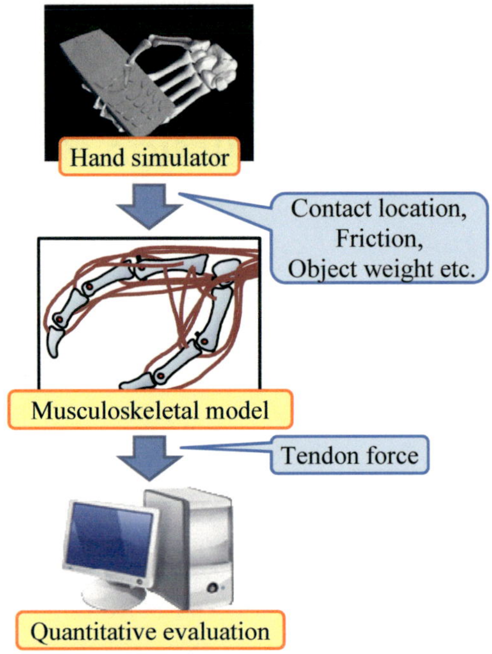

Fig. 1. Concept of the evaluation system

presented the concept of the evaluation of the pinching effort. We (Ikeda et al. (2009a) and Ikeda et al. (2009b)) have also evaluated the usability in the pinching activity by comparing the sensor data from the sensing hand with the human muscle activity.

In this chapter, we discuss the relationship between the pinching effort and the EMG data. Then we propose the evaluation method of the pinching effort using a tendon skeletal finger model. At the beginning of this chapter, the human pinching activity is analyzed to show that the tendon force reflect well the human sensation. Since we can not directly measure the tendon force in humans, we measure the surface EMG instead of the tendon force and compare the surface EMG with the questionnaire results in the human experiment. Second, we describe the detail of the tendon skeletal finger model and the pinching effort evaluation method. The score of pinching effort is calculated from the tendon forces which are estimated in a pinching simulation. The simulation result is compared with the human experiment result. These results show that the proposed method is useful for the quantitative evaluation of the pinching effort.

2. Human pinching experiment

2.1 Measurement system

Fig. 2 shows an overview of the experiment to measure human pinching activity. A capacitance triaxial kinesthetic sensor (PD3-32-05-80, Nitta) was put inside a holding cylinder to measure the pinching force. Disposable radiolucent electrodes (F-150S, Nihon Kohden) were put on the hand and the arm of the subject to measure the surface EMG of the FDS (flexor digitorum superficialis) muscle and the ADP (adductor pollicis muscle). The FDS muscle flexes the PIP joint of the index finger, and the ADP muscle adducts the CMC joint of the

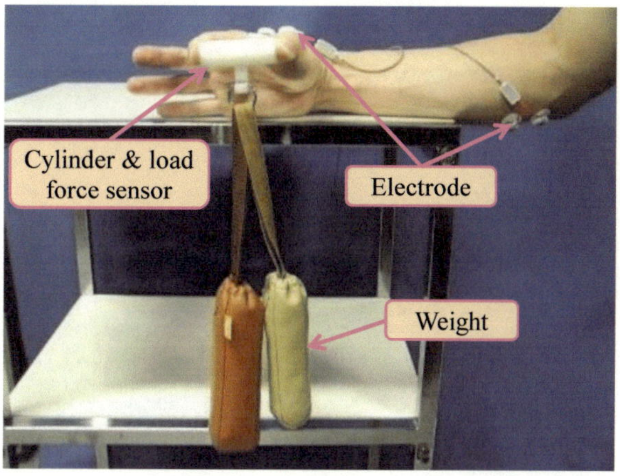

Fig. 2. Experiment overview of pinching an object

thumb. Fig. 3 shows the normal location of muscles in the forearm and the hand. The surface EMG were amplified by an EMG amplifier (EMG-021, Harada Electronics Industry) and stored in a PC through an A/D board (CSI-360116, Interface). In this chapter, the following processes are used for a quantitative analysis of the EMG signal:

1. Detrending: Remove, the DC (direct current) offset from the raw EMG signal
2. Rectification: Translates the EMG signal, that have been removed of the DC offset, to a positive polarity
3. Filtering: Smooth the rectified EMG signal using a low-pass filter ($4[Hz]$)
4. Integration: Calculate the integration value of the filtered EMG.
5. Normalization: Normalize the integrated EMG (EMG_{intg}) using a maximum/minimum EMG (EMG_{max} and EMG_{min}) value which are preliminary measured:

$$EMG_{norm} = \frac{EMG_{intg} - EMG_{min}}{EMG_{max} - EMG_{min}} + 1 \tag{1}$$

Fig. 4 shows the cylinders used in the experiment. These cylinders are made of ABS (acrylonitrile butadiene styrene) resin. Dimension of the cylinders are 20, 40, 60, 80 and 100 [mm] in length and 20 [mm] in diameter.

2.2 Experimental method

In our experiment, 300 and 600 [g] weights were used. Five healthy male subjects, average age: 24 years old and SD: 3.4, volunteered for the experiment. All subjects were given the experimental detail and they gave their consent to participate. The pinching activity was performed with their dominant arm. The arm of the subject was placed on a desk, and the middle, ring, and pinky finger were kept open so as not to influence the pinching activity. Subjects pinch in the length direction of the cylinder by using the index finger and thumb. Table 2 shows the average and standard deviation of the subjects' hand sizes. Fig. 5 shows the definition of the measured dimensions of the hand. The subjects' hand sizes were similar to the standard Japanese hand size.

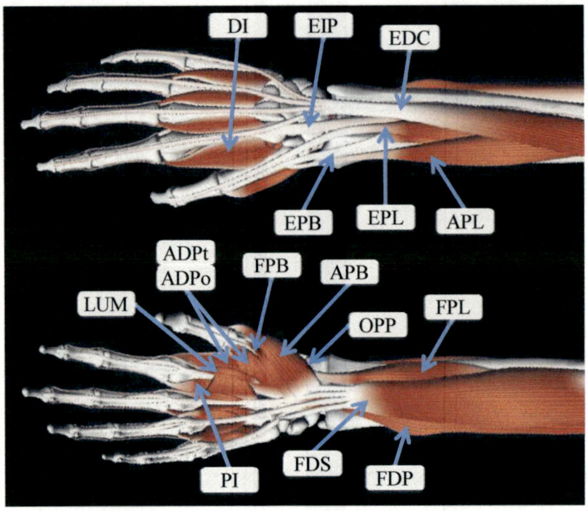

Fig. 3. Muscles that drive the index finger and the thumb (This figure is drawn with Kaitai Ensyo (gsport,inc.))

Index finger

FDP	Flexor Digitorum Profundus
FDS	Flexor Digitorum Superficialis
EIP	Extensor Indicis Proprius
EDC	Extensor Digitorum Proprius
LUM	Lumbricalis
DI	Dorsal Interosseous
PI	Palmar Interosseous

Thumb

FPL	Flexor Pollicis Longus
FPB	Flexor Pollicis Brevis
EPL	Extensor Pollicis Longus
EPB	Extensor Pollicis Brevis
APL	Abductor Pollicis Longus
APB	Abductor Pollicis Brevis
ADPt	The Transverse Head of The Adductor Pollicis
ADPo	The Oblique Head of The Adductor Pollicis
OPP	Opponents Pollicis

Table 1. List of muscle in the hand and the fore arm

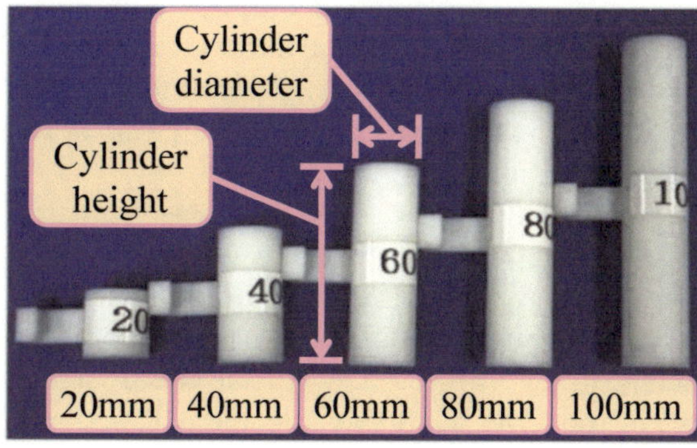

Fig. 4. Cylinder dimensions

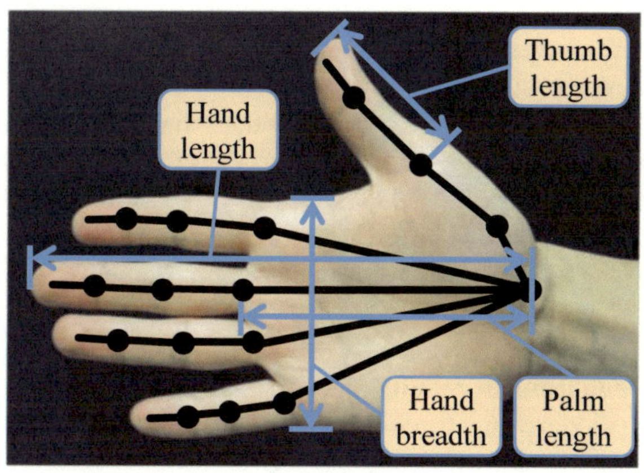

Fig. 5. Measured dimensions (see definitions of measurement on the website of Digital Human Research Center, AIST (http://www.dh.aist.go.jp/))

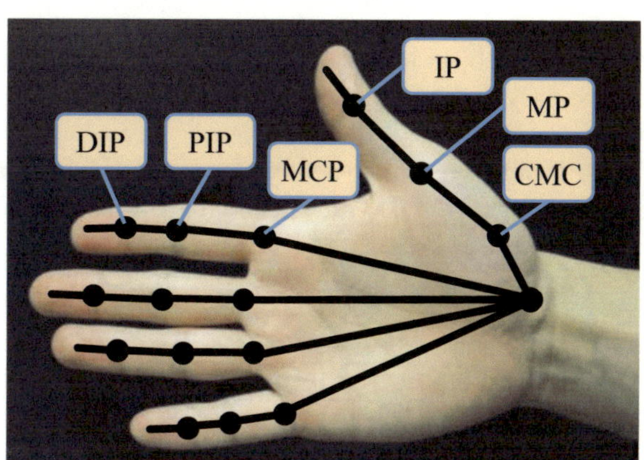

Fig. 6. Joint name of the index finger and the thumb

Before beginning the experiment, we explained its purpose to the subjects. In the experiment, the subjects pinched each cylinder and scored the effort level of the cylinder. The score had five levels from 1: "very easy to pinch" to 5: "very difficult to pinch". The subjects pinch the cylinders in arbitrary order and hold the cylinders for 15 [sec]. A two-minute interval was taken between each trial.

The subjects joint angles when pinching each cylinder was measured using a CyberGlove (CyberGlove Systems LLC). Fig. 6 shows the joint notation of the index finger and the thumb. We measure eight angles: the MCP (metacarpophalangeal: in the index finger) joint FE (flexion/extension direction), the MCP joint AA (adduction/abduction direction), the PIP (proximal interphalangeal) joint FE, the DIP (distal interphalangeal) joint FE, the CMC (carpometacarpal) joint FE, the CMC joint AA and the MP (metacarpophalangeal: in the thumb) joint FE. We can not measure the MP joint AA and the IP (Interphalangeal) joint FE because sensors were not present in the CyberGlove. The human joint angles are compared with simulation results.

2.3 Human experimental results

2.3.1 Questionnaire survey results

Fig. 7 shows the average and standard deviation of the scores. The curves in the figure are the approximate quadratic curves of the 300 and 600 [g] weights. The lowest score is observed in the 60 [mm] cylinder length for both the 300 and 600 [g] weights. On the other hand, higher score is observed when the cylinder length is 20 and 100 [mm] for both the 300 and 600 [g] weights. A possible reason is that the finger posture when pinching the middle length cylinder makes it easier to exert a pinching force.

2.3.2 Pinching force measurement results

Fig. 8 shows the typical pinching force when a subject pinches a cylinder. The dash line and the dot-dash line in the figure designate the theoretical force necessary to pinch the cylinders with 300 and 600 [g] weight, respectively. The theoretically necessary forces F_{theo} are calculated based on the friction coefficient μ between the finger and the cylinder:

$$F_{theo} = \mu M_{obj} \tag{2}$$

where M_{obj} is the weight of the object and $\mu = 0.5$. The measured force is somewhat larger than the theoretically necessary force because a human applies a safety margin in order to pinch an object tightly.

The highest pinching force is observed when a subject pinches the 100 [mm] cylinder for both weights. The possible reason is that the 100 [mm] is the hardest to pinch.

	Ave.	SD
Hand length [mm]	184.4	5.5
Palm length [mm]	104.6	4.7
Hand breadth [mm]	82.6	5.3
Thumb length [mm]	61.6	2.8

Table 2. Average and standard deviation of hand size (see definitions in Fig. 5)

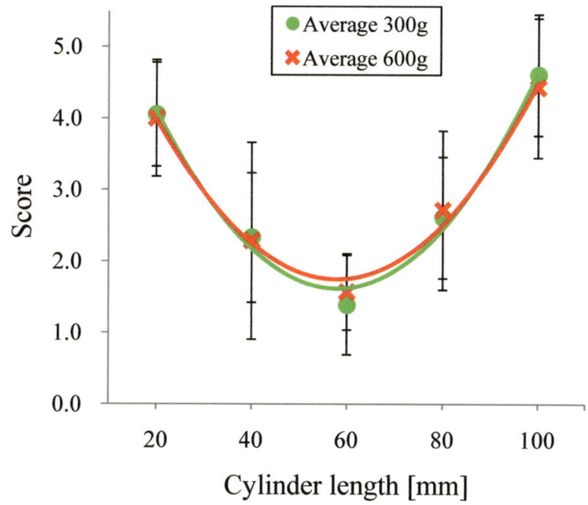

Fig. 7. Questionnaire results

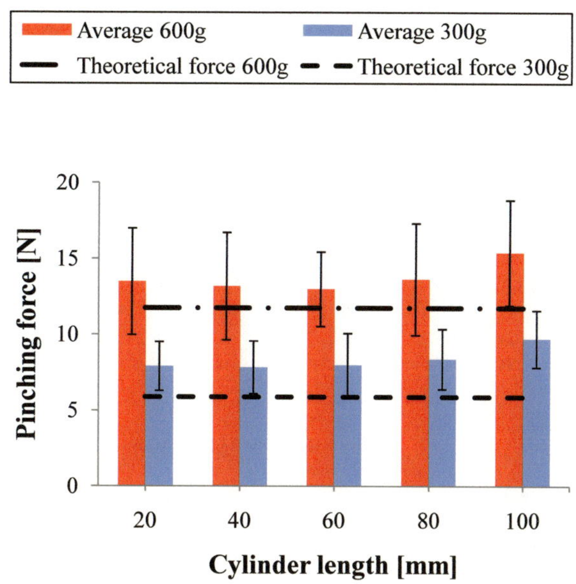

Fig. 8. Pinching force

2.3.3 Surface EMG measurement results

We evaluate the pinching effort from the EMG signal during the pinching activity. The EMG signal is normalized using the data process, shown in Sec. 2.1, because the amplitudes of the EMG signals are different between each subject.

Fig. 9 shows the normalized EMG related to the index finger and thumb when the cylinder weight is 300 [g], and Fig. 10 shows the normalized EMG when the cylinder weight is 600 [g]. The normalized EMG of the index finger FDS becomes lower according to the cylinder length, and the normalized EMG of the thumb ADPt becomes higher according to the cylinder length. The possible reason is that the finger posture when pinching a short cylinder makes it hard for

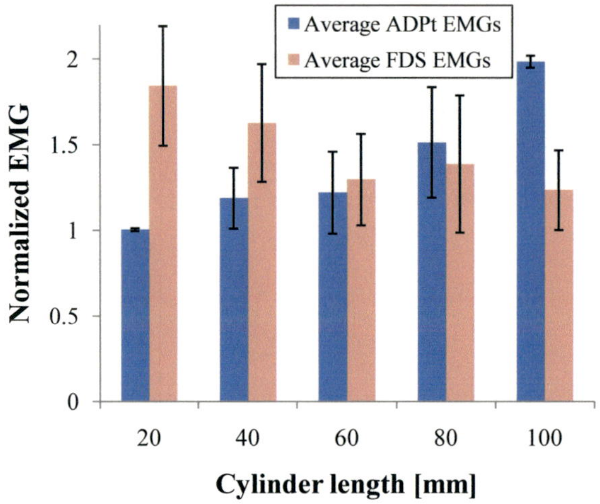

Fig. 9. Integrated EMG (300[g])

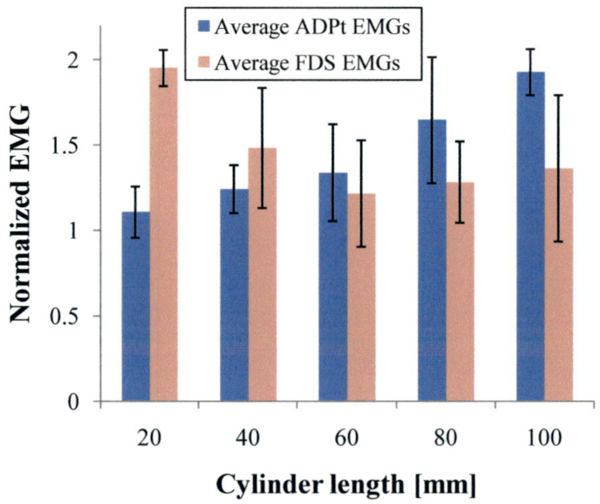

Fig. 10. Integrated EMG (600[g])

the index finger to exert a pinching force. On the other hand, when pinching a long cylinder, a large antagonist force is necessary to open the thumb widely, and thus the muscle activity of the thumb increases.

Fig. 11 shows the average EMG and the questionnaire score when the cylinder weight is 300 [g], and Fig. 12 shows the average EMG and the questionnaire score when the cylinder weight is 600 [g]. The lowest score is observed when the subject pinches the cylinder with the lowest EMG, and the highest score is observed when the subject pinches the cylinder with the highest EMG. The correlation coefficients between the average EMG and the questionnaire result are 0.86 at 300 [g] and 0.97 at 600 [g]. The p-values are 0.061 at 300 [g] and 0.005 at 600 [g]. Thus there are correlations between the surface EMG and the questionnaire result, but the p-value of 300 [g] result is high ($p > 0.05$). A possible reason is that the 300 [g] weight was too light to evaluate the pinching effort. These results signify that the integrated surface EMG is an important index to indicate pinching effort, pointing to the potential for

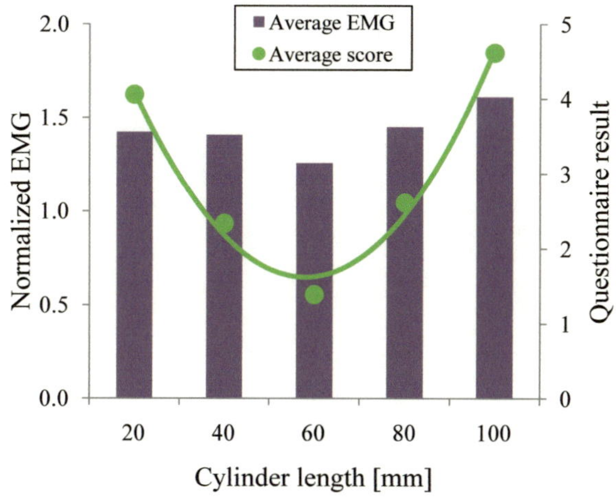

Fig. 11. Average EMG and questionnaire score (300[g])

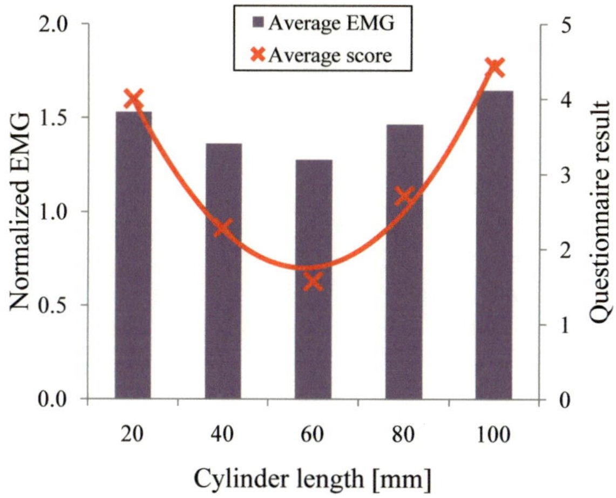

Fig. 12. Average EMG and questionnaire score (600[g])

quantitative evaluation using the muscle or tendon force. These results indicate a possibility that the quantitative evaluation using the muscle or tendon force.

3. Finger model

3.1 Tendon skeletal model

Fig. 13 shows the index finger and the thumb finger model. The index finger model consists of a fixed metacarpal and three phalanges. The DIP and PIP joints have 1 DOF (degree of freedom) for flexion/extension, and the MP joint has 2 DOF for flexion/extension and adduction/abduction. The thumb model contains a fixed trapezium bone and three phalanges. The IP joint has 1 DOF for flexion/extension, and the MP and CMC joints have 2 DOF for flexion/extension and adduction/abduction.

It is difficult to construct an anatomically accurate finger model because the human hand structure is very complex. Some research (Lee et al. (2008) and Deshpande et al. (2008))

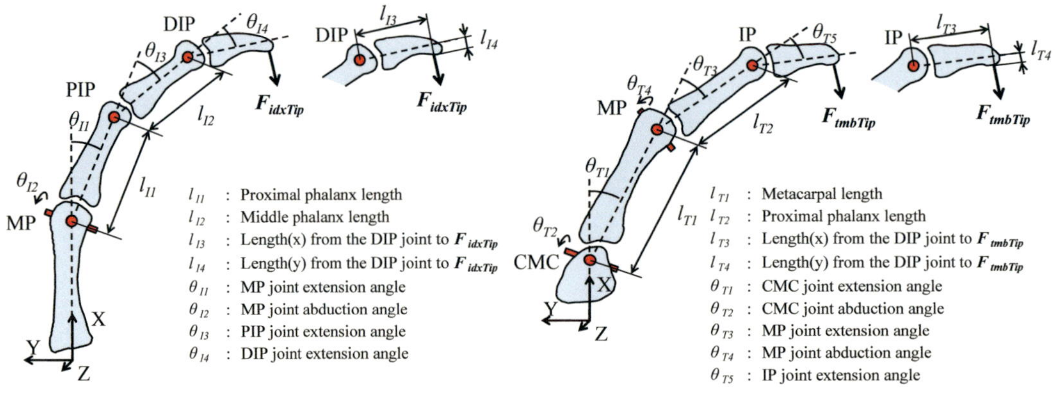

(a) Index finger model (b) Thumb model

Fig. 13. Index finger and thumb model

discussed the importance between the finger posture and the moment arm when exerting a fingertip force. Kamper et al. (2006) discussed importance of finger posture and moment arm when mapping from muscle activation to joint torque. The index finger joint torques $\boldsymbol{\tau}_{idx}$ and thumb joint torques $\boldsymbol{\tau}_{tmb}$ were calculated from the following equations:

$$\boldsymbol{\tau}_{idx} = \mathbf{M_{idx} F_{idxTendon}} \tag{3}$$

$$\boldsymbol{\tau}_{tmb} = \mathbf{M_{tmb} F_{tmbTendon}} \tag{4}$$

where $\boldsymbol{\tau}_{idx} = \left\{ \tau_{DIP}\ \tau_{PIP}\ \tau_{MCPa}\ \tau_{MCPf} \right\}^T$ is the vector of the index finger joint torques, $\mathbf{M_{idx}}$ is the matrix of the index finger moment arms at each joint, $\mathbf{F_{idxTendon}} = \{ f_{FDP}\ f_{FDS}\ f_{EIP}\ f_{EDC}\ f_{LUM}\ f_{DI}\ f_{PI} \}^T$ is the vector of the index finger tendon forces, $\boldsymbol{\tau}_{tmb} = \left\{ \tau_{IP}\ \tau_{MPa}\ \tau_{MPf}\ \tau_{CMCa}\ \tau_{CMCf} \right\}^T$ is the vector of the thumb joint torques, $\mathbf{M_{tmb}}$ is the vector of the thumb moment arms at each joint, and $\mathbf{F_{tmbTendon}} = \{ f_{FPL}\ f_{FPB}\ f_{EPL}\ f_{EPB}\ f_{APL}\ f_{APB}\ f_{ADPt}\ \ f_{ADPo}\ f_{OPP} \}^T$ is the vector of the thumb tendon forces.

3.2 Tendon moment arm

It is well known that the moment arm at each joint changes according to the joint angle. In this chapter, the moment arms $\mathbf{M_{idx}}$ and $\mathbf{M_{tmb}}$ are calculated by the quadratic approximation which is shown in Fig.14 and Fig.15. These profiles are given by the quadratic approximation based on the raw cadavers data that were measured by An et al. (1983) and Smutz et al. (1998). The tendon forces are calculated accurately using the variable moment arms.

3.3 Tendon force estimation

The joint torques $\boldsymbol{\tau}_{idx}$ and $\boldsymbol{\tau}_{tmb}$ can be calculated with Jacobian matrices:

$$\boldsymbol{\tau}_{idx} = \mathbf{J_{idx}^T F_{idxTip}} \tag{5}$$

$$\boldsymbol{\tau}_{tmb} = \mathbf{J_{tmb}^T F_{tmbTip}} \tag{6}$$

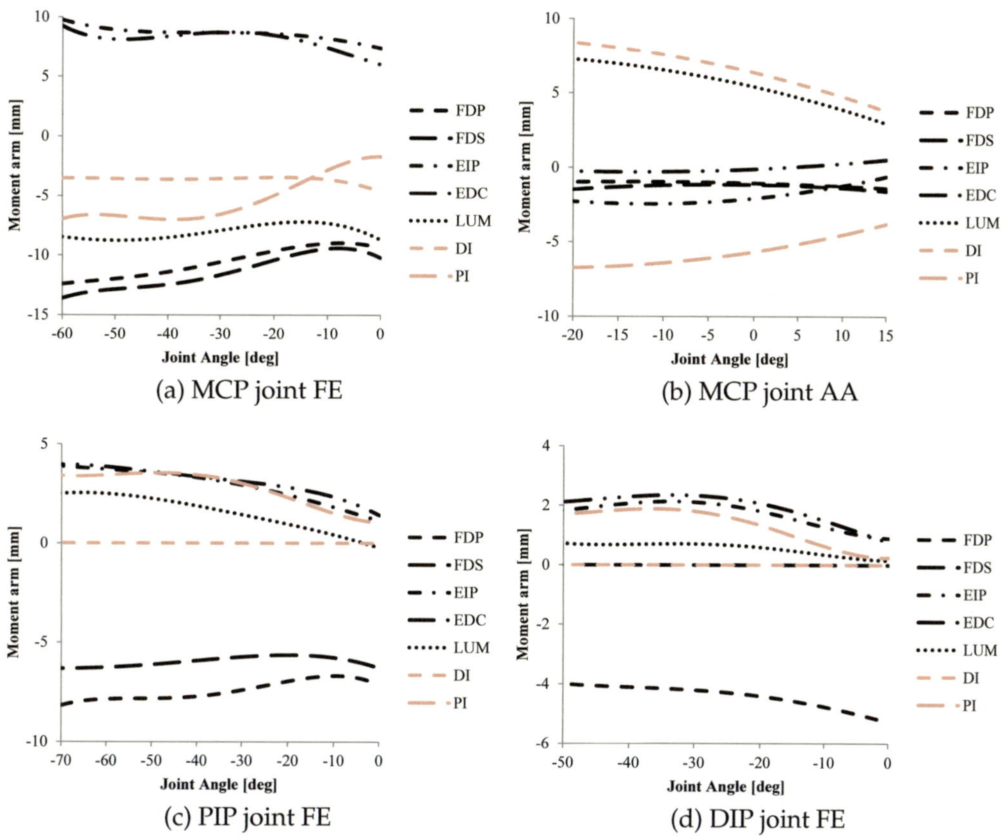

Fig. 14. Index finger moment arms

where $\mathbf{J_{idx}}$ is the index finger Jacobian matrix, $\mathbf{J_{tmb}}$ is the thumb Jacobian matrix, $\mathbf{F_{idxTip}} = \{ f_{Ix}\ f_{Iy}\ f_{Iz}\ \tau_{Ix}\ \tau_{Iy}\ \tau_{Iz} \}^T$ is the index fingertip force and torques, and $\mathbf{F_{tmbTip}} = \{ f_{Tx}\ f_{Ty}\ f_{Tz}\ \tau_{Tx}\ \tau_{Ty}\ \tau_{Tz} \}^T$ is the thumb fingertip force and torques. The following equations were obtained by substituting Eq. 3 to Eq. 6 (see definitions in Fig. 13):

$$\mathbf{F_{idxTip}} = \left(\mathbf{J_{idx}J_{idx}^T}\right)^{-1} \mathbf{J_{idx}M_{idx}F_{idxTendon}} \quad (7)$$

$$\mathbf{F_{tmbTip}} = \left(\mathbf{J_{tmb}J_{tmb}^T}\right)^{-1} \mathbf{J_{tmb}M_{tmb}F_{tmbTendon}}. \quad (8)$$

The tendon forces can be calculated from the fingertip forces based on Eq. 7 and Eq. 8. However, it is a redundant problem because 6 DOFs of the finger are driven by 7 tendons for the index finger, and 6 DOFs are driven by 9 tendons for the thumb. Therefore, the tendon

FDP	FDS	EIP	EDC	LUM	DI	PI	FPL	FPB	EPL	EPB	APL	APB	ADPt	ADPo	OPP
4.1	3.65	1.12	1.39	0.36	4.16	1.6	2.08	0.66	0.98	0.47	1.93	0.68	2.0	2.0	1.02

Table 3. PCSA (Physiological Cross Sectional Area) [cm^2] of each muscles (Valero-Cuevas et al. (1998) and Valero-Cuevas et al. (2003))

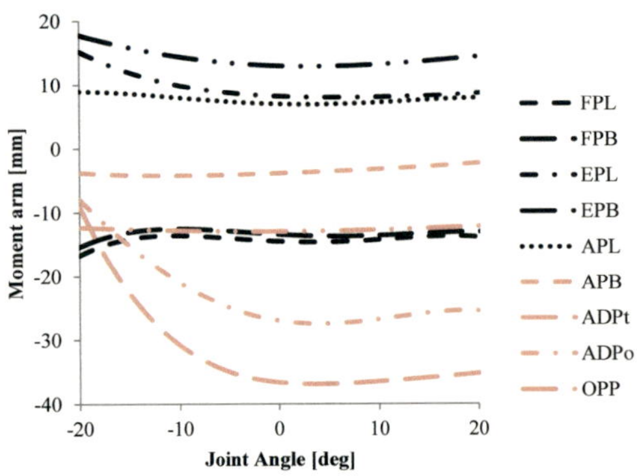

(a) CMC joint FE

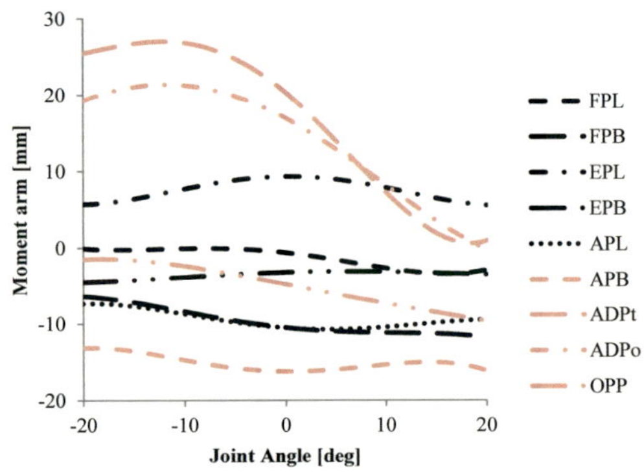

(b) CMC joint AA

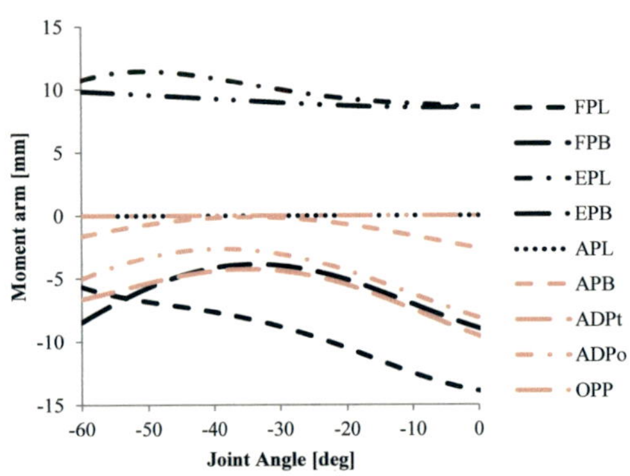

(c) MP joint FE

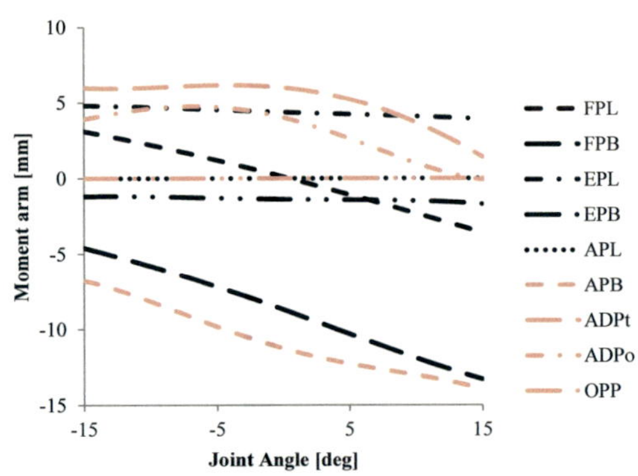

(d) MP joint AA

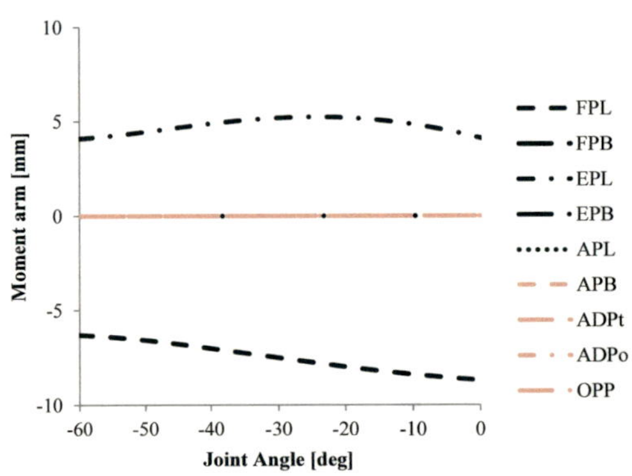

(e) IP joint FE

Fig. 15. Thumb moment arms

forces are derived by Crowninshield & Brand (1981) from the optimization calculation of the following equation:

$$u(F_{Tendon}) \triangleq \sum_{i=1}^{n} \left(\frac{f_i}{PCSA_i} \right)^2 \rightarrow \min \tag{9}$$

$$0 \leq f_i \leq f_{imax} \tag{10}$$

where $PCSA$ is a physiological cross sectional area of each muscle and f_{max} is a maximal force of each muscle that is determined by $PCSA$ and maximal muscle stress Zajac (1989). In this chapter, we used the $PCSA$ values of Cuevas *et al.* research Valero-Cuevas et al. (1998)Valero-Cuevas et al. (2003) (Table 3).

3.4 Score of the pinching effort

The pinching effort score is defined by following equation:

$$Score(F_{Tendon}) = \frac{1}{n} \sum_{i=1}^{n} \frac{f_i}{f_{imax}} \rightarrow \min \tag{11}$$

where n is the total number of tendons used for pinching an object. For example, when only the index finger used, n is 7, and when the index finger and the thumb used, n is 16. f_i is the tendon force of each tendon and f_{imax} is the maximum force that the muscle can exert to each tendon. The load ratio of each tendon f_i / f_{imax} denotes the force margin. Thus minimum score implies minimum load.

4. Cylinder pinching simulation

4.1 Condition of cylinder pinching simulation

Cylinder length 20, 40, 60, 80 or 100 [mm], diameter 20 [mm] and weight 600[g] are used in the simulation. The cylinder is pinched in the longitudinal direction by both the index finger and the thumb. Table 4 shows the finger model parameters and table 5 shows the limit angle of each joint. The finger link parameters are given based on the measurements of that of the subject. The contact points are the fingertip of each finger and the center of the cylinder. The friction coefficient is set as $\mu = 0.5$ and the fingertip force is set as 11.76 [N]. The vectors from the DIP/IP joint to the load point are $\mathbf{P_{idx}} = \{\, 10.0\ 5.0\ 0.0 \,\}^T$ and $\mathbf{P_{tmb}} = \{\, 17.0\ 5.0\ 0.0 \,\}^T$.

4.2 Simulation results of pinching cylinders

Fig. 16 shows the estimated tendon force for each of the index finger and the thumb when pinching the cylinders. The tendon forces of the thumb ADPt becomes higher according to the cylinder length. On the other hand, the tendon forces of the index finger FDS become lower according to the cylinder length. The pattern of these tendon forces is similar to the human muscle activity shown in Fig. 9 and Fig. 10. This suggests that the finger model can

l_{I1}	l_{I2}	l_{I3}	l_{I4}	l_{T1}	l_{T2}	l_{T3}	l_{T4}
39.0	25.0	10.0	5.0	45.0	32.0	17.0	5.0

Table 4. Finger link parameters [mm]

simulate the human muscle activity during the pinching activity. The score of each cylinder length was calculated from these tendon forces using Eq. 11.
Table 6 shows the simulated joint angles and measured joint angles of the human. In the simulation, the most efficient posture to exert fingertip force is when the AA directions of each joint are zero. The human finger postures are different from the simulation results (see θ_{I2} and θ_{T2} in table 6). This comes from the modeling and measurement errors. However, there are strong correlations between the simulated joint angles and the measured joint angles. Table 7 shows the correlation coefficients and p-value when pinching the 20 to 100 [mm] cylinder respectively. The average error of all the joint angles is 5.86 [deg] and the standard deviation of the error is 4.40 [deg]. These results show that the estimated finger posture is sufficient for pinching force estimation.

	flexion(adduction)	extension(abduction)
θ_{I1} [degree]	-60	0
θ_{I2} [degree]	-25	15
θ_{I3} [degree]	-75	0
θ_{I4} [degree]	-60	0

	flexion(adduction)	extension(abduction)
θ_{T1} [degree]	-20	25
θ_{T2} [degree]	-20	20
θ_{T3} [degree]	-60	10
θ_{T4} [degree]	-15	15
θ_{T5} [degree]	-60	20

Table 5. Limit angles of each joint

Cylinder length	θ_{I1}	θ_{I2}	θ_{I3}	θ_{I4}
20 [mm]	-60.0	0.0	-18.5	-11.9
40 [mm]	-51.2	0.0	-24.3	-17.0
60 [mm]	-37.8	0.0	-20.7	-21.5
80 [mm]	-19.5	0.0	-25.6	-26.5
100 [mm]	-2.3	0.0	-19.4	-29.7

Cylinder length	θ_{T1}	θ_{T2}	θ_{T3}	θ_{T4}	θ_{T5}
20 [mm]	-3.8	0.0	-3.0	0.0	-5.1
40 [mm]	4.0	0.0	-10.1	0.0	-7.2
60 [mm]	5.1	0.0	-0.1	0.0	-11.0
80 [mm]	9.3	0.0	-4.9	0.0	-11.2
100 [mm]	14.4	0.0	-3.1	0.0	10.8

Cylinder length	θ_{I1}	θ_{I2}	θ_{I3}	θ_{I4}
20 [mm]	-62.5	-6.8	-23.6	-5.6
40 [mm]	-51.6	-4.8	-27.0	-9.5
60 [mm]	-21.8	-0.6	-15.9	-17.6
80 [mm]	-8.1	-3.2	-18.3	-23.6
100 [mm]	14.2	-7.1	-17.3	-31.2

Cylinder length	θ_{T1}	θ_{T2}	θ_{T3}	θ_{T4}	θ_{T5}
20 [mm]	-4.5	8.5	-5.0	-	-
40 [mm]	0.4	14.8	-10.6	-	-
60 [mm]	12.3	-1.8	-10.6	-	-
80 [mm]	16.3	-7.3	-10.6	-	-
100 [mm]	15.5	-11.7	-11.0	-	-

Table 6. Simulated and measured joint angle ([deg])

	20 [mm]	40 [mm]	60 [mm]	80 [mm]	100 [mm]
Correlation coefficient	0.98	0.96	0.87	0.85	0.83
P-value	$\ll$0.001	<0.001	0.012	0.016	0.020

Table 7. The correlation coefficient of the joint angles

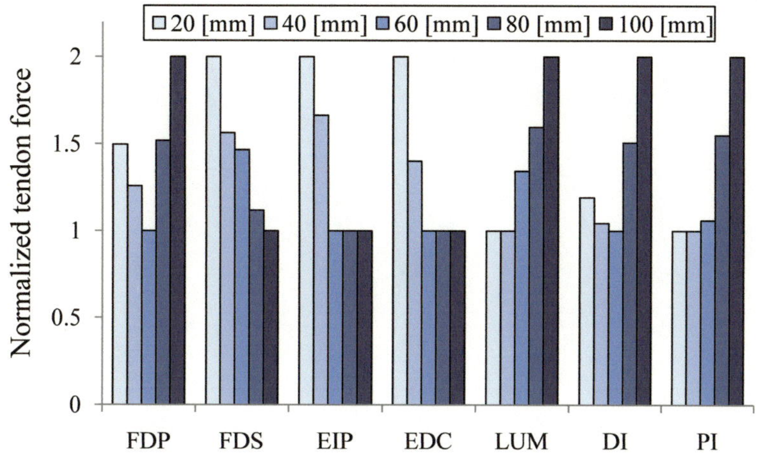

(a) Muscle of the index finger

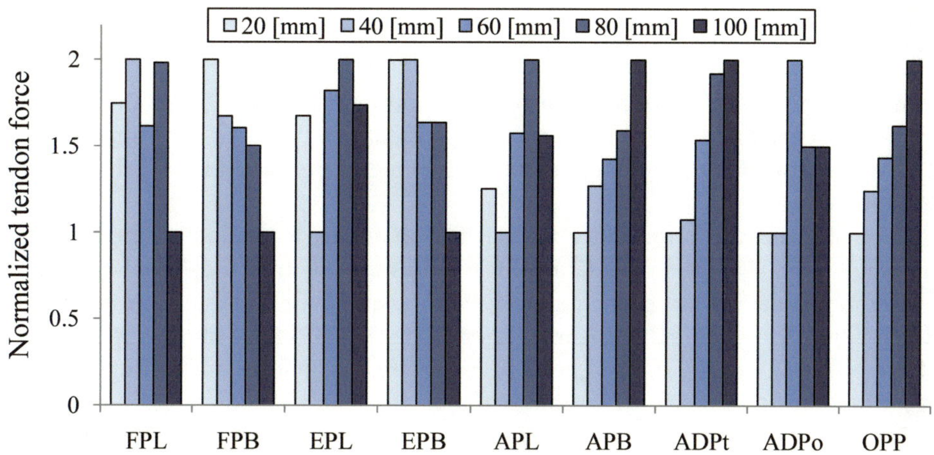

(b) Muscle of the thumb

Fig. 16. Simulation results

Fig. 17 shows the evaluated score by the simulation and human questionnaire results. The curves in the figure are the approximate quadratic curve of the results. The lowest score is observed in the 60 [mm] cylinder length. On the other hand, the highest score is observed in the 20 [mm] cylinder length. The simulated score pattern is similar to the human questionnaire score pattern. There is a strong correlation between the simulated score and the questionnaire score of human (the correlation coefficient is 0.97 and the p-value is 0.007). This indicates that the proposed method can reflect the human subjective pinching effort and our finger model is useful for the pinching effort evaluation.

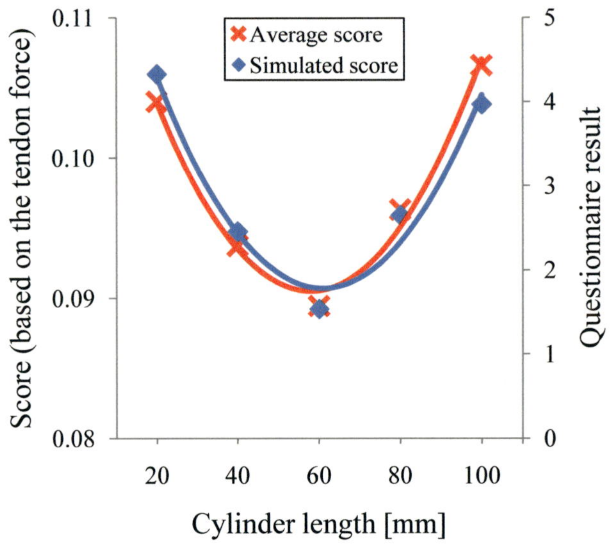

Fig. 17. Simulation scores

5. Conclusion

This research is aimed at the quantification of the product usability based on the estimated tendon force. At the first step of the quantitative evaluation, we tried to evaluate a pinching activity. We proposed the evaluation method of the pinching effort and show the effectiveness of the proposed method.

At first, we showed the importance of the tendon forces to evaluate pinching effort by human experiment. The experimental results of a human pinching a cylinder are shown: the subjective pinching effort, the pinching force, the human EMG, and the finger posture. These experimental results indicate that the integrated surface EMG is one of the important indexes to indicate pinching effort. This suggests a possibility for quantitative evaluation using the muscle or tendon force. Second, the index finger and thumb models that are used for the tendon force estimation are developed. The finger models mimic the human tendon skeletal structure. The simulation results of the pinching activity are compared with the sensory evaluation of subjects. The experimental results show that the simulation scores are similar to the questionnaire survey results and the estimated finger posture is also similar to the human finger posture. Our method can evaluate the pinching effort from the viewpoint of the muscle activity.

6. References

An, K. N., Chao, E. Y., Cooney, W. P. & Linscheid, R. L. (1979). Normative model of human hand for biomechanical analysis, *Journal of Biomechanics* 12(10): 775–88.

An, K. N., Ueba, Y., Chao, E. Y., Cooney, W. P. & Linscheid, R. L. (1983). Tendon excursion and moment arm of index finger muscles, *Journal of Biomechanics* 16(6): 419–25.

Brook, N., Mizrahi, J., Shoham, M. & Dayan, J. (1995). A biomechanical model of index finger dynamics, *Medical Engineering & Physics* 17(1): 54 – 63.

Crowninshield, R. D. & Brand, R. A. (1981). A physiologically based criterion of muscle force prediction in locomotion, *Journal of Biomechanics* 14(11): 793–801.

Deshpande, A. D., Balasubramanian, R., Lin, R., Dellon, B. T. & Matsuoka, Y. (2008). Understanding variable moment arms for the index finger mcp joints through the act hand, *The second IEEE/RAS-EMBS International Conference on Biomedical Robotics and Biomechatronics (BioRob2008)*, pp. 776–82.

Flanagan, J. R., Bowman, M. C. & Johansson, R. S. (2006). Control strategies in object manipulation tasks, *Current Opinion in Neurobiology* 16(6): 650–9.

Holzbaur, K. R. S., Murray, W. M. & Delp, S. L. (2005). A model of the upper extremity for simulating musculoskeletal surgery and analyzing neuromuscular control, *Annals of Biomedical Engineering* 33(6): 829–40.

Ikeda, A., Kurita, Y. & Ogasawara, T. (2008). Pinching motion evaluation using human like sensing device, *Proceedings of Joint 4th International Conference on Soft Computing and Intelligent Systems and 9th International Symposium on advanced Intelligent Systems (SCIS & ISIS 2008)*, pp. 1135–8.

Ikeda, A., Kurita, Y. & Ogasawara, T. (2009a). Evaluation of pinching effort by a tendon-driven robot hand, *Proceedings of 2009 IEEE International Conference on Robotics and Automation (IEEE ICRA 2009)*, pp. 3437–42.

Ikeda, A., Kurita, Y. & Ogasawara, T. (2009b). A tendon skeletal finger model for evaluation of pinching effort, *Proceedings of 2009 IEEE/RSJ International Conference on Intelligent Robots and Systems (IEEE IROS 2009)*, pp. 3691–6.

Kamper, D. G., Fischer, H. C. & Cruz, E. G. (2006). Impact of finger posture on mapping from muscle activation to joint torque, *Clinical Biomechanics* 21(4): 361–9.

Kong, Y. K. & Freivalds, A. (2003). Evaluation of meat-hook handle shapes, *International Journal of Industrial Ergonomics* 32(2): 13–23.

Lee, S. W., Chenb, H., Towlesa, J. D. & Kamper, D. G. (2008). Estimation of the effective static moment arms of the tendons in the index finger extensor mechanism, *Journal of Biomechanics* 41(7): 1567–73.

Nakamura, Y., Yamane, K., Fujita, Y. & Suzuki, I. (2005). Somatosensory computation for man-machine interface from motion capture data and musculoskeletal human model, *IEEE Transactions on Robotics* 21(1): 58–66.

Radhakrishnan, S. & Nagaravindra, M. (1993). Analysis of hand force in health and disease during maximum isometric grasping of cylinders, *Medical and Biological Engineering and Computing* 31(4): 372–6.

Smutz, W. P., Kongsayreepong, A., Hughes, R. E., Niebur, G., Cooney, W. P. & An, K. N. (1998). Mechanical advantage of the thumb muscles, *Journal of Biomechanics* 31(6): 565–70.

Sueda, S., Kaufman, A. & Pai, D. K. (2008). Musculotendon simulation for hand animation, *ACM Transactions on Graphics (Proceedings SIGGRAPH)* 27(3): 775–88.

Tada, M. & Pai, D. K. (2008). Finger shell: Predicting finger pad deformation under line loading, *Proceedings of the Symposium on Haptic Interfaces for Virtual Environment and Teleoperator Systems*, pp. 107–112.

Valero-Cuevas, F. J. (2005). An integrative approach to the biomechanical function and neuromuscular control of the fingers, *Journal of Biomechanics* 38(4): 673–84.

Valero-Cuevas, F. J., Johanson, M. E. & Towles, J. D. (2003). Towards a realistic biomechanical model of the thumb: the choice of kinematic description may be more critical than the solution method or the variability/uncertainty of musculoskeletal parameters, *Journal of Biomechanics* 36(7): 1019–30.

Valero-Cuevas, F. J., Zajac, F. E. & Burgar, C. G. (1998). Large index-fingertip forces are produced by subject-independent patterns of muscle excitation, *Journal of Biomechanics* 31(8): 693–703.

Zajac, F. E. (1989). Muscle and tendon: properties, models, scaling, and application to biomechanics and motor control, *Biomedical Engineering* 17(4): 359–411.

8

Electromyogram of the Cibarial Pump and the Feeding Process in Hematophagous Hemiptera

Ricardo N Araujo[1], Nelder F Gontijo[1], Alessandra A Guarneri[2], Alberto F Gontijo[3], Adriana C Soares[1] and Marcos H Pereira[1]
[1]*Departamento de Parasitologia, Instituto de Ciências Biológicas Universidade Federal de Minas Gerais*
[2]*Centro de Pesquisas René Rachou, Fiocruz*
[3]*Colégio Técnico da Universidade Federal de Minas Gerais; Belo Horizonte, Minas Gerais Brazil*

1. Introduction

The feeding process of hematophagous insects constitutes an important period in their life cycle. During this process, the insect is in close contact with its host, the blood required for reproduction and completion of insect development is obtained and pathogens can be transmitted. Several studies have focused on this period using different tools to monitor the details of feeding, with particular attention given to electromyograms of the cibarial pump. The cibarial pump is a structure associated with a complex of muscles located in the head of the insect. It controls the ingestion of blood from the host and transfers it to the gut. Monitoring of the frequency and shape of the electrical signals produced by this muscle complex enables the phases and parameters of the feeding process to be precisely determined and allows any disturbance or feature that may affect hematophagy to be evaluated. In this chapter we review technical and methodological issues that allow cibarial pump electromyograms to be used in studying the insect blood-feeding process and describe the results that may be obtained from such a system.

2. The feeding process in hematophagous hemiptera

Hemiptera is an order of insects comprising around 50,000–80,000 species with a variety of feeding habits. Hematophagy is seen in the hemipteran families Lygaeidae, Anthocoridae, Cimicidae, Polyctenidae and Reduviidae. The hematophagous species of the Reduviidae are included in the subfamily Triatominae. Triatomines and cimicids are the most studied hemipteran groups due to their medical importance. Species of both families live inside dwellings and feed on human blood (Schofield, 1995). The relatively large size of the hematophagous cimicids and triatomines facilitates their use in feeding behavior experiments. Moreover, colonies of the main species can be easily reared under laboratory conditions using several vertebrates as hosts.

Triatomines and cimicids are vessel-feeders or "solenophages", i.e., they obtain blood directly from the blood vessels (venules or arterioles) of vertebrate hosts (Lavoipierre et al., 1959). Their feeding process involves several steps, including puncturing of the host skin, a probing phase which consists of identification and canulation of a blood vessel, an engorgement phase, during which blood is removed from the host and transferred to the gut of the insect and finally cessation of feeding, when ingestion of blood stops and the mouthparts are removed from the host's skin. These processes differ slightly between triatomines and cimicids, due mainly to variations in gut physiology, mouthpart morphology and the amount and variety of biological molecules produced by the salivary glands and intestine. The main processes involved in the feeding of each group of insect are explained below.

a. Triatomines

The mouthparts of triatomines are composed of a three-segmented labium (or proboscis), a pair of mandibles and a pair of maxillae. Each maxilla articulates with the other and forms two canals: the alimentary canal through which blood passes and the salivary canal that conducts saliva to the feeding site (Figure 1). To initiate feeding, triatomines choose a suitable spot on the host skin where they anchor the feeding apparatus to the surface. They then use their mandibles (serrated structures contained in the mouthparts) to puncture the skin (Figure 2a). The long, flexible maxillae are introduced into the skin and initiate the probing phase, which is characterized by whip-like movements of these structures in the skin as the insect seeks a vessel to cannulate (Figure 2b) (Lavoipierre et al., 1959). At the same time, the cibarial pump produces periodic, isolated contractions that remove fluid samples for analysis by epipharingeal chemoreceptors (Smith & Friend, 1970). The probing phase lasts until the maxillae are able to cannulate the vessel (Figure 2c).

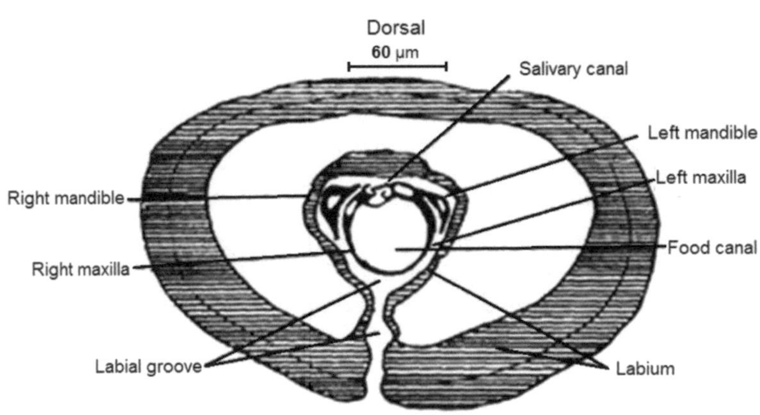

Fig. 1. Transverse section near the base of the proboscis of a fifth instar nymph of *Rhodnius prolixus* (redrawn from Lavoipierre et al., 1959).

The engorgement phase starts after the maxillae enter a blood vessel. This phase corresponds to the period when the insect extracts blood from the vessel through the mouthparts and transfers it to the gut. During this process, blood passes along the alimentary canal, through the foregut or esophagus to reach the anterior midgut, where it is stored. Pumping of blood involves a chambered structure associated with a complex of muscles located in the head of the insect, known as the cibarial pump. When the cibarial pump-associated muscles are contracted, a negative pressure is created in the chamber which draws blood up from inside the vessel. When the muscles relax, the chamber closes and pushes blood into the gut (Bennett-Clark, 1963). The contractions of the cibarial pump are sequential, repetitive and usually occur at regular intervals. This is the longest phase of the feeding process and can last from a few minutes to more than an hour, depending on the insect species, development stage and other characteristics of the insect and the host that may favor or delay the ingestion of blood.

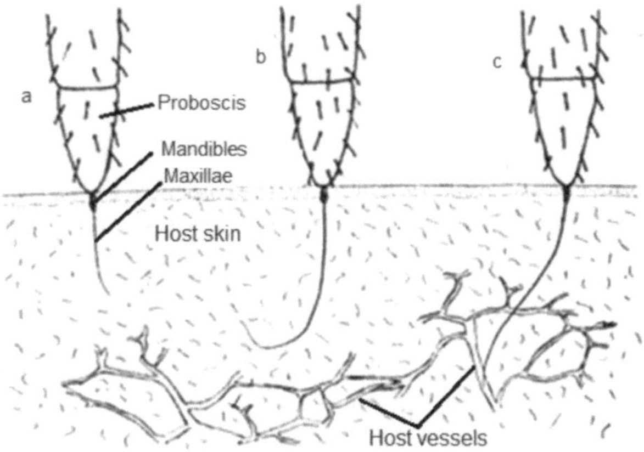

Fig. 2. Steps in the triatomine feeding process. a) puncture of the skin by the mandibles and introduction of the maxillae; b) whip-like movements of the maxillae in search of a blood vessel; c) cannulation of the blood vessel by the maxillae (redrawn from Lavoipierre et al., 1959).

b. Cimicids

The feeding process of cimicids is very similar to that of triatomines. Bedbugs (as these insects are popularly known) also have a feeding apparatus adapted to feed on fluids, with mouthparts consisting of several structures. A pair each of mandibles and maxillae (together forming a fascicle) align to form the alimentary and salivary canals (Figure 3). Although cimicids such as *Cimex* also take blood directly from the vessels of the host, their mandibles function in a different way from those of triatomines, penetrating deeply inside the dermis (Figure 4b) and supporting the maxillae which in cimicids they are the only structures that penetrate the blood vessel (Figure 4c) (Dickerson & Lavoipierre, 1959).

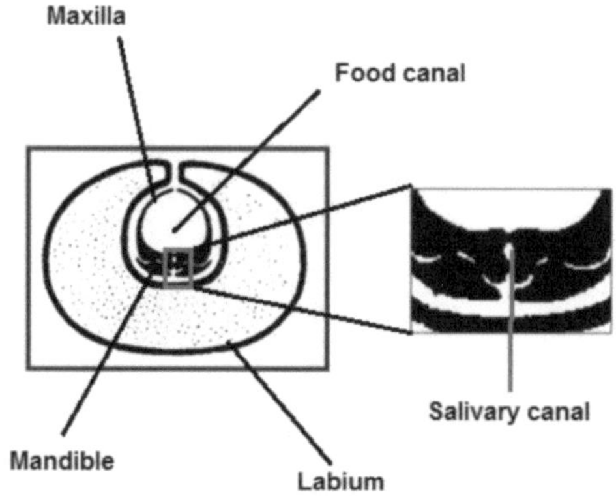

Fig. 3. Transverse section of the feeding apparatus of *Cimex lectularius* (redrawn from Schofield & Dolling, 1996).

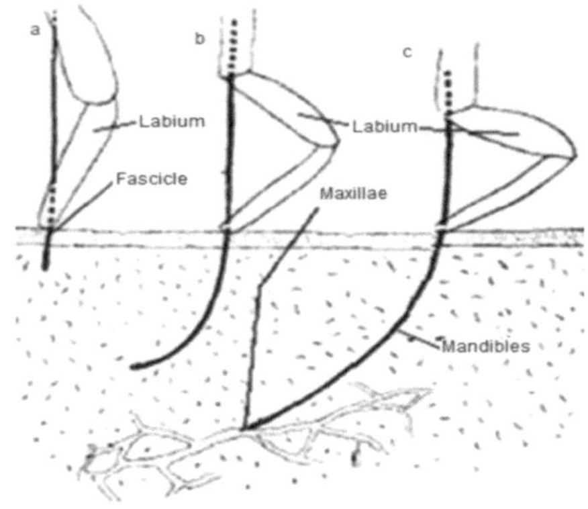

Fig. 4. Feeding behavior of the fascicle of *Cimex lectularius* in the host skin (redrawn from Dickerson & Lavoipierre, 1959). a) puncture of the skin by the mandibles; b) introduction of the fascicle into the dermis; c) mandibles give support to the maxillae that penetrate the blood vessel.

The feeding process of *Cimex lectularius* begins with the penetration of the fascicle into the host skin. The fascicle, which is highly flexible, carries out probing movements in all directions. These movements cease when a suitable vessel is found and cannulated (Figure 4). During these active movements of the fascicle, small hemorrhagic spots are formed (Dickerson & Lavoipierre, 1959). Based on histological observations, these hemorrhages led Gordon & Crewe (1948) to conclude that *Cimex* were telmatophagic or "pool feeders". However, Dickerson & Lavoipierre (1959) made direct observations with intravital microscopy and concluded that *Cimex* in fact feeds directly within the host blood vessel and is therefore solenophagic.
The engorgement phase in cimicids begins after probing movements have been completed. This phase is characterized by the rhythmic functioning of the cibarial pump, which promotes a negative pressure inside the blood vessel, propelling blood into the gut. The pump (Figure 5) is formed by a chamber with dorsal and lateral associated-muscles and is linked to the short esophagus (Snodgrass, 1944).

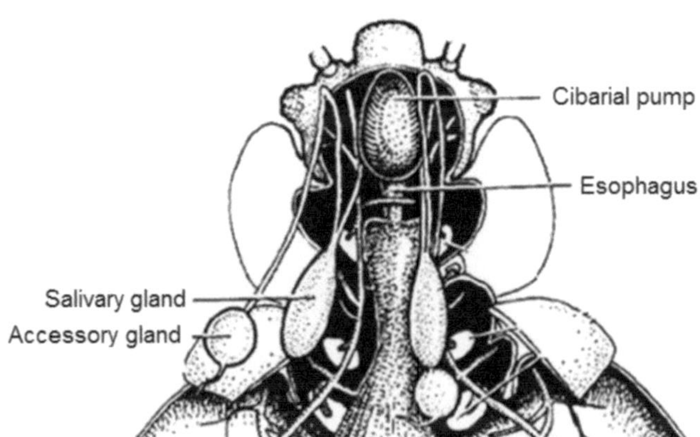

Fig. 5. Internal anatomy of the anterior part of *Cimex lectularius* (redrawn from Usinger, 1966)

3. Functional anatomy of the cibarial pump

The ingestion of blood by triatomines is promoted by the cibarial pump, which along with its associated musculature nearly fills the insect head capsule. The pump of a fifth instar nymph of *Rhodnius prolixus* consists of a rigid, ventrally positioned, U-shaped chamber, about 3.5 mm long by 0.28 mm wide and attached to an elastic ligament on either side which is more elastic and acts as a piston (Figure 6). The apical diameter of the chamber is about 10 µm. The pump is attached to the floor of the head by interstitial tissue. The piston is connected to the upper part of the head by two V-shaped muscle bundles. The first bundle is longer and is localized in the anterior part of the pump while the second is approximately seven times smaller and located distally (Figure 7) (Bennet-Clark, 1963). The pump is filled through contraction of these muscles and emptied by the retraction of the piston by means of the contraction of a ligament (Snodgrass, 1935; Smith, 1985), aid by the pre-cibarial valve and its associated muscles (Backus & McLean, 1982; McLean & Kinsey, 1984).

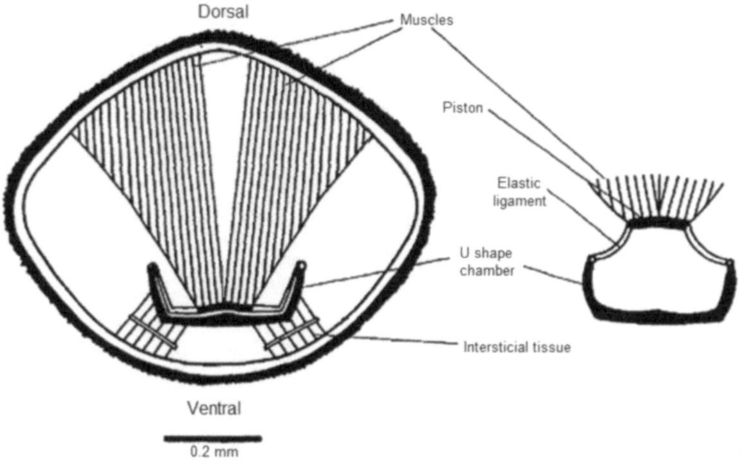

Fig. 6. Transverse cross-section of the head of a fifth instar nymph of *Rhodnius prolixus* showing the U-shape of the cibarial pump and the associated muscles contracted and relaxed (redrawn from Bennet-Clark, 1963).

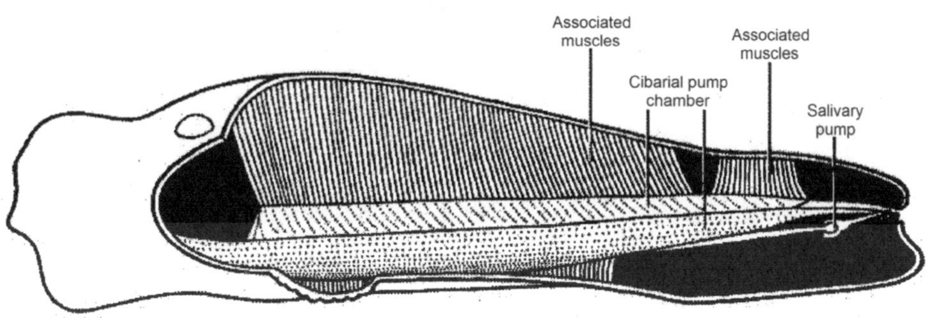

Fig. 7. Longitudinal cross-section of the head of a fifth instar nymph of *Rhodnius prolixus* head showing the cibarial pump and associated muscles (redrawn from Perez, 1969).

The cibarial pump supplies the force to move blood from the vessel to the insect midgut. A fifth instar nymph of *R. prolixus* consumes approximately 300 μL of blood in 5 minutes, which suggests (based on conservative calculations), that the cibarial pump produces a negative pressure of over 1-2 atmospheres during feeding (Bennet-Clark, 1963). During the engorgement phase, muscles associated with the cibarial pump contract sequentially and repetitively to allow ingestion of blood by the bug. Throughout the feeding period, the frequency of contractions can vary from 6 Hz (in periods when blood is easily ingested) to less that 1 Hz (when the insect is having problems in obtaining blood from the vessel).

4. History of the use of electrical recording in the study of triatomine blood-feeding behavior

The standard technique for studying feeding behavior in triatomines was developed in the 1970's by Smith & Friend, based on the models already used for studies of aphids (McLean & Kinsey, 1964; Tjallingii, 1985). Smith & Friend (1970) observed the action of the cibarial pump using an electrical resistance technique, carrying out modifications in order to capture clear signals. One of these was to avoid the use of a voltage source in series with the animal; a signal of sufficient strength could be obtained by simply connecting two platinum electrodes (one each on the thorax and bloodmeal), to the input of a Grass Pi5 high input-impedance preamplifier (Smith, 1979). A further modification was to record from the brass mesh on which the animal rested during feeding, rather than from an electrode in the thorax. This modification enabled signals to be acquired from the cibarial pump of early instar nymphs, which are too small to allow an electrode to be affixed to the thorax. Although this produced a much noisier signal due to the additional resistive pathway through the animal and movements of the tarsi, filtering the output of the preamplifier with a step band-pass filter (General Radio Type 1952 Universal Filter), usually allowed the pump strokes (though not the shape of the resistance changes) to be distinguished from the noise. A bandwidth of about 30-200 Hz was usually employed. Most records were obtained in this manner, since it involved no manipulation of the animals and these would therefore feed more readily. A storage oscilloscope and/or a Brush Mark 280 pen recorder were used to observe the shape and duration of changes in signal associated with pumping. The signal triggered the sweep of a second oscilloscope to record the number of strokes of the cibarial pump, as well as the pumping frequency. A signal derived from the sweep circuit was then used as the input to a rate meter and a pulse counter. The output of the rate meter was recorded on a chart recorder. The origin of the voltage changes recorded is unknown. They may represent impedance changes, in association with a voltage source such as a junction potential between electrodes and the hemocoele or diet, or else they reflect the current produced by activity of the pump muscle, in a manner analogous to that of an electrocardiogram.

In the following discussion, we describe a new system derived from that created by Smith & Friend that can be used to record and analyze the electrical signals produced by the cibarial pump during the insect feeding process. We also show how the use of this technology, together with live microscopy (intravital microscopy) of the cibarial pump, led to the conclusion that the electrical signals produced are related to the activity of muscles associated with the pump.

5. Acquisition system and treatment of the electrical signals produced during the feeding process

The acquisition system is based on the connection of one electrode to the insect, another to the host, and both to a detection system (Figure 8). The electrodes consist of fine wires, usually gold with a diameter of 90 μm and are connected to the back of the insect (Figure 9) and to the host skin with a small piece of tape. Contact between the electrode and insect/host is increased by using a conductive electrolytic gel (Regisgraf-Gel®).

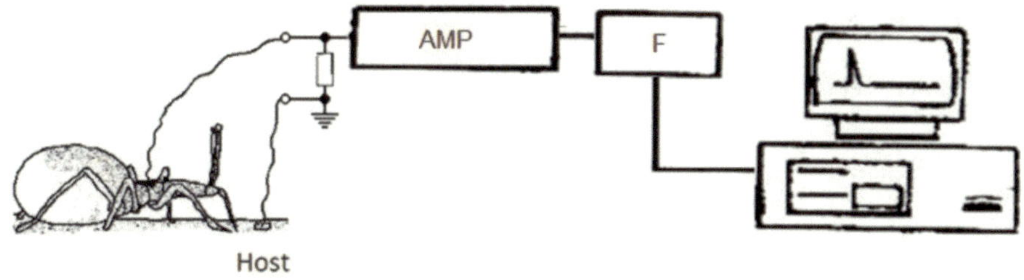

Fig. 8. Basic system and connections to detect the electrical signals produced by the cibarial pump of insects. AMP - amplifier; F- filter.

Provided insects remain immobile during the feeding process, the only relevant muscles that contract are those associated with the cibarial pump, allowing their electrical signals to be detected. However, insects have an exoskeleton made of chitin which has a very high electrical resistance. Thus an amplifier of high input impedance and high gain is required to pick up electrical signals, which have a peak-to-peak order of magnitude of 1 mVpp, from the suction process (Prutchi & Norris, 2005). These two properties favor the uptake of 60 Hz noise from the power grid, as well as of radiofrequency signals in general. Shield cables and amplifier configurations with a high common-mode rejection rate should therefore be used. Another problem that must be overcome in the amplifier is the DC voltage signals generated by the electrolytic potential of fine wire in contact with the conductive gel. This voltage can vary with the type of metal used to make the electrode, the type of the gel used, and also the local temperature. DC voltage changes of electrodes are slow (in the order of seconds) and must be automatically compensated by the amplifier.

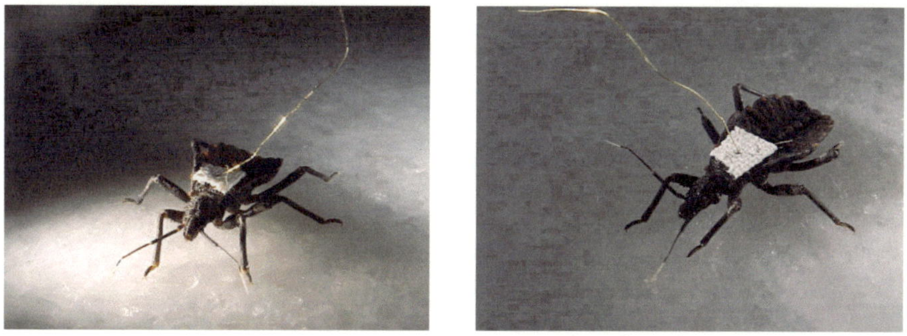

Fig. 9. Gold wire electrodes fixed on the back of an insect used to pick up electrical signals during the feeding process.

For assays with artificial feeders, the electrode is immersed directly in the diet. When insects are placed on a metal mesh rather than fixing electrodes to the thorax, the metal mesh should also be moistened with the electrolytic gel.
Operational amplifiers with J-FET (TL071) are used in the input of the acquisition system. These have high impedance (~$10^{12}\Omega$) and form a traditional instrumentation amplifier configuration (Figure 10). A 47MΩ resistor defines the impedance in the entrance of the amplifier, and avoids overcharging the signal from the surface of the insect. Although we would have preferred to use differential entrances directly on the body of the insect to increase the common mode rejection rate, this type of configuration was not viable due to difficulties in fixing the electrode to the ventral surface of the insect and the interference that this would cause to the feeding process.
A RC low-pass first-order filter with cut-off frequency of approximately 16 kHz was set into the amplifier input to prevent entry of radiofrequencies eventually picked up by the wires. Any DC voltage in the non-inverting input tends to appear amplified in the output of the block, being due to feedback to the inverting input by a passive RC filter with a high time constant. After some seconds, the DC signal is minimized in the output, since it will appear simultaneously in both inverting and non-inverting input.
After the amplifier block, there are three filtering circuits: a notch section centered on 60 Hz and two sections of a second order Butterworth filter (Figure 10). The final blocks are the digitalization of the signals and their visualization using a control software. The digitalizing interface has a 12-bit digital-analog converter, with adjustable sampling rate. The control software establishes the input sensibility and the sampling frequency. The output signal is shown in Figure 11.
The components were assembled in a fiberglass printed circuit board and packed in a metallic box with good electromagnetic shielding. The circuit was fed by 9V batteries to avoid the entrance of 60 Hz noise from any rectified power supply. The input and output of the apparatus used shielded wires with grounded outer sheaths. Ω

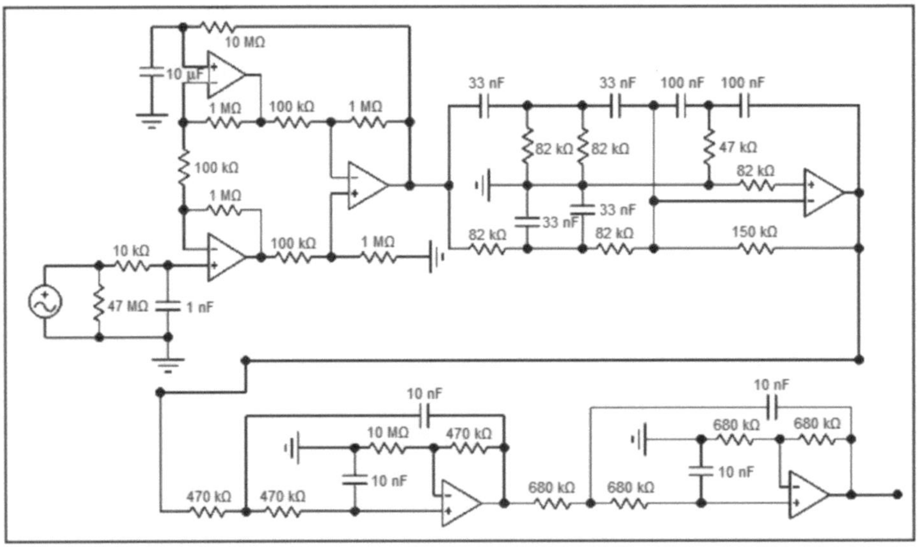

Fig. 10. Sketch of the amplifier and low-pass filter.

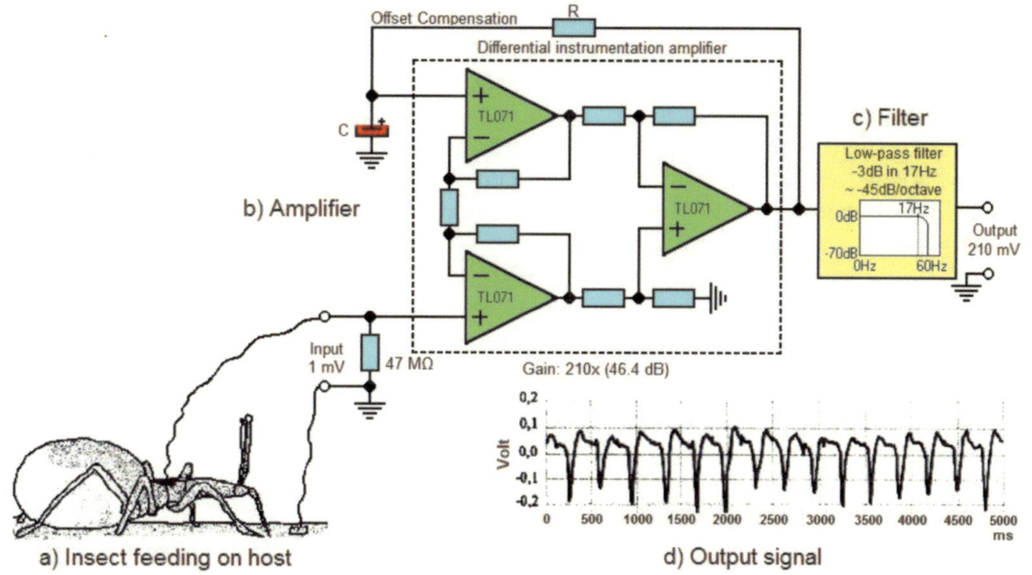

Fig. 11. General sketch of the electronically monitoring of the cibarial pump. (a) the signals produced are collected by gold wires fixed onto the dorsal surface of the insect and on the host skin; (b) the signals are amplified 210 times, (c) signals are filtered by a low-pass filters and digitalized by a AC-100 plate connected to a computer, (d) signal's mV variation are shown on the computer screen. TL071 - Operational amplifiers with J-FET; R - resistor; C-capacitor.

The control software operates in two modes - i.e., data acquisition mode and analysis & visualization. In the data acquisition mode some parameters are adjusted before the acquisition of the signal such as the sensibility, sampling rate and the scale of the on-screen abscissa. The conversion and time recording start on zero and the converted data are recorded on a matrix with 360,000 positions and shown on the screen. Acquisition time varies from 30 minutes (at the highest sampling rate - 200 samples/second) to 5 hours (at the lowest acquisition rate - 20 samples/second).

When data acquisition ends, the user should change to the analysis and visualization mode, where the recorded data can be visualized as desired. The data can be saved in the hardware or a disc, generating a *name.dat* file, which can be launched or transferred to external software for analysis.

Analysis of the signals collected can be manually or automatically analyzed, each of them important in verifying different parameters of the feeding process. For manual analysis the user should load the *.dat* file and visualize the format of the signals throughout the experiment. Automatic analysis can be performed in the software MATLAB® (MathWorks Inc.) or the very similar Octave (http://www.octave.org), using the functions "fft" and "specgram" (MathWorks, 1995). The function "fft(a,n)" calculates the discrete Fourier transformation of vector "a", computed with the algorithm of the rapid Fourier transform. The Fourier transformation can be used to find the harmonic components of the frequencies from a signal of physiological origin in relation to time. The "n" parameter specifies the number of points or samples used in the FFT.

The function "specgram" calculates the discrete Fourier transformation from a signal stored in the vector "a" using the sliding window technique (Figure 12). The spectrogram represents the magnitude of this function. In cases where the insects alter the contracting profile during feeding, computing a more localized FFT by considering only the subset of points from a small window that slides along vector "a" allows visualization of the feeding behavior versus time in relation to the harmonic content of the signals collected. The line below shows a command to the function "specgram" containing a higher number of configuration parameters:

B = specgram (a, nfft, Fs, window, noverlap, 'dflag');

The number of points (nfft) that comprise the window can be adjusted by the user as well as the superposition between windows.

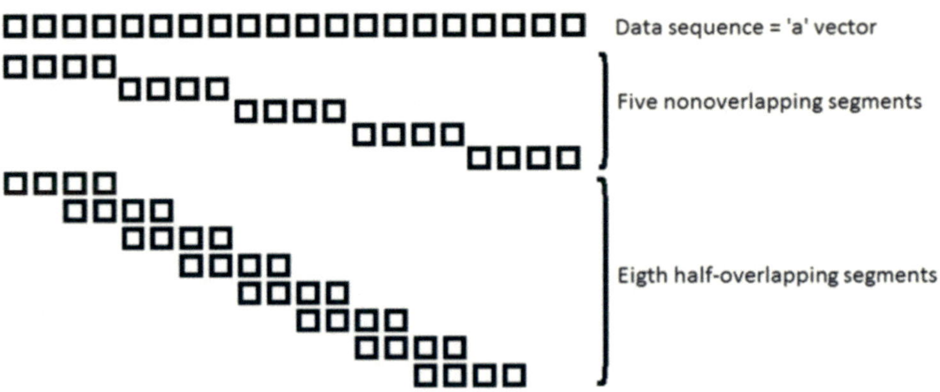

Fig. 12. Sliding window technique used in the "specgram" function.

Since each value of the vector "a" only supplies information on the signal amplitude throughout successive sampling, the temporal dimension of the experiment is lost. The parameter Fs informs the function of the sampling frequency used to obtain the data. The value T=1/Fs provides the time interval between samples. These adjustments set the vertical axis of the spectrogram to the correct Hz scale and the horizontal axis to time in seconds.

The output graphic shows the intensity of the components of the frequencies based on color tones (Figure 13). The weakest and strongest intensity signals are represented by blue and red tones, respectively.

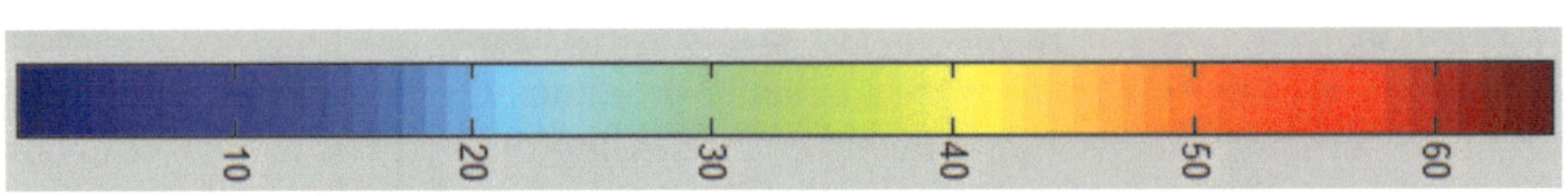

Fig. 13. Colors in the graph generated by function "specgram" indicate the intensity of the signals.

Rapid Fourier transformation can only be done in periodic signals and the points from the block of data may not satisfy this requirement. A conformant function then forces the signal into periodic by multiplying the samples by a window whose main characteristic is that it begins and ends with values close to zero. This technique inserts distortions in the real signal spectrum, hence the importance of the type of window function to be multiplied.

The parameter 'window' specifies the type and size (number of points) of the multiplier function. There are several window functions, including boxcar, bartlett, hamming, hanning, kaiser, etc. The length of the window function should be lower than or equal to nfft. Figure 14 shows three examples of windows, each with 65 points.

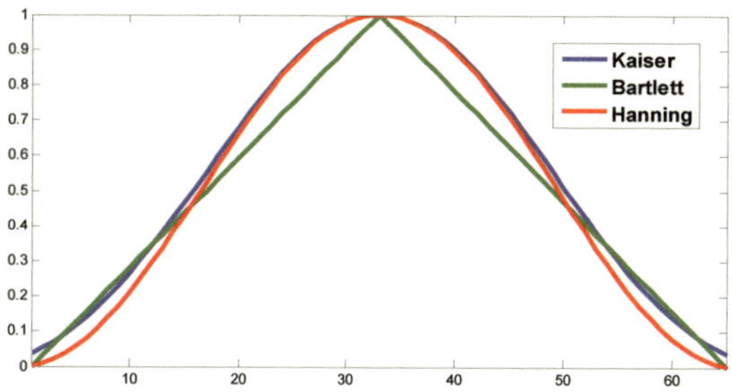

Fig. 14. Examples of windows used to convert signals to periodic.

Figures 15 to 20 show the steps followed by the functions "fft" and "specgram" to process the signals collected during blood-feeding. Figure 15 presents a small extension of the signals of the electromyogram with 1,024 points from the middle of an experiment. Figure 16 shows the extension of the signals after the elimination of the average value ("detrend" function).

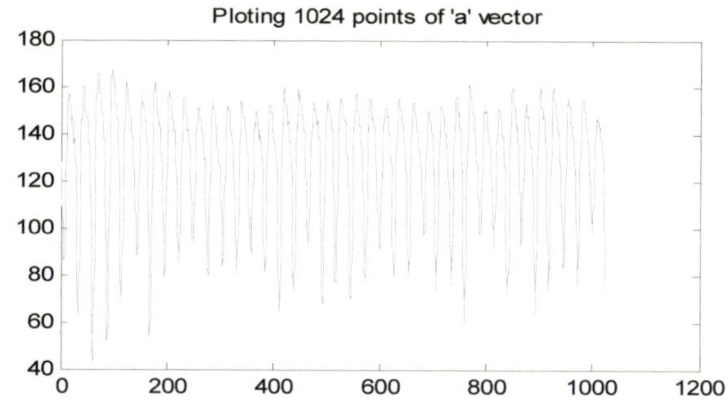

Fig. 15. 1024 points from vector "a".

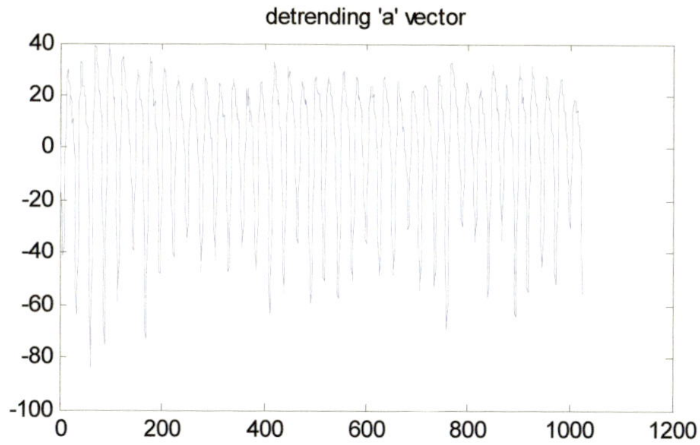

Fig. 16. Elimination of the average value from "a".

Figure 17 shows the shape of the Hanning window that will be multiplied by the pre-processed signal shown in Figure 16. Figure 18 shows the profile of the windowed signal after multiplication by the Hanning window.

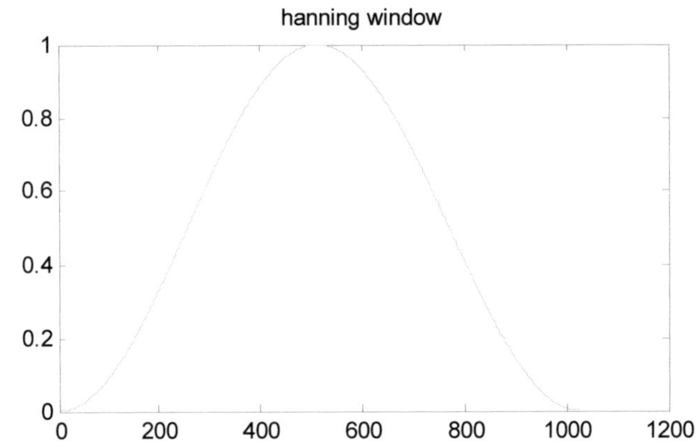

Fig. 17. Format of the Hanning window.

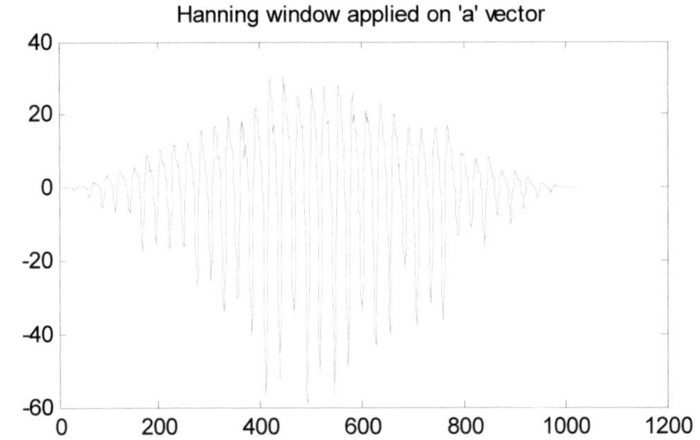

Fig. 18. Hanning window applied to the block of data.

Figure 19 shows the spectrum generated by the FFT with peaks of energy localized in well-defined frequencies. The peak marked with a red dot (7.5659 Hz) is the fundamental frequency of the signal collected. The second and third peaks represent the harmonic frequencies of the fundamental frequency.
Finally, Figure 20 shows the spectrogram of the entire experiment, which has a duration of approximately 15 minutes. There is no signal at the first seconds because the triatomine has yet to make contact with the host. Probing begins, followed by the engorgement phase which is characterized by a strong and stable signal with well-defined frequencies. The energy of the signal collected is strongly concentrated within two or three harmonic frequencies. Small frequency variation can be perceived over time. At the end of the experiment, the signal resumes presenting disturbances and noises that remove part of the energy from the harmonic frequencies, visible as a blurred spectrum.

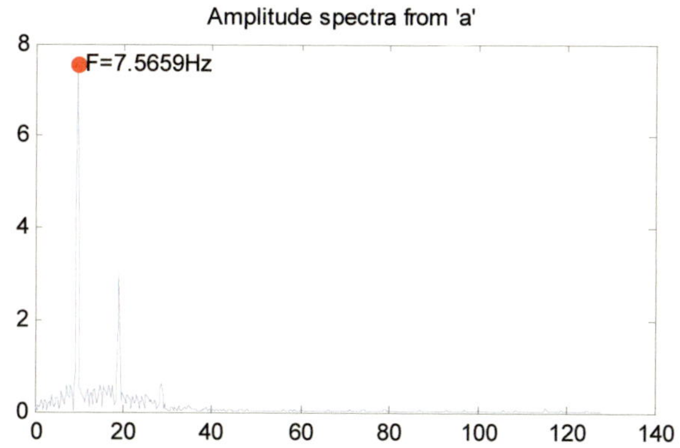

Fig. 19. Identification of the fundamental frequency of the signal analyzed.

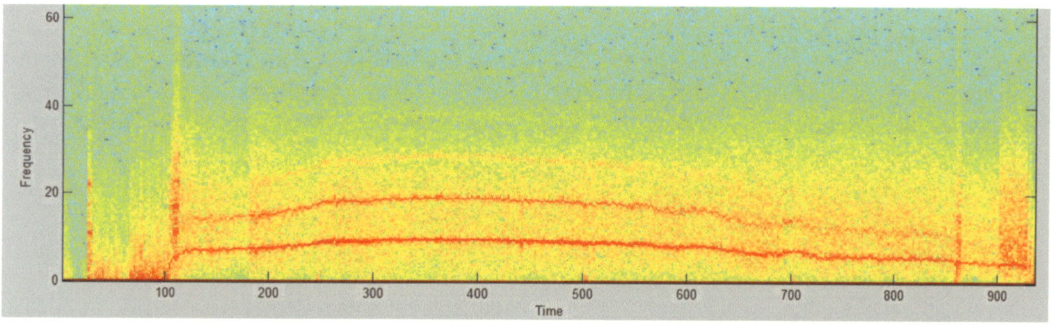

Fig. 20. Spectrogram of the entire experiment, which has a duration of approximately 15 minutes.

The more vertical and rapid the rise and fall of the analyzed signal, the more harmonic frequencies will be found along the vertical axis of the spectrogram. This means that the cibarial pump-associated muscles are receiving more electrical excitations and are working at higher intensity.

Figure 21 shows another experiment where the signal presents higher harmonic frequencies with greater amounts of energy.

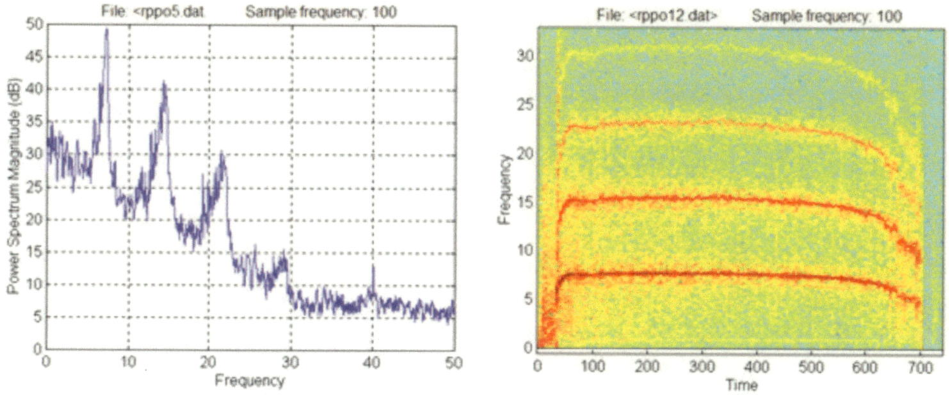

Fig. 21. Spectral content and spectrogram of a signal richer in harmonic frequencies.

6. Intravital microscopy of the cibarial pump and simultaneous recording of electrical signals

It is of paramount importance to confirm that the electrical signals shown above are indeed related to contraction of the cibarial pump muscles. This was done by means of experiments that record the electromyogram of the cibarial pump simultaneously with intravital microscopy of the cibarial pump. Images of the head of the bug during the feeding process were recorded using a digital camera connected to a stereomicroscope (Wild Heerbrug M5-89797). White light was directed onto the insect head to increase its transparency, facilitating observations of the cibarial pump in action. The images produced were analyzed using ImageJ software (Abramoff et al., 2004; Rasband, 2007). They were converted to 8 bits and the software used to calculate the dark area for each frame of the recorded videos (~25 frames/s). The values were transferred to Microsoft Excel and SigmaPlot 2002 for Windows Version 8.0 for analysis and graphic construction (Alves et al., 2011). Contrasting areas in the images (2D images) were measured during the feeding process for the area surrounding the cibarial pump in the head of the bug as an indicator of filling of the pump with blood, related to muscular contractions (Figure 22). Using this technique the chamber of an empty cibarial pump can easily be differentiated from the other structures of the insect head, whereas a blood-filled pump shows the same intensity as other structures of the head.

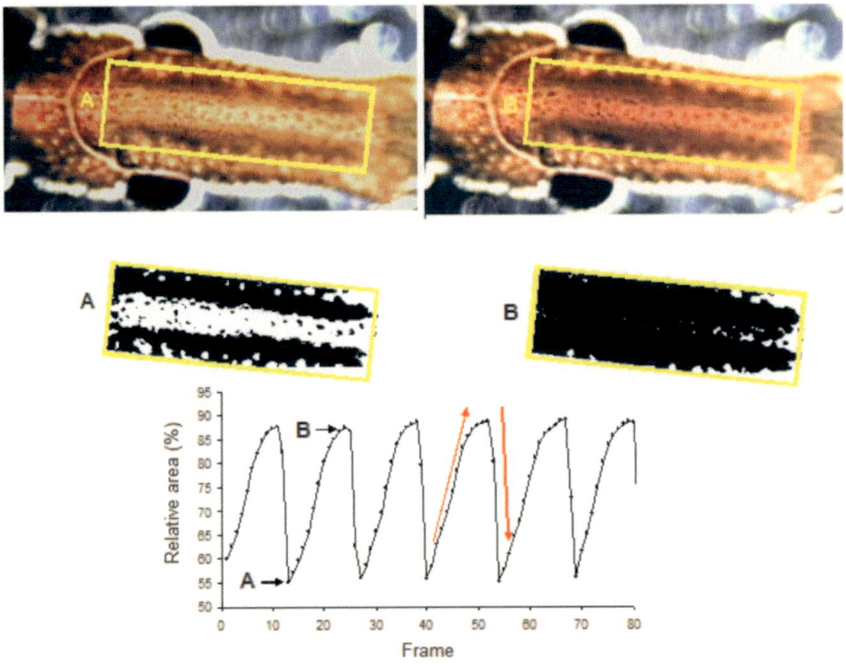

Fig. 22. Analyses of the cibarial pump images recorded by intravital microscopy of fifth instar of *Rhodnius prolixus* during blood feeding. Upper panel: Images with selected area (rectangle) indicating the cibarial pump when empty (A) or filled with blood (B). Lower panel: Images of the selected areas converted to 8 bits. The graph shows % variation in the area occupied by blood inside the cibarial pump over time (25 frames/second). Arrows indicate the region of the graph that represents the closing (A) and opening (B) of the pump.

When the graphs constructed from intravital microscopy of the insect head and the electromyogram of the cibarial pump are analyzed together, a strict synchrony can be observed between the electrical signals recorded and the filling of the pump chamber with blood (Figure 23) confirming that the electrical signals recorded are truly produced by cibarial pump-associated muscles.

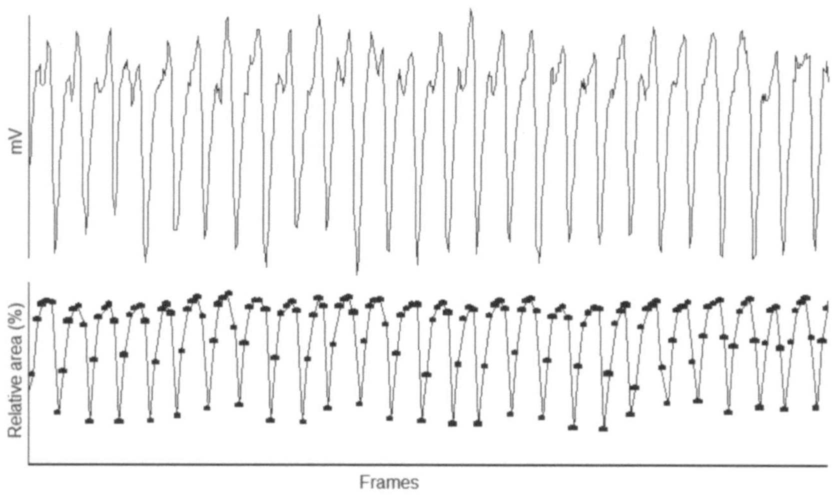

Fig. 23. Simultaneous monitoring of electrical activity (mV) and the flow of blood through the cibarial pump (relative area based on analyses of intravital microscopy images of the cibarial pump) of fifth instar nymphs of *Rhodnius prolixus* during the engorgement phase.

7. Profile of the signals produced during the feeding process and their meaning

The electrical signals produced by the cibarial pump can be selected and precisely monitored in such a way that the profiles obtained allowed delineation of each phase of the feeding process and calculation of the level of effort / difficulty in pumping blood. The signals detected before the bite show a somewhat regular profile with a small variation in mV (Figure 24). The bite is characterized by a sudden decrease in the mV, followed by a strong variation in mV characteristic of the probing phase (Figure 24). During the probing phase, some isolated, clearly formed signals can be seen, typical of those emitted by contractions of the cibarial pump. These isolated signals are attributed to "tasting" of the diet by the bug (Smith & Friend, 1970; Smith, 1979). It is assumed that during tasting, the insect ingests a sample for analysis by the gustatory sensilla, which can identify whether any of the vessel's content is spread on the tissues due to increased permeability and extravasations of liquid.

Once a suitable vessel is found, probing ceases and the engorgement phase begins. This is characterized by a change in the signal profile from strong irregular variations of mV to variations with similar intensity and regular intervals presenting distinct, regularly distributed mV peaks (Figure 25). The engorgement phase is considered to have begun when a sequence of ten regular peaks is detected.

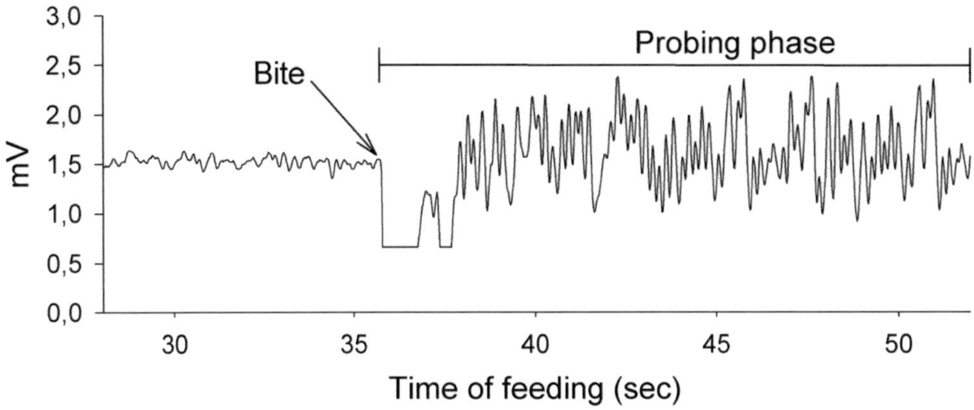

Fig. 24. Profiles observed before the bite and during the probing phase (modified from Araujo et al., 2009b).

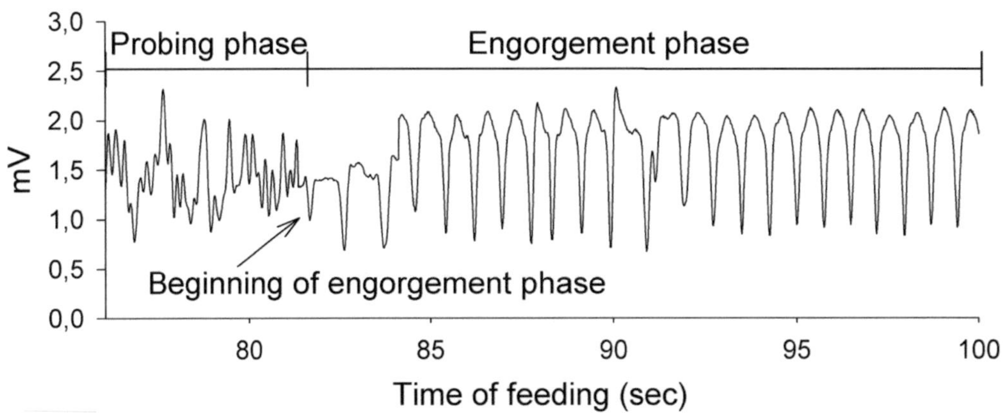

Fig. 25. Profiles observed during probing and beginning of the engorgement phase of *Cimex lectularius* feeding on mice (modified from Araujo et al., 2009b).

The engorgement phase can last from a few minutes (< 10 min) to more than one hour. The end of this phase is characterized by a sudden stop in the variation of the mV, resulting in a profile similar to the one seen before the bite, indicating that the insect has removed its mouthparts from the host (Figure 26).

The phases identified above can be added to other information to compose a set of important parameters used to study the feeding process. As well as noting the duration of blood-feeding, beginning of the engorgement phase and the end of the feeding process, the insects should be weighed before and after the observations in order to determine the weight gain (WG, defined as final minus initial weight). Based on the cibarial pump records, the total contact time (TCT) is defined as the time during which the insect mouthparts remain inserted into the host skin. Non-ingestive time (NIT) is the sum of the cumulative probing time (CPT) plus interruption time (IT). CPT is defined as the time from initial insertion of the mouthparts into the host up to the beginning of the engorgement phase. If the insect ceases probing and resumes blood-feeding elsewhere, the first probing time is added to the second and so on. IT is defined as the time during which the insects are not pumping blood after the engorgement phase has begun. The quantity of liquid ingested per cibarial pump contraction (QLC) is obtained by dividing the WG by the total number of cibarial pump contractions during engorgement. Pump frequency (F) represents the total number of cibarial pump contractions divided by the functioning time of the cibarial pump. Ingestion rate (IR, mg/min) is calculated by multiplying QLC by F. The total number of bites (B) and the number of interruptions to feeding (I) during the whole process are also noted.

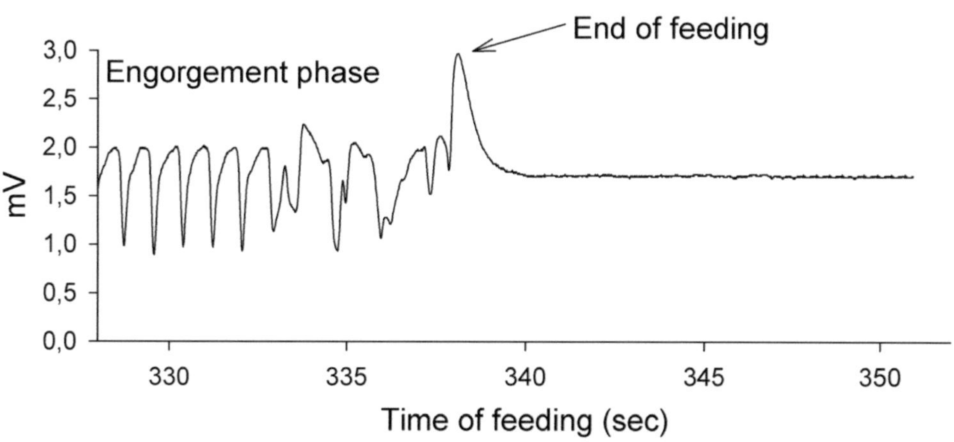

Fig. 26. Profiles observed at the end of the feeding of *Cimex lectularius* on mice showing the moment the mouthparts are removed from the host (modified from Araujo et al., 2009b).

The different profiles of the electrical signals can indicate other features that may be occurring during the engorgement phase. Parameters such as the negative pressure produced by the cibarial pump, dimensions of the food canal, blood viscosity, and the size of host red cells as well as their capacity to deform can influence both the ingestion rate (Kingsolver & Daniel, 1995) and the functioning of the cibarial pump. All these influences modify the profile of the electrical signals of the cibarial pump, reflect the performance of the bug during feeding and may indicate impediments to bloodmeal ingestion. An insect with high feeding performance shows electrical signals with regular peaks throughout the entire process (Figure 27a). Insects that impeded during feeding present a different electrical profile, in which the contractions are arrhythmic and the electrical signals have irregular shapes (duplicate peaks or intermediary forms between one or two peaks) (Figure 27b). The duplicate peaks seen in the cibarial pump contractions of bugs presenting difficulties in feeding may be explained by a lack of synchrony between the two bundles of the cibarial pump-associated muscles. These two electrical profiles can be seen at different moments in the same insect. Performance is usually higher at the onset of feeding, the electrical signal at the end, being disrupted, with a low pumping frequency.

A better overview of the whole feeding process is obtained using the matlab environment to analyze the profiles obtained by the electrical signals. The analyses facilitate the identification of all the above parameters and the variation of the cibarial pump frequency during the engorgement phase can be seen more easily (Figure 28). Insects with good performance are able to keep the cibarial pump working at high frequencies (~4 - 5.5 Hz) during engorgement (Figure 28a). Insects with low performance usually are unable to keep the cibarial pump operating at high frequencies for more than the first third of the process, after which some problems are seen such as a reduction in the signal frequency, interruptions and irregular signals (seen as a blurred spectrum) (Figure 28b).

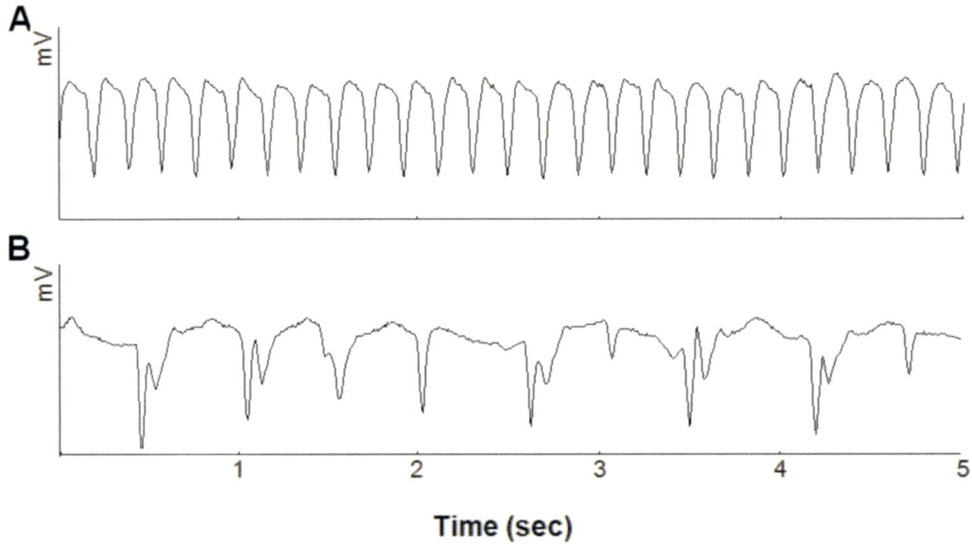

Fig. 27. Electrical profile of the engorgement phase from high (A) and low (B) performance feeding periods.

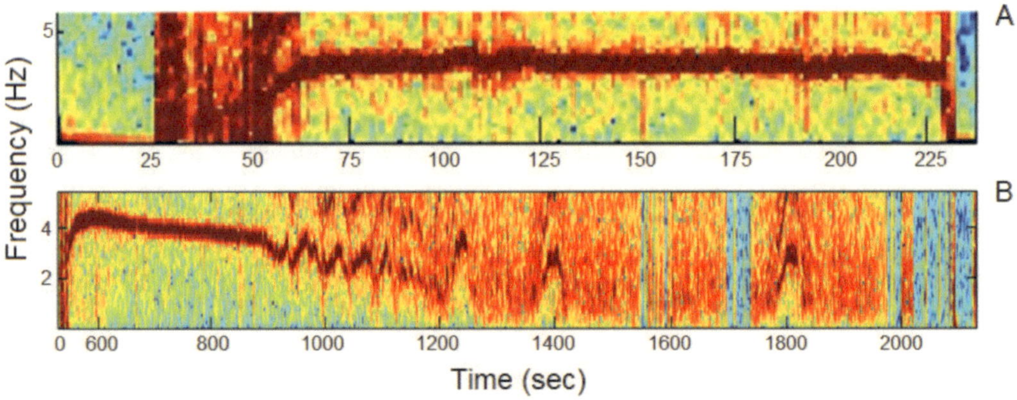

Fig. 28. General view of the whole feeding process of *Cimex lectularius* feeding on mice. A) high performance during the whole feeding process; B) low performance during the last two-thirds of engorgement.

8. Electromyogram studies of the cibarial pump

The analysis of feeding parameters based on cibarial pump electromyograms of different triatomine species feeding on pigeons, mice, humans or artificial feeders has provided sufficient information for us to know whether any differences were due the host type (Guarneri et al., 2000), triatomine species (Sant'Anna et al., 2001) or developmental stage (Guarneri et al., 2003) or to molecules produced in the salivary glands (Araujo et al., 2009a) or intestine (Araujo et al., 2007) of the insect. The QLC and maximum pumping frequency (obtained from experiments using artificial feeders) are related to the intrinsic morphlogical characteristics of the insect mouthparts. Based on the electrical signal methodology, several studies have demonstrated total ingestion rate (IR) to be the main parameter that determines contact time between a particular triatomine species and an immobilized host. IR values for fifth instar nymphs of the species studied to date vary from 3.1 mg/min for *R. neglectus* feeding on mice to 25.20 mg/min for *T. infestans* feeding on pigeons (Sant'Anna et al., 2001; Guarneri et al., 2000) (Table 1). The highest IR values for feeding on mice are observed for *T. infestans* (15.0 mg/min) and *R. prolixus* (11.9 mg/min) which are the most important vectors of *Trypanosoma cruzi* (etiological agent of Chagas' disease) in South and Central America, respectively (Guarneri et al., 2000; Sant'Anna et al., 2001). IR also varies considerably between different nymphal instars of the same species, for example, from 0.4 mg/min for first instars to 11.3 mg/min for fifth instars of *T. brasiliensis* feeding on humans (Guarneri et al., 2003). These differences in the IR observed during the post-embryonic development of triatomines are correlated to the QLC in the nymphal instar (Figure 30). It is noteworthy that males and females are sexually dimorphic with regard to cibarial pump volume. The higher QLC in females provides better performance than that seen in males, possibly an adaptation to increase their fitness in situations of higher competition.

Species	Pigeon	Mouse
T. infestans [a]	25.2 ± 6.0	15.0 ± 4.9
T. brasiliensis [a]	14.5 ± 5.6	10.8 ± 4.7
T. pseudomaculata [a]	5.0 ± 2.6	3.3 ± 0.9
R. prolixus [b]	19.5 ± 5.0	11.9 ± 3.8
R. neglectus [b]	5.7 ± 1.8	3.1 ± 1.6
R. robustus [b]	13.3 ± 6.2	7.4 ± 4.2
R. nasutus [b]	8.3 ± 3.9	8.5 ± 3.5

[a] Guarneri, 1999; [b] Sant'Anna et al., 2001.

Table 1. Mean values and standard deviation of the ingestion rate (mg/min) for different triatomine species feeding on pigeon or mouse.

Unlike IR, parameters such as F and NIT are influenced by the host physiology. Most of the triatomine species feeding on mice have a lower F value than those feeding on pigeons, whereas NIT values are variable. However, except for *R. nasutus*, triatomines feeding on mice usually have a longer NIT (Sant'Anna et al., 2001). This might be related to haemostatic differences between birds and mammals. Birds have thrombocytes that perform a similar function to mammalian platelets but are less effective. They also seem to lack some coagulation factors, particularly in the intrinsic pathway (Lewis, 1996).

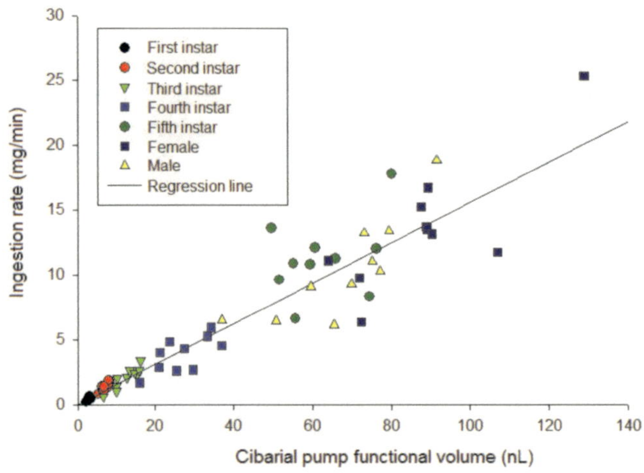

Fig. 29. Correlation between cibarial pump functional volume and ingestion rate of different developing instars of *Triatoma brasiliensis* feeding on humans.

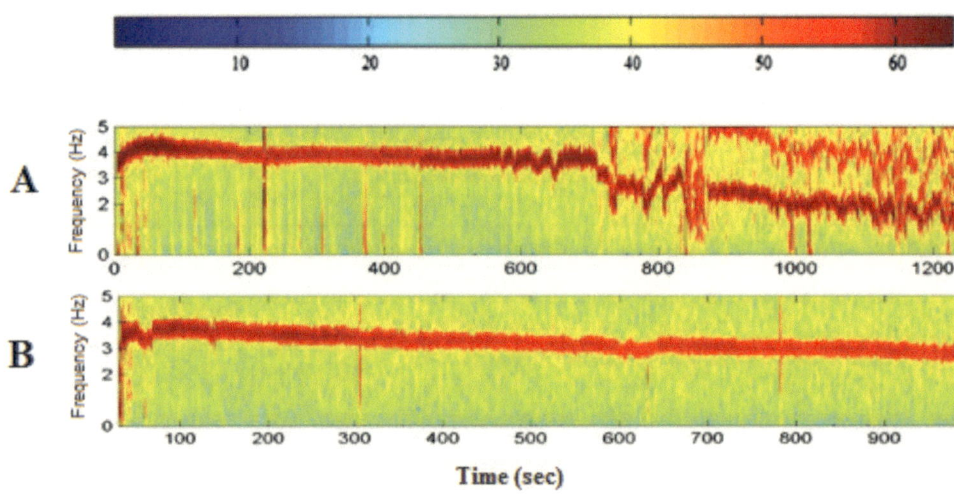

Fig. 30. Frequency spectrum over time produced by the cibarial pump contractions from *Triatoma brasiliensis* fed on the lateral tail vein of anesthetized mice. (A) *T. brasiliensis* feeding on non-treated mice; (B) *T. brasiliensis* feeding on mice treated with heparin. The colors represent the magnitude of occurrence of each frequency in the scale presented at the top of the figure.

Recent studies have shown that the coagulation process in the anterior midgut (crop) environment considerably influences feeding performance (Araujo et al., 2007; Paim et al., 2011). Insects that had their intestinal anticoagulant knocked down by RNA interference or by ingestion of exogenous thrombin had significantly lower total ingestion rate and weigh gain. The simplest explanation for the lower volumes ingested is that blood in the midgut must remain in a liquid state during feeding, or else backpressure induced by increased viscosity will prevent successful pumping of blood into the midgut (Araujo et al., 2007). As confirmation of the importance of the intestinal anticoagulants, Paim et al. (2011) demonstrated that *T. brasiliensis* fails to maintain the cibarial pump frequency during the whole feeding process, even under the most favorable conditions (e.g. when feeding on large-caliber vessels). This difficulty disappears when the host is previously treated with a systemic anticoagulant (Figure 29).

9. References

Abramoff, M.D., Magalhaes, P.J. & Ram, S.J. (2004). Image processing with ImageJ. *Biophot Int*, Vol. 11, pp. (36-42).

Alves, C.L., Araujo, R.N., Gontijo, N.F. & Pereira, M.H. (2011). Importance and physiological effects of hemolymphagy in triatomines (Hemiptera: Reduviidae). *J Med Entomol*, Vol. 48, pp. (372-381).

Araujo, R.N., Soares, A.C., Paim, R.M., Gontijo, N.F., Gontijo, A.F., Lehane, M.J. & Pereira, M.H. (2009a). The role of salivary nitrophorins in the ingestion of blood by the triatomine bug *Rhodnius prolixus* (Reduviidae: Triatominae). *Insect Biochem Mol Biol*, Vol. 39, pp. (83-89).

Araujo, R.N., Costa, F.S., Gontijo, N.F., Gonçalves, T.C.M. & Pereira, M.H. (2009b). The feeding process of *Cimex lectularius* (Linnaeus 1758) and *Cimex hemipterus* (Fabricius 1803) on different bloodmeal sources. *J Insect Physiol*, Vol. 55, pp. (1151-1157).

Backus, E.A. & McLean, D.L. (1982). The sensory systems and feeding behavior of leafhoppers. I. The aster leafhopper, *Macrosteles fascifrons* Stål (Homoptera: Cicadellidae). *J Morphol*, Vol. 172, pp. (361-379).

Bennet-Clark, H.C. (1963). Negative pressures produced in the cibarial pump of the blood sucking bug *Rhodnius prolixus*. *J Exp Biol*, Vol. 40, pp. (223-229).

Dickerson, G. & Lavoipierre, M.M. (1959). Studies on the methods of feeding of bloodsucking arthropods. II. The method of feeding adopted by the bed-bug (*Cimex lectularius*) when obtaining a blood-meal from the mammalian host. *Ann Trop Med Parasitol*, Vol. 53, pp. (347-357).

Gordon, R.M. & Crewe, W. (1948). The mechanisms by which mosquitoes and tsetse-flies obtain their blood-meal, the histology of the lesions produced, and the subsequent reactions of the mammalian host; together with some observations on the feeding of *Chrysops* and *Cimex*. *Ann Trop Med Parasitol*, Vol. 42, pp. (334-356).

Guarneri, A.A. (1999). Influência da fonte alimentar no potencial biológico de triatomíneos. Master's dissertation, Universidade Federal de Minas Gerais, Belo Horizonte, Brazil.

Guarneri, A.A., Diotaiuti, L., Gontijo, N.F., Gontijo, A.F. & Pereira, M.H. (2000). Comparison of feeding behaviour of *Triatoma infestans*, *Triatoma brasiliensis* and *Triatoma pseudomaculata* in different hosts by electronic monitoring of the cibarial pump. *J Insect Physiol*, Vol. 46, pp. (1121-1127).

Guarneri, A.A., Diotaiuti, L., Gontijo, N.F., Gontijo, A.F. & Pereira, M.H. (2003). Bloodfeeding performance of nymphs and adults of *Triatoma brasiliensis* on human hosts. *Acta Trop*, Vol. 87, pp. (361-370).

Kingsolver, J.G. & Daniel, T.L. (1995). Mechanics of food handling by fluid-feeding insects. In *Regulatory Mechanisms in Insect Feeding* (Chapman, R.F. and De Boer, G., eds), pp. 32-73, Chapman & Hall.

Lavoipierre, M.M.J., Dickerson, G. & Gordon, R.M. (1959). Studies on the methods of feeding of blood-sucking arthropods. I — The manner in which triatomine bugs obtain their blood-meal, as observed in the tissues of the living rodent, with some remarks on the effects of the bite on human volunteers. *Ann Trop Med Parasitol,* Vol. 53, pp. (235–252).

Lewis, J.H. (1996). *Comparative hemostasis in vertebrates.* Plenum Press, New York.

MathWorks (1995) *Simulink(TM), Dynamic System Simulation Software,* The MathWorks Inc., Natick, MA, USA.

McLean, D.L. & Kinsey, M.G. (1964). A technique for electrically recording aphid feeding and salivation. *Nature,* Vol. 202, pp. (1358-1359).

Paim, R.M., Araújo, R.N., Soares, A.C., Lemos, L.C., Tanaka, A.S., Gontijo, N.F., Lehane, M.J. & Pereira, M.H. (2011). Influence of the intestinal anticoagulant in the feeding performance of triatomine bugs (Hemiptera; Reduviidae). *Int J Parasitol,* Vol. 39, pp. (83-89).

Pérez, J.R. (1969). Estudio sobre la anatomía de *Rhodnius prolixus. Rev Venez Sanid Assist Soc,* Vol. 34, pp. (10-98).

Rasband, W.S., ImageJ, U. S. National Institutes of Health, Bethesda, Maryland, USA. http://imagej.nih.gov/ij/, 1997-2011.

Prutchi, D. & Norris, M. (2005). *Design and Development of Medical Electronic Instrumentation: A Practical Perspective of the Design, Construction, and Test of Medical Devices,* John Wiley & Sons Inc, Hoboken, New Jersey.

Sant'Anna, M.R.V., Diotaiuti, L., Gontijo, A.F., Gontijo, N.F. & Pereira, M.H. (2001). Feeding behaviour of morphologically similar *Rhodnius* species: influence of medical characteristics and salivary function. *J Insect Physiol.* Vol. 47, pp. (1459–1465).

Schofield, C.J. (1994). *Triatominae: Biologia y control.* Eurocommunica Publications, West Sussex.

Schofield, C.J. (1995). Overview - Biosystematics of the Reduviidae. *Proceedings of International Workshop on Population Genetics and Control of TriatomiLnae,* Santo Domingo de los Colorados, Ecuador, 1995, Sep. 24-28.

Schofield, C. J. & Dolling, W. R. (1996). Bedbugs and kissing-bugs (bloodsucking Hemiptera). In: *Medical Insects and Arachnids,* Lane, R. P. & Crosskey, R. W., pp. (483-516), Chapman & Hall, London.

Smith, J.J.B. (1979). Effect of diet viscosity on the operation of the pharyngeal pump in the blood-feeding bug Rhodnius prolixus. *J Exp Biol,* Vol. 82, pp. (93–104).

Smith, J.J.B. & Friend, W.G. (1970). Feeding in *Rhodnius prolixus*: responses to artificial diets as revealed by changes in electrical resistance. *J Insect Physiol,* Vol. 16, pp. (1709–1720).

Snodgrass, R.E. (1935). *Principles of insect morfology.* MacGraw-Hill Book Company Inc., 667. pp. (319) Figs. New York.

Snodgrass, R.E. (1944). The anatomy of the Mallophaga. *Occas Papers Cal Acad Sci,* Vol. 6, pp. (145-229).

Soares, A.C., Carvalho-Tavares, J., Gontijo, N.de.F., dos Santos, V.C., Teixeira, M.M. & Pereira, M.H. (2006). Salivation pattern of *Rhodnius prolixus* (Reduviidae; Triatominae) in mouse skin. *J Insect Physiol,* Vol. 52, pp. (468–472).

Tjallingii, W.F. (1985). Electrical nature of recorded signals during stylet penetration by aphids. *Entomol Exp Appl,* Vol. 38, pp. (177-186).

Usinger, R.L. (1966). Monograph of Cimicidae, Vol. 7. The Thomas Say Foundation, Baltimore.

Part 4

Pelvic Floor Muscle Function from Electromyograms

9

Anal Sphincter Electromyogram for Dysfunction of Lower Urinary Tract and Pelvic Floor

Chuangyu Qu, Dangfeng Xu, Cunzhou Wang,
Jie Chen, Lei Yin and Xingang Cui
Department of Urology, Changzheng Hospital
Second Military Medical University
China

1. Introduction

The electromyogram (EMG) is a diagnostic tool that measures and records the electrical activity produced by skeletal muscles. The anal sphincter and urethral external sphincter are skeletal muscle in nature. There are two kinds of EMG in widespread use in the field of urodynamic investigation: surface (patch) and intramuscular (fine-wire) EMG. In our laboratory, the fine-wire electrode is introduced by aid of a needle, we called it needle-guided wire electrode, or simply as wire electrode (Xu et al, 2007). Sphincter EMG studies the bioelectric potentials generated in the distal striated sphincter mechanism. Such studies are performed at two different levels of sophistication, each with distinct goals and requiring different instrumentation. The first, termed kinesiologic studies, are commonly performed in the urodynamic laboratory and simply examine sphincter activity during bladder filling and voiding. The second are neurophysiologic tests, which require considerable expertise and elaborate equipment and are designed to examine the integrity of innervation of the muscle. However, clinically the most important information obtained from sphincter EMG is whether there is coordination or discoordination between the external sphincter and the bladder. Surface patch electrodes are placed on the skin/mucosa overlying the muscle of interest and thus pick up the potentials produced by various muscles in the vicinity. Wire electrodes are preferable because they are placed directly into the muscle of interest, allowing for the detection of activity in individual motor units. EMG of the anal sphincter derived from transdermal route, being combined with simultaneous recording of uroflow rate, and bladder, abdominal pressure and then detrusor pressure (=bladder pressure–abdominal pressure) during both bladder storage and voiding phases, can give rise to a general essential data about functional states of the main elements (i.e. detrusor and sphincter) of lower urinary tract and the pelvic floor.

Sphincter dysfunction, either overactive or underactive, may occur in patients with either neurogenic or non-neurogenic lower urinary tract dysfunctions (LUTD). Recently, the European Association of Urology published its guideline (2008 version) on neurogenic LUTD, which is categorized into detrusor and sphincter levels, and the location of lesions is no longer emphasized (Stöhrer et al, 2009). Although several classification systems have been proposed for neurogenic LUTD, the recommendations for a functional classification for motor function are based on urodynamic and clinical findings. According to the functional state of detrusor and sphincter (whether it is overactive, normo-active or underactive), they are permutated and combinated following the principle of mathematics, and eight groups of neurogenic LUTD are classified thereafter (Table 1): overacive detrusor (3 groups, combined with overactive, normo-active, or underactive sphincter, respectively); underactive detrusor (3 groups, combined with overactive, normo-active, or underactive sphincter, respectively); and normo-active detrusor (2 groups, combined with only overactive, or underactive sphincter, respectively).

Type No	States of the functional elements of the lower urinary tract		Location of the lesion
	Detrusor	Sphincter	
1	**Overactive**	**Overactive**	Spinal
2	**Overactive**	Normo-active	Suprapontine
3	**Overactive**	Underactive	Lumbosacral
4	Underactive	**Overactive**	Lumbosacral
5	Underactive	Normo-active	Lumbosacral
6	Underactive	Underactive	Subsacral
7	Normo-active	**Overactive**	Sphincter only
8	Normo-active	Underactive	Sphincter only

Table 1. The European Association of Urology (EAU)-Madersbacher classification system of neurogenic LUTD.

In both congenital and acquired neurogenic LUTD, early diagnosis and treatment are essential because irreversible changes within the lower urinary tract may occur, even when the related neuropathologic signs are normal. Additionally, neurogenic LUTD can, by itself, be the presenting feature of neurologic pathology. The classification of the disease cannot be defined purely by site of the neurogenic lesion. Typically, the detrusor should be overactive for those with suprasacral lesions or upper motor neuron lesions, and be underactive for those with sacral or hyposacral, or lower motor neuron lesions. However, most patients may presented not typically with a combination of both storage and voiding symptoms, which may be due to multiple spinal cord injury, incomplete spinal cord injury or non-traumatic spinal cord lesion. A comprehensive urodynamic investigation protocol including EMG is mandatory to reveal the dominant character. We have also found some cases who presented with clinical, urodynamic and EMG abnormality, whereas their MRI and surgical exploration were negative. The neurogenic lesion developed at follow-up, and the lesion usually was unresectable at that time.

In the absence of neurologic disease, one cannot use the term detrusor-sphincter dyssynergia to describe EMG finding of sphincter overactivity. Instead, the term non-neurogenic neurogenic bladder, pelvic floor hypertonicity or dysfunctional voiding is used (Hinman, 1986; Deindl et al, 1998; Carlson et al, 2001). Sphincter functional state represents the state of the pelvic floor because of its ability of phasic functional change. Generally, sphincter overactivity is a behavioral problem and is often seen in children with voiding dysfunction and in neurologically normal women with voiding problems (Carlson et al, 2001; Goldman & Zimmern, 2006; Kuo, 2010). We have identified this phenomenon in Chinese women with urinary frequency and poor-weak flow, and the prevalence of this

disorder is more than 30%. Most of those women had a history of such behavioral problem as voluntary withholding of urination in individuals who work long hours, or voiding in an unnatural position, i.e., with her haunch hanged up for avoidance of touching commode.
Furthermore, sphincter overactivity not only implies some degree of functional obstruction, but also co-exists with overactive bladder (OAB) or stress urinary incontinence (SUI). The intrinsic mechanism may be related with guarding or continence reflex of the sacral spinal cord (Kamo et al, 2004). When the bladder is filled to near capacity or following a sudden increase in intravesical pressure, pudendal motorneuron firing occurs. Urodynamic and EMG data indicate that a rise in maximal urethral pressure corresponds to increased EMG activity of the striated muscles of the pelvic floor. This phenomenon has been termed the guarding or continence reflex and represents a somatic mechanism for increasing urethral resistance. The firing of the pudendal motorneuron may also be induced by detrusor overactivity, more leaked urine into the proximal urethra in female patients with SUI, inhibited by more urine into the lower part of the ureter or acute anal stretch (Akkad et al, 2007; Chen et al, 2007; Chen et al, 2008; Xu et al, 2010). Voluntary overactivity of this reflex can result in obstruction of the lower urinary tract and differentiating voluntary contraction of this sphincter from detrusor sphincter dyssynergia can be difficult. Close examination of the onset of sphincter activity relative to the rise in intravesical pressure can help distinguish a guarding reflex from true detrusor sphincter dyssynergia (Rudy & Woodside, 1991). There were 3 characteristic urodynamic features in this patient population that were distinct from those seen in patients with true detrusor-external sphincter dyssynergia: (1) quieting of the external sphincter EMG immediately prior to the onset of a detrusor contraction, (2) quieting of the EMG during the upslope of a detrusor contraction, and (3) augmented EMG activity during the downslope of the detrusor contraction. Although both involve incoordinate bladder and pelvic floor/external sphincter activity, a simple cystometrogram (CMG) with EMG may allow reliable differentiation between true detrusor-external sphincter dyssynergia and non-neurogenic neurogenic bladder.
Differentiating voluntary contraction of the sphincter from detrusor sphincter dyssynergia or dysfunctional voiding is not as important clinically as someone declared previously. If the recipient is a healthy volunteer, the finding may be voluntary contraction of the sphincter. If the recipient is a patient and he or she has symptoms related to lower urinary tract, we would rather consider it as dysfunctional voiding in neurological intact ones, or neurogenic detrusor sphincter dyssynergia in patients whose neurogenic system is involved. The real intention of the guarding reflex is beneficial for the subject. It is associated with unbalance between the detrusor and sphincter, and perhaps it is already a pathologic change when the reflex is fortified too much, such as in patients complained of OAB or SUI. The most important question that urodynamic personnel should answer is whether the finding is an artifact or abnormal sign.
EMG artifacts were so common in adults that EMG signals should be interpreted with great caution previously, and they could be very frustrating and difficult to deal with especially when EMG studies was performed using surface patch electrodes. At present, especially when wire electrode is widely used in practice in this institution, the situation is not as what they addressed and sphincter state whether normal or overactive, could be displayed very distinctly (see below).
This Chapter deals with the utilization of the EMG signal (with needle electrodes) from the anal sphincter as an indicator of dysfunction of the lower urinary tract. The major impact is that anal sphincter EMG may serve to present the functional state of the urethral sphincter.

At the following description text, we are going to express our thinking and measures about this subject.

2. Consideration

Urodynamic study (Life-Tech Urovision Janus and MMS Solar) involving more than 7000 patients with LUTD have been conducted with wire electrode EMG and gained better results since 2002 in this institution. Other equipments (Laborie, Nidoc, Dantec and Duet) have also been used since 1985. The aetiology and causes underlying various LUTD were explored, and then allow management decisions to be made. Apart from the guidelines the company proposed, some modifications were undertaken. The surface patch electrode was forsaked from the very beginning. The main reason was that it cannot be pasted on the perianal skin firmly. The wire of the electrode was first exerted out from inside of the needle hole (Fig. 1,b), and in our modification it was inserted into the needle hole from outside inside (Fig. 1 c, d). The most brittle part of wire is the site of reflexion, and if this happened, the debris will remain in the needle tube, not fall into the surrounding tissue.

2.1 Technological consideration: Electrocircuit system as a whole

EMG artifacts may be caused by multiple sources including the patient and the urodynamics suite itself. Electrical signals from other electrical equipment such as lights, transformers, electrocautery units, or the fluoroscopy equipment can all contribute. Other sources of artifact include improper grounding, defective insulation, and movement of the patient (Webster & Guralnick, 2002). Apart from the usually mentioned factors leading to weak signals or artifacts, including electrodes being placed too far from the sphincter, becoming wet, having too low gain or falling off the patient (Blaivas et al, 2007), other factors associated with technical consideration should be more important thereafter. From the point of electrology, the EMG recording system of the equipment, the cables, the wires and the muscles between two electrode tips compose an electrocircuit system. The internal or external factors of the system, such as its integrity, consistency, environmental temperature, humidity, the bio-electric resistance of the tissues tested in between and distance length between the electrodes, may influence the tracing outcomes. External moving force against the needle or breaking off of the closed circuit of the system should also be considered. The static bio-electric resistance between the two poles are dependent on the medium in between. In our series of 152 patients measured at a radian of 1.0 π between the two poles, resistances were 6.30±2.10 kΩ (3.0~12.0), 7.74±2.97 kΩ (1.5~16.0), 2150.66±1733.58 kΩ (100~8000) for saline, muscle and skin respectively (Cui et al., 2009). Apparently, the resistance of muscle was higher than saline and lower than skin (P=0.001). Most EMG recording artifacts are secondary to a recorded potential that does not arise from the depolarization of the striated muscle to be studied. EMG raw signals, expressed in micro-volts, were obtained directly from the electronic circuitry and were not normalized. For example, when surface patch is used, the potential may come from the levator ani muscles or other pelvic floor muscles. If these factors are all OK and within normal limits, abnormal findings on the screen may imply pathological significance, and cannot be blamed ad libitum as artifacts.

From our experience, nearly 70%-80% so-called "artifacts" or bad recordings of EMG came actually from an open circuit, not from a closed circuit, of the electrocircuit system (Fig. 2). Open circuit means some thing wrong, usually break or bad conduct, occurred in the electrocircuit system. Closed circuit means an intact electrocircuit system, The normal EMG tracings are continuous and consecutive, strengthening in the storage phase and relaxing in the voiding phase. It had better response to cough or other physiological actions. At the beginning of CMG, before bladder filling begins, the patient is asked to demonstrate volitional control of the sphincter by actively contracting and relaxing it. The ability to do this implies intact pyramidal tracts. Next, the bladder control reflex is tested by squeezing the glans penis or clitoris or pulling on the Foley catheter. A burst of EMG activity is a positive result and implies an intact sacral arc. Bladder filling then begins; and, as it proceeds, there is a progressive recruitment of sphincter activity, demonstrated by increased amplitude and frequency of firing. Just before the onset of voiding, sphincter activity ceases and remains so for the duration of micturition. Once the bladder is empty, sphincter EMG activity resumes.

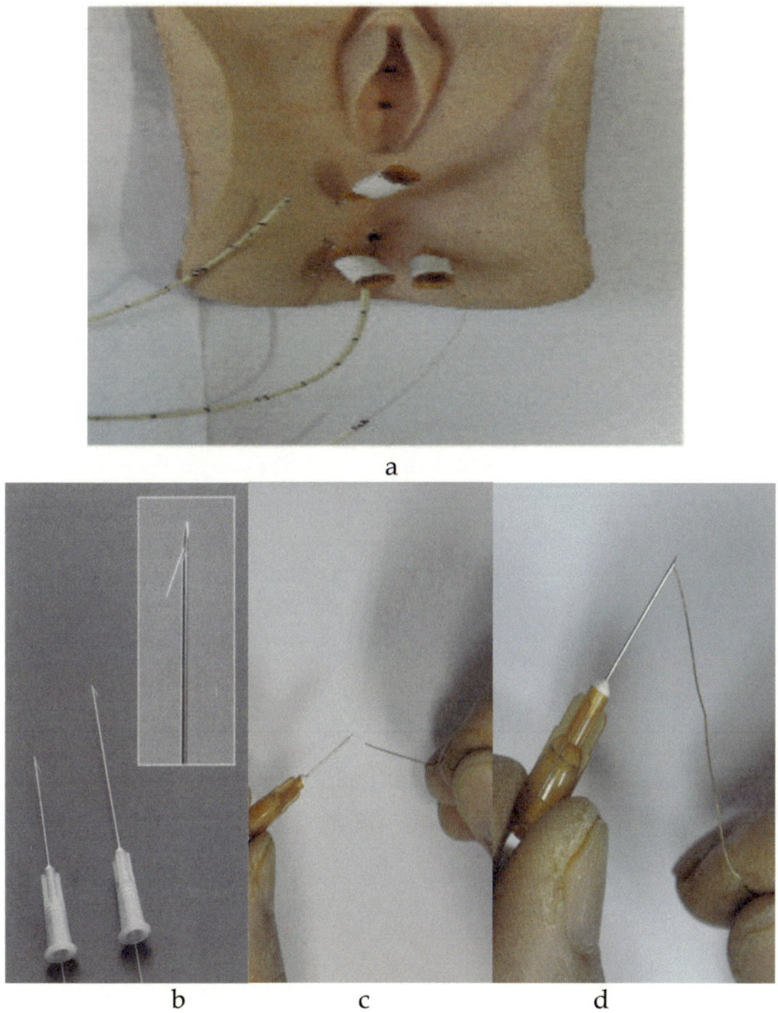

Fig. 1. Needle-guided wire electrodes and its modification: the original design with wire inserted into needle from needle tail then inside outside (b), modified design with wire inserted into needle head from outside inside (c, d), and the modified needles puncturing into the anal skin at 3, 9 and 10:30 o'clock (a).

When needle-guided wire electrodes are used, the raw signals of the anal sphincter coming from half circle of the anus are expressed on the urodynamic screen in a condense fashion (20 sec/grid). Their potential amplitude could be measured: the more sphincter it includes, the higher the amplitude. Concentric electrodes and oscillometer were used to measure motor unit potentials (MUP), and signals came from only a granule-size sphincter were displayed on the oscillometer in a faster velocity (20 ms/grid). So the former was a continuous trace and latter was wave-like or ECG-like. However, due to changes in location, orientation or other factors, it is not possible to point the difference. The electrocircuit was secured making sure that the equipment was in good condition, the wires in unbroken and no tarnishing state, the inserted needles free from outside interference and so on. Otherwise, the trace would be abnormal and referred to as "artifact". The crenate-like EMG trace in Fig 2a came from the screen before the wire was inserted into the anus with the wire disparted. The lower amplitude trace in Fig 2b came from the screen before the wire was inserted into the anus with the wires linked together. The intermittent, crenate-like, sawtooth-like, or wave-like EMGs in Fig. 2c and d show that something went wrong (wire is broken or the needle guided the wire is compressed by lateral force) in the circuit during examination. By re-doing or changing of the wire electrode, the trace became normal.

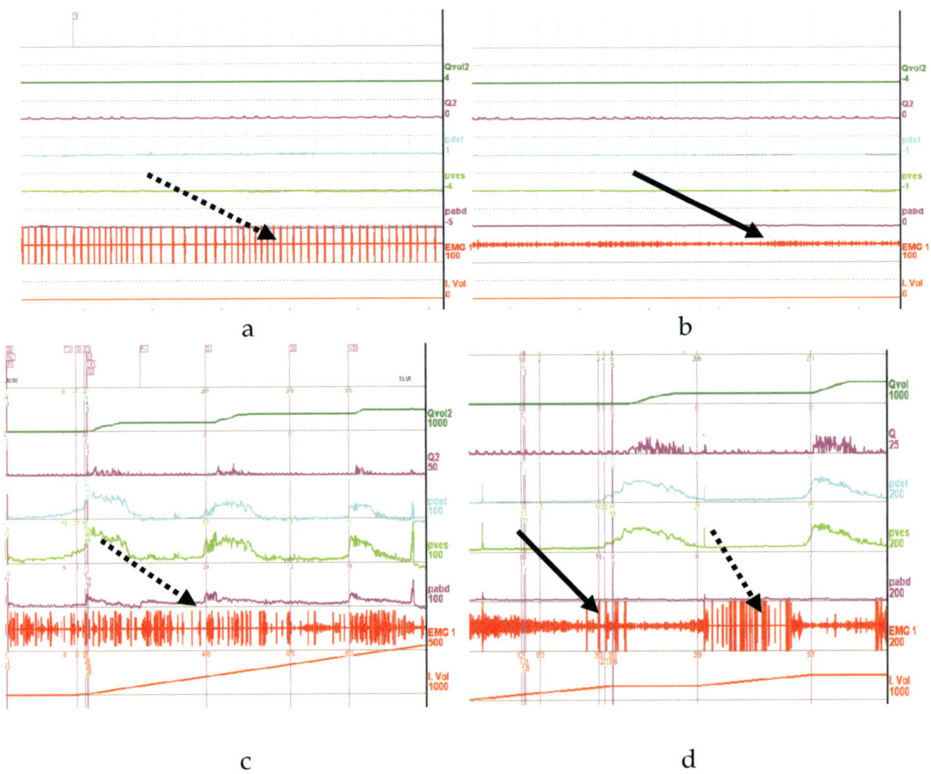

Fig. 2. Urodynamic and EMG trace recordings displaying anal sphincter EMG: the electrocircuit system is in open circuit (a) or in closed circuit (b), without insertion of the wire or urodynamic investigation. Bad recordings of EMG during urodynamic investigation: intermittent trace from beginning to end as dashed arrows indicated (c), or in the intermediate phase due to external depressing force toward the needle, which turned normal (as solid arrows indicated) after revision of the needle direction (d).

2.1.1 Wire or patch electrodes

Compared with the perineal surface patch electrodes which are widely used in most labs in Europe and United States, the only shortcoming of the needle-guided wire electrode is a slight pain associated with needle puncturing. The surface electrode is easy to fall off, having low sensitivity and poor reliability. Although patients have a greater tolerance for surface EMG electrodes, the reliability of the latter when compared to needle-guided wire electrode or even concentric needle electrode (CNE) is doubtful. Volume conduction results in the compounding of motor unit signals from all the muscles of the perineal body, makes signals from an individual muscle difficult to identify. Given the differing innervation of the levator ani muscles and the external urethral sphincter it is unlikely that EMG activity of the levator ani muscles recorded with surface electrode adequately reflects motor unit activity of the external urethral sphincter. As the ways of expression are concerned, CNE inserted into the rhabdosphincter close to the urethral orifice are superior to surface electrodes patched close to the anus for EMG documentation of urethral sphincter relaxation during voiding (Mahajan et al, 2006). A study was conducted to compare interpretations of EMG recordings from surface electrodes with those from urethral CNEs during voiding. Consenting women underwent urodynamic testing with a 30 G, 3.8 cm CNE at the 12 o'clock position in the striated urethral sphincter muscle, and with surface electrodes placed at the 2 and 10 o'clock positions around the anus. Pressure-flow studies (PFS) were conducted with simultaneous input from both EMG electrodes. Representative, de-identified paper copies of EMG signals were assembled by chronology and electrode type. Six examiners unaware of the patient details were asked to determine if the tracings were interpretable and whether there was quiescence of the urethral sphincter motor unit during voiding. The consistency between the interpretations of each tracing was assessed using McNemar and κ statistics. Twenty-two women undergoing urodynamic testing for incontinence (16), voiding dysfunction (two) or urinary retention (four) participated in the study. CNE tracings were consistently more interpretable than surface electrode tracings (mean 89% vs 67%). When tracings were interpretable, a significantly higher percentage of CNE EMG tracings (mean 79%) had urethral sphincter motor unit quiescence than surface electrod EMG tracings (mean 28%). The κ values for agreement among the reviewers' interpretations were highly variable and none were statistically significant. Reviewers unanimously agreed on only 12 of the 44 tracings, and 11 of these showed quiescence when using a CNE. CNEs were more often interpretable than surface electrodes for determining motor unit quiescence during voiding. CNE EMG appeared to have greater clinical utility for central reading than surface electrodes (Mahajan et al, 2006).

2.1 2 Radian and its influence on the amplitude of potentials

Surface electrodes are placed at the 2 and 10 o'clock positions around the anus, and the needle-guided wire electrodes we used, representing two poles of the circuit, are placed at the 3 and 9 o'clock position around the anus. CNE has two poles indeed too, but the distance of them is almost neglectable and it describes less myoelectric information than those with longer distance. Two wire electrodes at radian distance of 0.25 π, 0.75 π, or 1.0 π prevail over CNE in potential amplitude and the potential increased in accordance with the radian as our experiment displayed. This experiment was conducted in this institution on patients suffered from LUTD to study the role of radian distance of the wire-electrodes and its impact on the amplitude and quality of EMG (Cui et al., 2009). Between September 2008 and January 2009, a total of 152 patients with LUTD underwent comprehensive urodynamic study. Each underwent three sessions of CMG, EMG and PFS with one of the 3 radians when EMG was conducted. The electrodes were randomly placed at radians of 0.25 п (9-10:30 o'clock), 0.75 п (10:30-3 o'clock), or 1.0 п (3-9 o'clock) (Fig. 3. a). The electro-potentials during storage and voiding phases were measured separately, recorded and analyzed according to their disclosed radians. Mean electro-potentials during storage phase were 13.6±6.2, 23.2±11.8, 30.6±14.2μV at 0.25п, 0.75п, or 1.0п respectively (F=86.94, P=0.000) as to the whole group. When the data were further analyzed according to their gender, age or original disease, this gradually increased trend still remained (Table 2). The result was that the potentials of the storage phase were influenced by the radians of the electrodes either in total, or in different genders, age subgroups or original diseases. There was a positive relation between them, either in total or divided by gender, age or original diseases. It could be ratiocinated that wire electrodes with three radian distances (0.25, 0.75 or 1.0 п) should be better than the CNE. These data suggest that the use of either 1.0, 0.75 or 0.25 п for use as an EMG standardization criterion will do and is warranted, and that the 1.0 п is the best. Whereas there were no significant differences during voiding phase in the mean electro-potentials between the patients with or without sphincter overactivity (Table 3). It seems

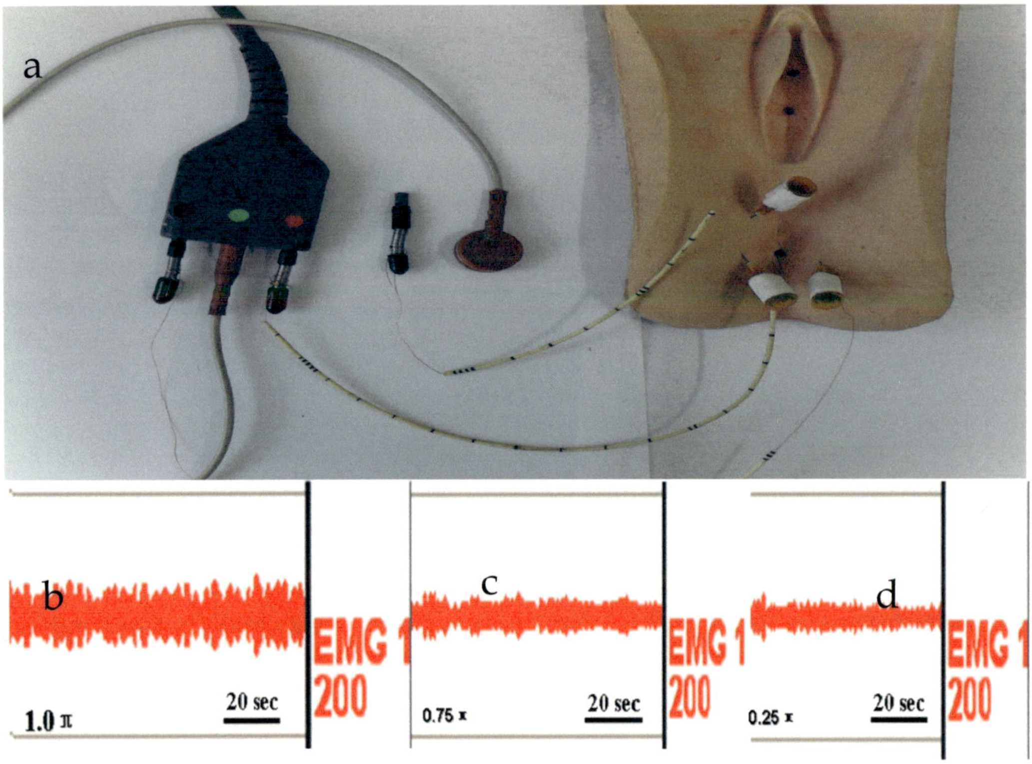

Fig. 3. The design of the experiment: an EMG cable with three interfaces (black, green and red, the green interface for grounding), three electrode adapters and three end needle-guided wires directly acupunctured into the anal sphincter at 3, 9, and 10:30 o'clock positions around anus (a), the EMG tracings during storage phase with radian of 1.0 п (b), 0.75 п (c), and 0.25 п (d) in a patient.

that the sphincters during the voiding phase are relaxed as loosely in patients with intact detrusor-sphincter relation and contracted as tightly in patients with sphincter overactivity as possible irrespective of distance or radian between the two electrodes (Fig. 4). Using Solar from MMS (Netherlands), we can also record simutanously detrusor sphincter synergia or dyssynergia as Janus from Life-tech (USA) in same patients (Fig 4)

Variables	Data of electro-potentials at different orientations (expressed in radians and degrees in parentheses)			*F* value	*P* value
	0.25 π (45°)	**0.75 π (135°)**	**1.0 π (180°)**		
In general (n=152)					
Data	13.60±6.20 (4.60-33.00)	23.20±11.82 (5.20-85.00)	30.57±14.18 (6.40-127.6)	86.94	<0.001
Influence factor analysis					
Sex					
Male (n=79)	14.86±6.90 (6.20-33.0)	25.84±14.01 (9.8-85.00)	32.49±16.61 (9.80-12.76)	36.14	<0.001
Female (n=73)	12.24±5.06 (4.60-24.2)	20.35±8.04 (5.20-45.00)	28.48±10.70 (6.40-127.6)	70.49	<0.001
Age					
<30 (n=18)	14.36±4.58 (8.8-24.2)	26.96±11.54 (14.2-61.4)	35.74±14.62 (20.2-79.6)	16.95	<0.001
30~ (n=15)	12.43±6.77 (5.4-30.4)	22.32±10.22 (8.2-52.4)	26.89±13.57 (9.8-52.8)	7.36	<0.001
40~(n=22)	13.42±6.18 (7.0-33.00)	20.31±8.19 (8.8-41.4)	29.37±12.48 (11.6-53.0)	16.19	<0.001
50~(n=36)	13.81±6.24 (4.6-28.6)	24.05±15.34 (5.2-85.0)	31.21±11.41 (6.4-55.0)	20.42	<0.001
60~(n=20)	13.25±6.46 (5.0-28.2)	23.19±9.60 (7.8-39.2)	28.46±8.14 (16.0-41.8)	17.90	<0.001
70~(n=41)	13.79±6.75 (5.0-32.4)	22.69±11.72 (6.0-73.0)	30.74±18.88 (13.2-127.6)	16.38	<0.001
Original disease					
BOO(n=52)	14.10±6.15 (6.2-32.4)	24.27±14.09 (9.8-85.0)	31.93±17.18 (13.4-127.6)	34.19	<0.001
DV(n=57)	12.77±6.17 (5.0-33.0)	22.11±11.12 (5.2-61.4)	28.86±12.83 (6.4-79.6)	16.42	<0.001
UAB(n=30)	14.54±6.65 (6.0-28.6)	22.82±10.53 (8.8-57.4)	28.97±11.50 (9.8-57.8)	24.24	<0.001
SUI(n=13)	13.09±5.72 (4.6-21.4)	24.62±7.55 (12.4-37.6)	36.26±11.23 (20.0-53.0)	24.24	<0.001

BOO, bladder outlet obstruction; DV, dysfunctional voiding; SUI, stress urinary incontinence; UAB, underactive bladder.

Table 2. Comparison of electro-potentials of anal sphincter at storage phase among different location radians of the electrodes μV, mean±SD (range)

Variables	Data of electro-potentials at different orientations (expressed in radians and degrees in parentheses)			*F* value	*P* value
	0.25 π (45°)	**0.75 π (135°)**	**1.0 π (180°)**		
Influence factor analysis (n=122)					
Original disease					
Without sphincter overactivity (n=65)	14.54±6.78 (4.0-34.0)	15.55±7.90 (5.0-40.0)	16.91±6.93 (4.0-34.0)	1.76	0.17
BOO(n=52)	13.48±6.20 (4.0-30.0)	13.98±6.17 (5.0-30.0)	15.75±6.57 (4.0-31.0)	1.85	0.16
SUI(n=13)	18.77±7.57 (8.0-34.0)	21.85±10.85 (10.0-40.0)	21.54±6.57 (13.0-34.0)	0.51	0.60
Sphincter overactivity DV(n=57)	87.18±66.31 (7.0-300.0)	95.40±70.26 (10.0-300.0)	102.79±80.55 (11.0-400.0)	0.66	0.52

BOO, bladder outlet obstruction; DV, dysfunctional voiding; SUI, stress urinary incontinence; UAB, underactive bladder.

Table 3. Comparison of electro-potentials of anal sphincter at voiding phase among different location radians of the electrodes μV, mean±SD (range)

2.1.3 Use of TL value

To compare the values of EMG potential at different time, for example, before start of voiding or during maximal flow rate (i.e., Qmax), a derived parameter, TL value, was introduced (Xu, et al., 2007, 2010). TL value is a derived parameter used to measure the degree of detrusor-sphincter synergia. In digitalization terms, sphincter overactivity or dysfunctional voiding was expressed with a quantitative analysis of the potentials using the parameter of tense/loose (TL) value. TL value is derived from sphincter EMG as a format of (lg [potentials before voiding/at Qmax]) with a positive number (>0) as normal level and a negative number (<0) indicating sphincter overactivity during voiding. By this parameter, information of sphincter EMG could be utilized maximally. However, this parameter is possible only after consecutive and satisfactory recording of EMG tracing alongside with CMG and PFS recording during monitoring of the storage and voiding process. In laboratories where EMG signals are recorded poorly or given up, this value is not available. Indirect parameters, such as PdetQmax (≥20 cmH2O), Qmax (<12 mL/s) and increased EMG were used in the diagnosis of dysfunctional voiding (Wang & Chen, 2003). PdetQmax means the detrusor pressure at maximum flow rate in the voiding phase. The diagnosis of dysfunctional voiding was made when there was an increased external sphincter activity during voluntary voiding in neurologically intact people, as evidenced by EMG tracing and/or fluoroscopy, with a sustained detrusor contraction (Carlson et al, 2001, Chuang & Kuo, 2007, Kuo, 2010). If the TL value is measured in these figures, a minus value will be obtained too.

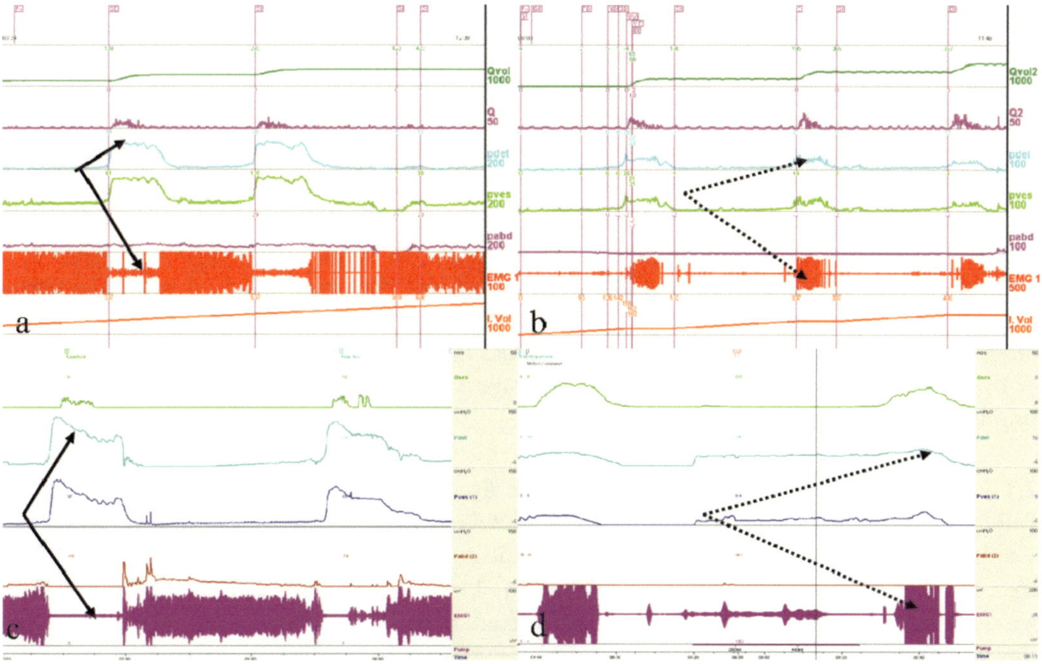

Fig. 4. Simutaneous recording of CMG, EMG and PFS using different facilities (Life-Tech and MMS) in female patients displaying bladder outlet obstruction and detrusor external sphincter synergia as indicated by solid arrows (a, c), and dysfunctional voiding or sphincter overactivity as indicated by dashed arrows (b, d) with radian of 1.0 π.

Another special type of dysfunctional voiding is Fowler's syndrome in women, which has three characteristic features: sphincter overactivity, detrusor underactivity, and polycystic ovary (Fowler et al., 1988; Fowler, 2003). In Fowler's syndrome urinary retention is associated with a primary abnormality of the striated urethral sphincter, characterized by an abnormal sphincter EMG signal displaying 'complex repetitive discharges' and elevated maximum urethral closure pressure (MUCP). Many of the young women with this disorder manifest features of polycystic ovaries, suggesting that it is due to a hormonally sensitive channelopathy. A normal mechanism for suppression of incontinence involving the striated urethral sphincter becomes exaggerated in Fowler's syndrome and prevents voiding. Reports of increased urethral pressure and sphincter volume corroborate the concept that inappropriate sphincter contraction causes the urinary retention, leading to detrusor failure with loss of bladder sensation (Wiseman et al., 2001). Six female patients with Fowler's syndrome in whom sacral neuromodulation restored their ability to void underwent functional brain magnetic resonance imaging immediately after neuromodulation and when untreated (Kavia et al, 2010). The most striking results were the widespread negative responses to bladder infusion, which were quite different from the activations seen in 'normal' individuals. The function of visceral sensation in the right insula representating brain responses to bladder filling was abnormal (negative) when the bladders in the patients with Fowler's syndrome were empty. Increase of bladder volume and neuromodulation treatment reduced the extent of negative neural responses, and normal (positive) responses in the periaqueductal grey strengthened, whether used alone or together. They concluded that the primary abnormality of the syndrome is an overactive urethra that generates abnormally strong inhibitory afferent signals, so effectively blocking bladder afferent activity at the sacral level and deactivating the periaqueductal grey and higher centres (Kavia et al, 2010). This central reflex and sacral guarding reflex have the same nature. The constraction of the pelvic floor-external sphincter complex is a normal response to control urgent urination and results in a reflex inhibition of the detrusor. When this action becomes habitual with time or exaggerated, as in patients with dysfunctional voiding or Fowler's syndrome, abnormal dyscoordination carries over to voluntary voiding, resulting in sphincter overactivity, intermittent urinary stream and post-void residual urine (McGuire, 1984, as cited in Carlson et al, 2001). We think a negative TL value is also a criteria for the diagnosis of Fowler's syndrome. Abnormal EMG findings may imply neural, psychological, or behavioural dysfunction from central, peripheral, regional or reflexual origin. It certainly provides the directions for further research.

2.1.4 EMG, MUP and other neurophysiologic examination

Failure of the sphincter to relax or stay completely relaxed during micturition is abnormal. The inappropriate sphincter activity during voiding has a variety of patterns, ranging from crescendo contraction to failure of relaxation. In neurologic conditions, abnormal EMG waveforms, in addition to detrusor-sphincter dyssynergia, are seen. These include fibrillation potentials, complex polyphasic potentials, and complex repetitive discharges, but they require more specialized equipment for their demonstration (Aminoff, 2007; Nandedkar et al, 1986). Due to the limited utility of clinical examination (Agur et al, 2009; Warren et al, 2011), urodynamics and imaging studies to demonstrate a neurogenic etiology of the LUTD, the role of clinical neurophysiologic methods remains important. For evaluation of patients with neurogenic LUTD a number of neurophysiologic methods have been used, including motor unit potential (MUP), interference pattern, nerve conduction, evoked potential, and sacral reflex analysis (Finsterer, 2001; Podnar, 2007).

Nerve conduction studies are performed by the stimulation of a peripheral nerve and the monitoring of the time taken for a response to occur in its innervated muscle. The time from stimulation to response is termed the latency. Nerve conduction studies are tests of the integrity of a reflex arc and can be relatively sensitive indicators of the presence of neurologic disease. In urologic practice, these studies are most often performed as bladder-cortex reflex latency determinations. They require elaborate instrumentation and careful user interpretation. Abnormal responses occur in a variety of situations and are particularly diagnostic in patients with diabetes and peripheral neuropathies. In patients with conus medullaris or cauda equina lesions, normal, prolonged, or absent latencies may be found, and asymmetrical responses are not uncommon. Patients with suprasacral lesions may have normal or low latencies (26 to 30 msec) because of loss of inhibitory neural pathways from higher centers (Webster & Guralnick, 2002).

Evoked response studies are means to assess afferent neuronal pathways by applying a stimulus to a peripheral nerve (e.g., dorsal penile nerve/pudendal nerve) and recording the cortical response. As such, they are used to test the integrity of peripheral, spinal, and central nervous system pathways. They also require sophisticated instrumentation using averaging techniques, and their performance is confined to specialized centers (Aminoff, 2007).

Sphincter EMG derived from concentric needle electrodes comes from muscle fibres within 0.5 mm of tip of the needle. The analysis of the EMG data using this type of electrode shown on an oscillometer with a speed of 10 ms/div (much faster as compared with a speed of 10-20 s/div in urodynamic study) is known as MUP (Podnar et al, 2000; Podnar, 2007). Those from two wire electrodes inserted in the same position as the anal surface electrode comes from half of the sphincter muscle fibres as whole. So the EMG trace is smooth and constant with strain or coughing-induced strengthening. If a MUP means electronic activity of a small group of motor units of the sphincter, then sphincter EMG gained from needle guided-wire electrodes means highly concentrated MUP. The former is just like a piece of roasted mutton, and the latter is a long string of roasted mutton. Three quantitative MUP analysis techniques (manual-MUP, single-MUP and multi-MUP), with similar sensitivities for detecting reinnervation changes, are available (Podnar et al, 2000; Podnar, 2007).

Normally, potentials generated during sphincter activity may be recorded with a specialized concentric needle electrode inserted directly into the muscle to be tested, and the MUP recorded from the distal urethral sphincter muscle has a biphasic or triphasic waveform with an amplitude of 50 to 300 mV and a firing frequency of 10 to 100 discharges per second. Simplistically, when the motoneuron or nerve to a muscle is damaged, those muscle fibers that have lost their innervation become reinnervated by adjacent healthy nerves. The resultant MUP changes from a simple waveform to one that is larger in amplitude, complexity, and duration; these are termed polyphasic potentials. At least five deflections on the tracing must be present for a MUP to be called polyphasic (Abrams et al, 1988). These are thought to represent the increased number of muscle fibers per motor unit that follows reinnervation. Normal muscle may have up to 15% of its activity in the form of such polyphasic potentials; however, when the amount of polyphasic activity is significantly greater than this, neuropathy is implied. Other findings that suggest neuropathy include fibrillation potentials, which are spontaneous, low-amplitude potentials of short duration, and positive sharp waves, which are biphasic potentials. Neurophysiologic studies require more sophisticated instrumentation and investigator expertise and are designed to actually diagnose and characterize the presence of neuropathy or myopathy. MUPs in health and disease differ, and, within certain limitations, the expert observer may use these studies to determine whether neuropathy is present. Neurophysiologic studies are beyond the expertise of most urodynamic laboratories and are uncommonly indicated. Their role is in diagnosis of occult neuropathy or myopathy. In the patient with overt neurologic findings who has bladder dysfunction, neurogenic bladder dysfunction can be deduced without further study. In such cases, a kinesiologic study to identify the pattern of dysfunction is all that is indicated. MUP studies find their role in the evaluation of the patient with bladder dysfunction of unknown cause in whom neuropathy is suspected. They are also used in medicolegal situations in an attempt to correlate voiding symptoms and sexual dysfunction with prior injuries.

Furthermore, MUP may be preferable for ongoing study on underactivity of detrusor or sphincter (Takahash et al, 2000; Jiang et al, 2009a, 2009b, 2010). Today, this abnormality is associated with intrinsic sphincter deficiency (ISD) in patients with SUI, intermittent or constant urinary incontinence after spinal shock in patients suffered from spinal cord injury, multiple system atrophy (MSA) or multiple sclerosis. Unilateral needle EMG of the subcutaneous external anal sphincter muscle, including quantitative MUP analysis is clearly indicated in patients with suspected MSA, particularly in its early stages when the diagnosis is unclear. If the test is normal, but the diagnosis remains unclear, it might be of value to repeat the test later (Libelius & Johansson, 2000, as cited in Podnar, 2007). The main urodynamic finding is lowered MUCP or Valsavour leak point pressure in patients with SUI. There would be subtle myogenic injuries occurred in skeletal sphincter as Takahash found in patients with type 3 SUI (ISD) (Takahash et al, 2000). In order to determine the EMG features of the striated urethral sphincter in patients with type 3 SUI, Takahash et al performed EMG and MUP analysis of the striated urethral sphincter muscle and urodynamic studies in a total of 51 women, 41 female patients with type 3 SUI and 10 women with normal urinary control. MUP of SUI patients showed significantly shorter duration, lower amplitude, and larger number of phases compared with those in the control group. Thirty (73%) of the SUI patients showed an obvious low amplitude (less than 350 mV)/short duration (less than 4.5 milliseconds)/polyphasic pattern and early recruitment of interference activity with low amplitude at voluntary contraction of the striated sphincter, both indicating existence of myogenic damages. These patients showing myogenic damages had significantly lower Valsavour leak point pressure and more leakage in the pad-weigh test compared with the SUI patients without myogenic damage findings. These results suggested that myogenic-dominant damages of the striated urethral sphincter may contribute to the etiology of ISD in most patients with type 3 SUI (Takahash et al, 2000).

2.2 Clinical consideration and EMG significance

It is very important to check the functions of detrusor-sphincter and their relationship with patients with LUTS. If the patients have both detrusor and sphincter intact and in harmony, treatment for other organic or functional disorder, for example, outlet obstruction and lower compliance, is then feasible. From this point of view, excellent measurement of EMG widens the scope of LUTS.

Kinesiologic or EMG studies do not diagnose neuropathy but may characterize its effects. They are indicated in any patient in whom there is a suspicion of discoordination between the sphincter and the bladder. Thus, patients with spinal cord injury, with neurologic disorders (e.g., Parkinson's disease, spinal dysraphism, multiple sclerosis, and MSA), or with voiding dysfunction after radical pelvic surgery or spinal surgery; children with voiding dysfunction and upper tract changes; and young women with urinary retention are appropriate candidates. In this last group, there is evidence that involuntary muscle fiber activity preventing sphincter relaxation may have a hormonal etiology associated with polycystic ovarian disease (Fowler, 1988; Fowler et al., 2003). However, EMG should be interpreted in light of the patient's symptoms, physical findings, and urologic and urodynamic investigations (Abrams et al., 1988; Goldman, 2006; Griffiths et al., 1997). Except in patients with an unusual voiding history, a standard neurologic evaluation of the perineum and lower extremities is usually adequate to exclude most neurologic problems (O'Donnell et al., 1998, as cited in Webster & Guralnick, 2002). Thus, there is limited role for EMG or kinesiologic studies in the routine urodynamic evaluation of incontinent or obstructed patients in whom neuropathy is not suggested by other clinical findings. Furthermore, often video-urodynamic studies provide as much information as is needed in determining the coordination between bladder and sphincter (which can be viewed fluoroscopically) and allow management decisions to be made (Shah, 1994; McGuire et al, 1996, as cited in Webster & Guralnick, 2002). However, if detrusor is relevant to sphincter urodynamically, it is very helpful to use standard urodynamics to evaluate synergia or dyssynergia, in coordination or discoordination. We think video-urodynamics should be used for more sophisticated cases.

2.2.1 Baclofen as a useful agents for patients with dysfunctional voiding

In patients who complained of symptoms of frequency or urge may actually suffer from sphincter overactivity or dysfunctional voiding, to which baclofen (a GABA-ergic receptor agonist) may be administered as a rational option and obtain good response in this case. It was quantitatively analyzed using the TL value, which was successfully applied in a series of assessment. We had conducted a randomized double-blind placebo-controlled crossover trial in 60 women with dysfunctional voiding and LUTD from January 2003 to January 2006; patients were randomly assigned either baclofen 10 mg three times daily, then matching placebo for 4 weeks, or matching placebo then baclofen 10 mg three times daily for 4 weeks, separated by a 2-week washout period. Voiding diaries and multichannel urodynamics (at baseline, 4 and 10 weeks) were used to record the changes of voids/24 h and urodynamic variables. The efficacy analysis of the treatment showed that baclofen was associated with significantly fewer voids/24 h than placebo (mean difference from baseline 5.53 vs 2.70; P=0.001) and a significant increase in TL value (mean difference from baseline, −1.78 vs 0.01, P=0.001). A 4-week course of baclofen significantly reduced the number of voids/24 h and increased the TL value in women with dysfunctional voiding confirmed by anal sphincter EMG with wire electrode. Female patient with dysfunctional voiding (Fig. 5 a) received 4-week course of baclofen and her dysfunctional voiding disappeared at follow-up urodynamics (Fig. 5 b). These encouraging results suggest that baclofen could be used to treat dysfunctional voiding in women (Xu et al., 2007).

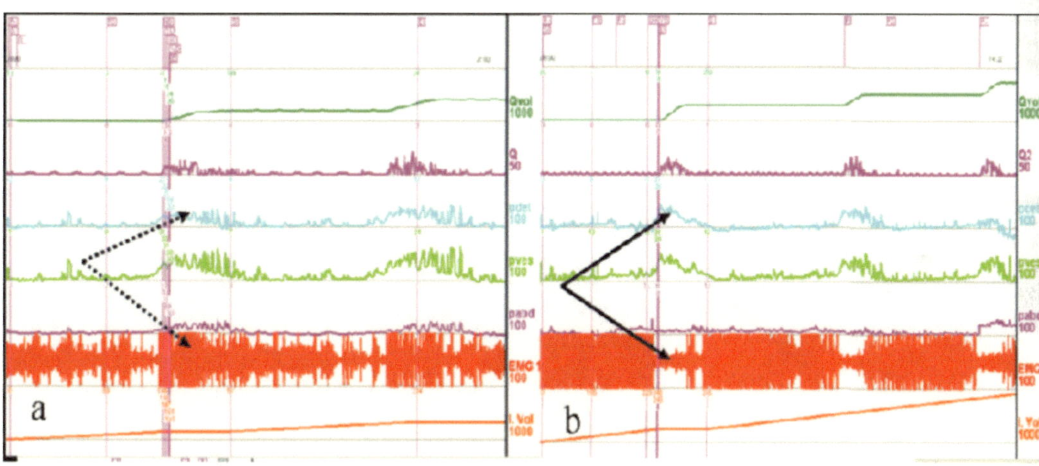

Fig. 5. A female patients aged 42 years old, who complained of urinary frequency for 3 years, was diagnosed as having dysfunctional voiding with a TL value of -0.65 as indicated by dashed arrows (a), and her symptoms improved significantly with a TL value of 0.67 as indicated by solid arrows after 4 weeks of treatment with baclofen during the follow-up urodynamic evaluation (b).

2.2.2 Dysfunctional voiding associated with SUI in female patients with shortened urethral functional profile length and its impact on outcome of tension-free vaginal tape procedure

In order to determine the prevalence of dysfunctional voiding in female SUI and its modification after tension-free vaginal tape (TVT) procedure, three hundred and sixty women with SUI were enrolled and underwent urodynamics from 2002 to 2008. Dysfunctional voiding was determined when non-neurogenic detrusor-sphincter dyssynergia occurred during voluntary voiding (Fig 6 b). It was further quantitatively analyzed using the tense/loose value, a parameter derived from external anal sphincter EMG. The distribution of other urodynamic variables was also evaluated. One hundred and fifty patients underwent the TVT procedure and forty of them were studied with urodynamics after anti-incontinence surgery of TVT during follow up. Overall, dysfunctional voiding was diagnosed in ninety-nine patients (Fig 6 b), with a prevalence of 27.5%. The functional profile length in SUI women with dysfunctional voiding was significantly shorter than that in SUI women without dysfunctional voiding (Fig 6 a) (3.13±0.76 vs 3.32±0.65, $P = 0.017$). After the TVT procedure, the recovery of SUI between cases with and without dysfunctional voiding showed no significant difference. The rate of dysfunctional voiding state change after the surgery, namely from with to without dysfunctional voiding or from without to with dysfunctional voiding, significantly differed between the female patients with and without dysfunctional voiding (66.7% vs 3.6%, $P < 0.05$) during follow up. The dysfunctional voiding improved after the surgery in SUI women with dysfunctional voiding. Dysfunctional voiding might represent a coexistent finding in women with SUI. The main difference of women with SUI and dysfunctional voiding, as compared with those without dysfunctional voiding, was a shortened functional profile length. In such cases, TVT procedure could improve dysfunctional voiding along with the treatment of SUI (Xu et al., 2010).

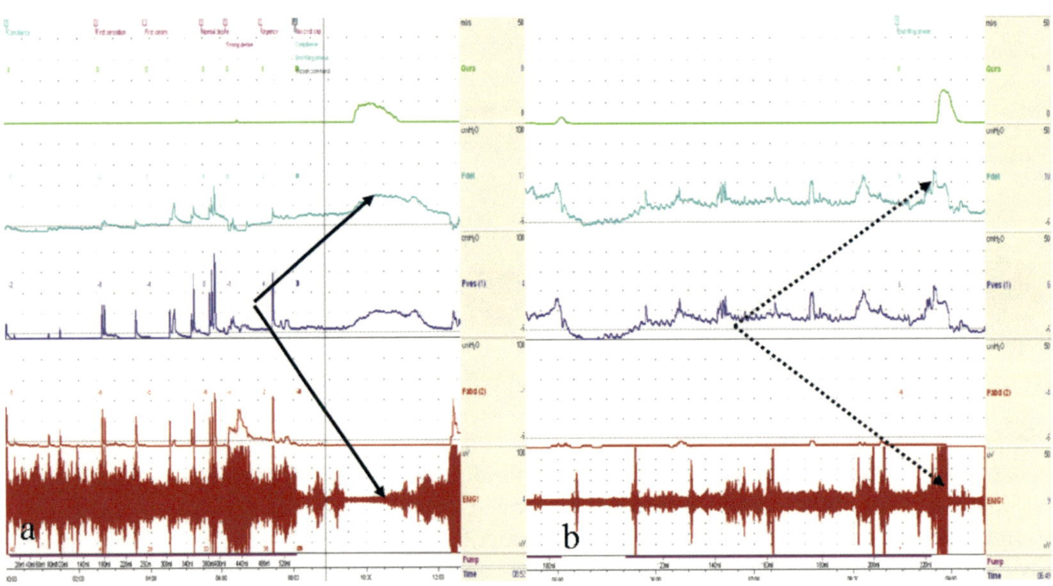

Fig. 6. Urodynamic studies on a female patient with stress urinary incontinence (SUI) without dysfunctional voiding as indicated by solid arrows (DV) (a) and another female patient with SUI and DV as indicated by dashed arrows (b) before the tension-free vaginal tape (TVT) procedure.

2.2.3 Timely selection of necessary surgical intervention for obstructed patients with decreased bladder compliance and intact detrusor contractility

Men older than 45 years old used to select conservative treatments (α-blockade, or 5α-reductase inhibitant, etc.) to treat their lower urinary tract obstructive symptoms, such as frequency, dysuria, and even nocturnal diuresis. If they complained of daily or nocturnal enuresis, the symptoms may be worse than before. This is a critical time point for them. Surgical intervention may be mandatory. Although the voiding reflex remains or detrusor is intact, the detrusor function has declined gradually since incontinence occurs. Between May 2002 and March 2009, a total of 4500 patients underwent urodynamic examination (Life-Tech Urovision Janus V) in this institute. Among them, 1500 male patients old than 45 years with obstructive symptoms were analysed. Among them, there were 15 patients with lower compliance and intact detrusor, and 15 patients with lower compliance and detrusor underactivity enrolled into this trial. Their urodynamics and surgical outcome were compared between the two groups. Routine endoscopic surgeries were carried out for them and those with lower compliance and intact detrusor gained better recovery thereafter as compared with those with detrusor underactivity (Xu et al., 2009) (Fig 7). The main improvement was disappearance of enuresis and increased peak flow rates during follow-up. The patients with detrusor underactivity improved slowly and 33% of them received self-catheterization or urodiversion operation at last. Male patients older than 45 years old complained of obstructive symptoms and nocturnal enuresis should routinely take comprehensive urodynamics. If they were diagnosed with decreased bladder compliance and intact detrusor, surgical intervention is a mandatory option. If they accept the surgical option, their prognosis is very well as compared with those with detrusor underactivity.

2.2.4 Lower compliance at second-half storage phase as main cause of hydroureteronephrosis in patients with diabetes insipidus

Nephrogenic diabetes insipidus with dilatation of upper urinary tract and bladder is rarely reported. Urinary tract dilatation and bladder dysfunction, usually in the form of a large, atonic bladder, are commonly believed to be secondary to high urine output. Low bladder compliance means an abnormal volume and pressure relationship, and an incremental rise in bladder pressure during the bladder filling. It is well known that at the time bladder capacity decreases, intravesical pressure increases, and the risk of upper deterioration increases. Hypocompliance is usually thought to be the range from 1.0 to 20.0 mL/cmH2O. Though the exact cause of hypocompliance is not known, it may be caused by changes in the elastic and viscoelastic properties of the bladder, changes in detrusor muscle tone, or combinations of the two (Park, 2010). The lower bladder compliance patterns could be classified into three groups (Cho et al., 2009). Group A (gradual increase) had the highest correlation with the presence of spinal cord injury. Group B (terminal increase) patients had a history of direct pelvic treatment such as radical prostatectomy and pelvic irradiation. Group C (abrupt increase and plateau) was positively correlated with the presence of detrusor overactivity and nocturnal enuresis. We found that children with polyuria, nocturnal enuresis and MRI-confirmed pituitary abnormality (hypointensities on T1-weighted MRI) and diabetes insipidus usually had hydroureteronephrosis, enlarged bladder capacity and lower bladder compliance at second-half storage phase. Their bladder compliance pattern belonged to terminal increase type as classified by Cho et al. Their detrusor and sphincter function had to be evaluated carefully as the first procedure. If the detrusor could contract and sphincter could relax during the voiding phase, the prognosis is good (Fig. 8), and vice versa. Che et al described 5 patients with nephrogenic diabetes insipidus whose first presentation was bilateral hydroureteronephrosis and chronic renal insufficiency (Che et al, 2009). Between May 2005 and March 2009, 5 boys came to our clinic with complaint of polydipsia and polyuria (4), bilateral flank pain (2), and fatigue (2). Ultrasonic scan found bilateral hydroureteronephrosis in all 5 patients and blood creatinine test showed renal insufficiency. Fluid deprivation test were performed and according to the results they were diagnosed as nephrogenic diabetes insipidus. All patients were catheterized for 7 to 18 days till blood creatinine level decreased as normal. Urodynamics showed that the mean values of the bladder capacity, detrusor pressure at the mid and end of filling, maximum flow rate (Qmax), and PVR were 760 ml, 15.0 and 40.5 cm H2O, 30.8 ml/s, and 436.3 ml, respectively. These results reminded us all these patients had a lower

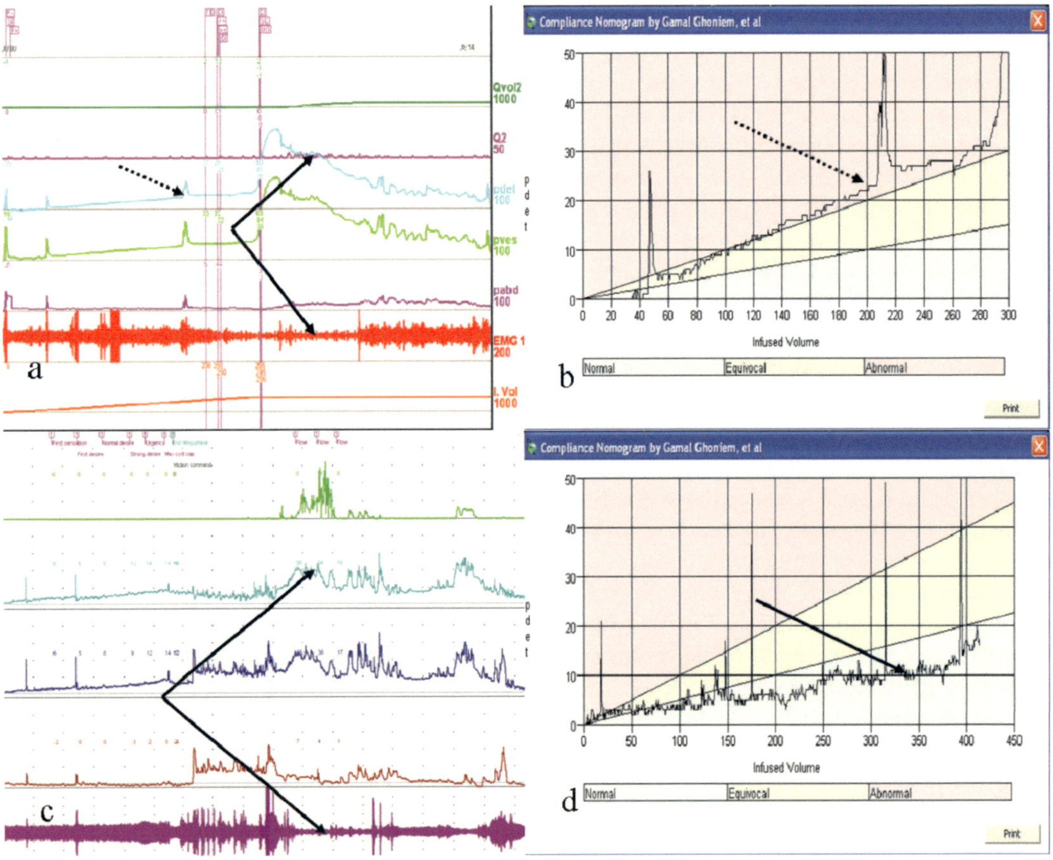

Fig. 7. A male patient aged 65 years old, who complained of poor-weak flow and urinary frequency for 5 years and nocturial enuresis for the last 5 months, was confirmed as having bladder outlet obstruction and lower bladder compliance as indicated by dashed arrow, however, his detrusor and sphincter function was still intact with detrusor-sphincter synergia as indicated by solid arrows (a, b), and his symptoms at follow-up recovered 6 months after a successful TURP with a normal flow rate and compliance thereafter as indicated by solid arrow (c, d).

compliance at second-half storage phase. Given that the detrusor and sphincter function well as displayed on EMG, operation or desmopressin are rational option for patients with obstruction or diabetes insipidus. The patients had taken desmopressin acetate (0.1 mg, 1/d), emphatic and timed voiding for three months, and then all symptoms were improved slightly. And after a follow of 4 to 12 months, renal function remained normal and PVR was reduced. Nephrogenic diabetes insipidus should be considered in patients with dilatation of the urinary tract and polyuria. A lower compliance at second-half storage phase may contribute to the dilatation of urinary tract. Normal detrusor contractility with large PVR is a unique manifestation of this condition.

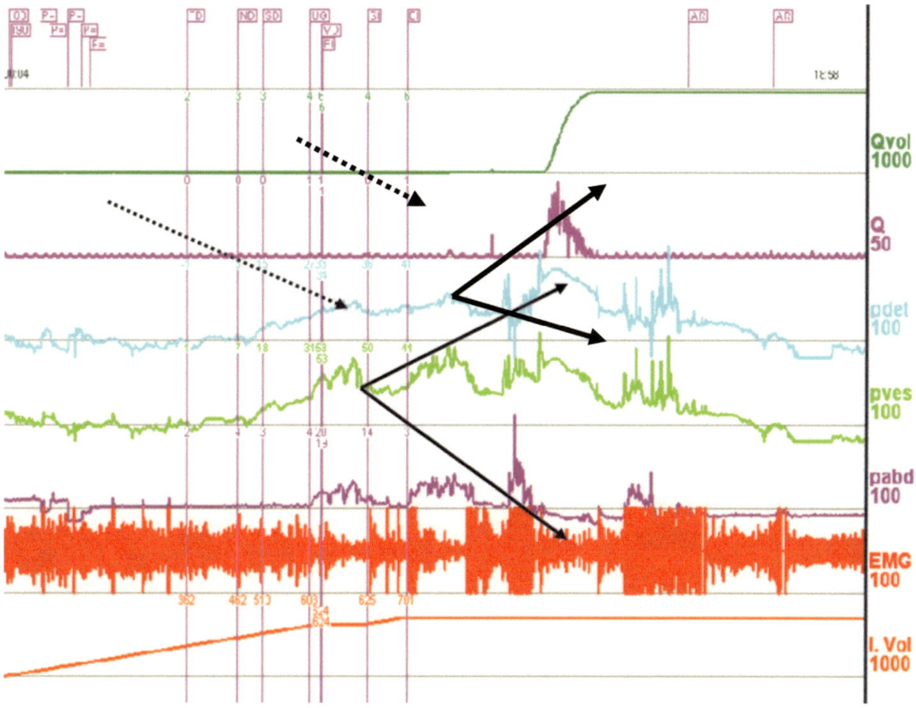

Fig. 8. A male patient aged 15 years old, complaining of pelvic pain and polyuria for more than 5 years, was found with hydroureteronephrosis and atrophy of the posterior lobe of the pituitary gland (hypointensitites on T1-weighted MRI of the pituitary gland). His functional bladder capacity reached 800 ml, and lower bladder compliance was terminal at a bladder volume of 400 ml as indicated by dashed arrow, whereas his detrusor contracted and sphincter relaxed normally when he initiated a voiding reflex as indicated by solid arrows.

2.2.5 Validation of somatic-autonomic nerve anastomosis or artificial somatic-autonomic reflex pathway for the purpose of re-establishing bladder function

In the field of neurogenic LUTD, abnormal changes of EMG should not be neglected as well. So far different opinions exist about the so-called "artificial somatic-autonomic reflex pathway" for patients complained of dysuria and incontinence after spinal cord injury or with spina bifida. Whether the operation succeeds or not depends upon exhibition of detrusor contraction and still remaining of detrusor and external sphincter dyssynergia. Theoretically, this type of neuro-anastomosis could not reverse dyssynergia. There were three kinds of neuro-anastomosis for patients with neurogenic LUTD due to spinal cord injury in China (with intercostals nerve: one author; with ventral roots of the lumbar or sacral nerves: two authors) (Fig. 9). They are: intercostal nerve anastomosed to pudendal nerve (Zhang & Zhao, 1993), T10 or T11 ventral root above the lesion anastomosed to the S2 ventral roots for complete conus medullaris injury with atonia bladder or detrusor underactivity, or S1 ventral root under the lesion anastomosed to the S2 or S3 ventral roots for hyperreflexic neurogenic bladder and external sphincter dyssynergia caused by complete suprasacral SCI (Lin et al., 2008a, 2008b, 2009, 2010); L5 ventral root under the lesion anastomosed to S2 or S3 ventral roots for hyperreflexic neurogenic bladder and external sphincter dyssynergia (Xiao et al., 2005; Xiao, 2006).

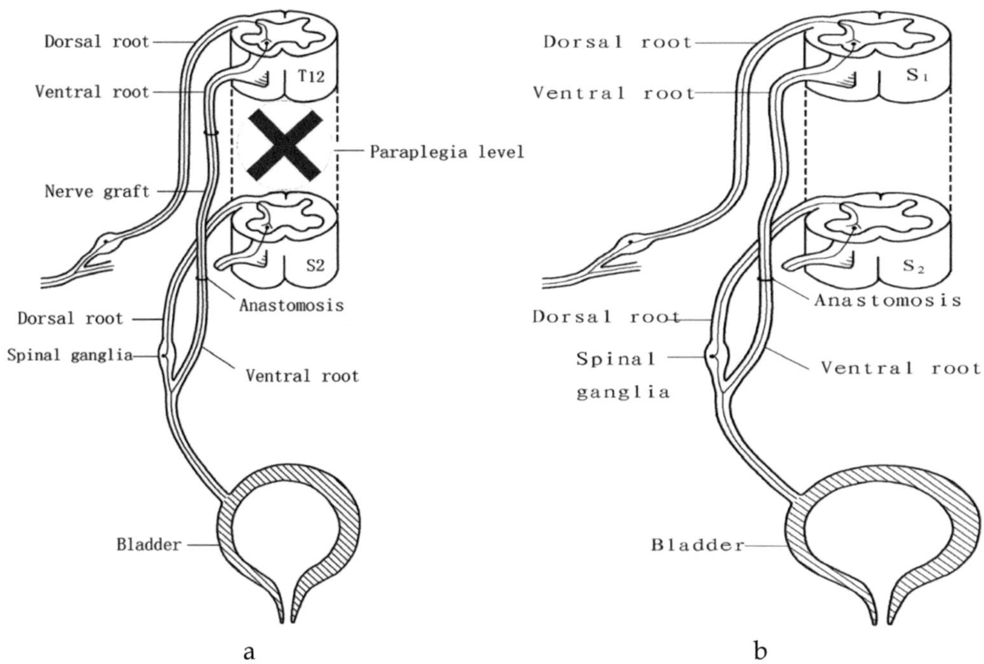

Fig. 9. Creation of microsurgical anastomoses between T12 and S2 ventral roots (a). Drawing showing creation of microsurgical anastomoses between S-1 and S-2 ventral roots (b). Reproduced from Lin and Hou (2010, *Neurosurgery* 66: 948-952; 2009, *Journal of Neurosurgery of Spine* 10: 452-457) with permission.

We have shown the detrusor contraction and sphincter overactivity in some patients suffered from spinal cord injury who received a successful procedure of artificial somatic-autonomic reflex pathway (T10 anastomosed to S2) for bladder control in this institution. One of them with neurogenic detrusor underactivity and sphincter overactivity due to L1 fracture received operation of neuroanastomosis nine years ago. Her spontaneous voiding pattern recovered 1 year later and continued to be normal thereafter. Urodynamic follow-up data showed clearly detrusor contraction and some degree of external sphincter dyssynergia (Fig 10). Whereas in the papers of other authors, who used surface patch electrode, which was inferior to CNE for EMG documentation of urethral sphincter relaxation during voiding phase (Mahajan et al., 2006), the so-called "satisfactory voluntary voiding with detrusor contraction" could still be debated and improved (Xiao, 2006).

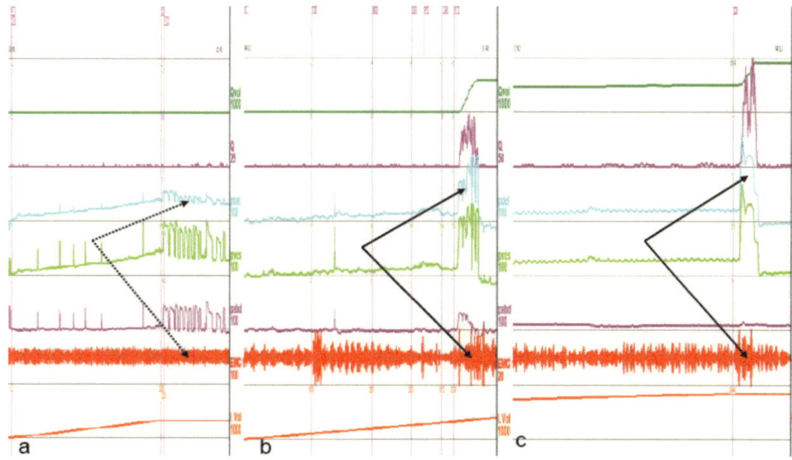

Fig. 10. A female patient aged 46 years old, complained of paraplegia due to fracture of L1 for 9 yeas, urodynamic study before the procedure (a), 5 years (b) and 9 years (c) after successful artificial somatic-autonomic reflex pathway procedure showed that detrusor was underactive before the operation (as dashed arrows indicated), and after the procedure, detrusor became contractile and detrusor-sphincter dyssynergia still remained (as solid arrows indicated). Voluntary voiding and bladder emptying was satisfactory with detrusor contraction and without abdominal straining. EMG, electromyogram; I. Vol, infused volume; Pabd, abdominal pressure; Pdet, detrusor pressure; Pves, vesical pressure; Q, flow rate; Qvol, uro volume.

2.2.6 Detrusor underactivity and symptomless detrusor underactivity

Detrusor underactivity (DUA) is recently known as underactive bladder, which is a diagnosis made on a simultaneous PFS and EMG (Chancellor & Kaufman, 2008; Thomas, et al., 2005). Such condition is characterized by a low sustained or wave-like contraction and is associated with poor flow or no flow at all. The ICS defines DUA as "a detrusor contraction of inadequate magnitude and/or duration to effect complete bladder emptying in the absence of urethral obstruction" (Griffiths et al., 1997). During conventional urodynamic measurements, adequate emptying of the bladder, without a detrusor contraction is possible in two ways. Firstly, in females who can have a very good relaxation of the pelvic floor; in this case, hardly any detrusor contraction is needed for complete voiding (Fig. 11a). These patients are considered to be 'normal', or belongs to symptomless detrusor underactivity. Secondly, in patients using abdominal straining without simultaneous sphincter relaxation to empty their bladder (Fig. 11b). These cases are considered to be 'abnormal'. (van Koeveringe et al., 2009). In a comparative study, ambulatory urodynamic measurements/monitoring was conducted in 25 patients categorized as suspected acontractile bladder by conventional urodynamic measurements. Of the 25 patients with a suspected acontractile detrusor based on the conventional urodynamic measurements data, 21 patients had multiple detrusor contractions during voiding attempts on ambulatory urodynamic measurements during normal daily life activities. Four patients even showed overactive detrusor contractions on their ambulatory urodynamic measurements. This implies that the symptoms of these patients must have been due to other factors such as pelvic muscular nonrelaxation, psychological reasons or obstruction. Only in 17% (four of 24 cases) the acontractile bladder was confirmed by ambulatory urodynamic measurements. (van Koeveringe et al., 2009). In order to display abdominal straining, the anal catheter must be fixed firmly so as to avoid its exodus from the anus. The female patient had better to change the position from supine to sitting. Sitting position was more normal than supine. (Xu et al., 2009, a).

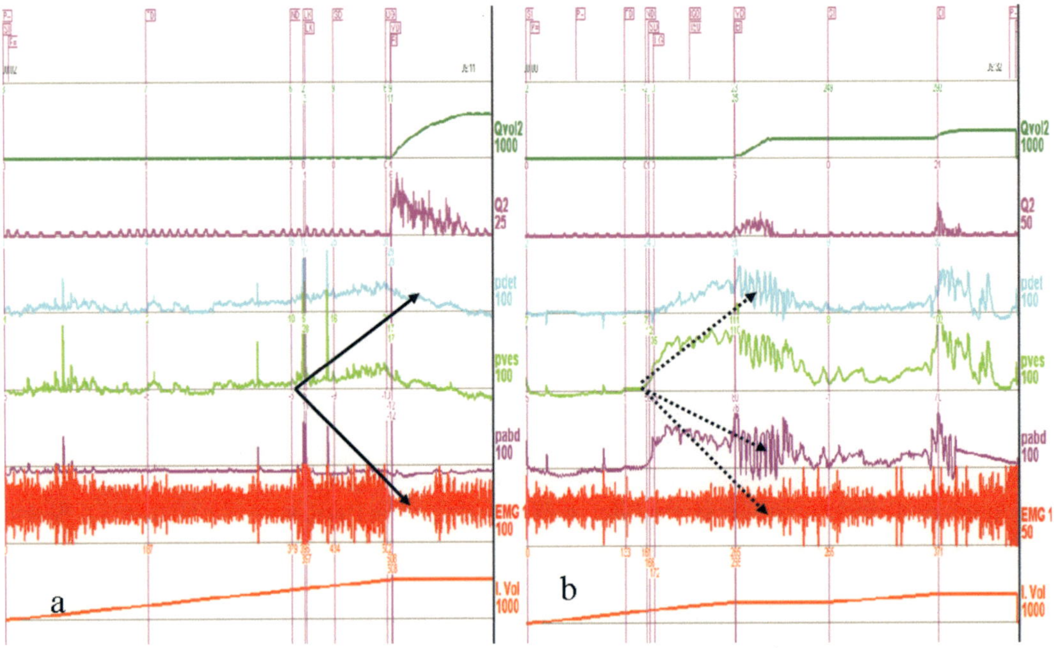

a b

Fig. 11. Detrusor underactivity in women: a female patient aged 50 years old, complained of urine loss with cough/laugh for 3 months. She finished urination fluently even without detrusor contraction and her sphincter relaxation was complete as indicated by solid arrows (a), another female aged 73 years old, complained of poor-weak flow and pain with voiding for 4 years (b). She was found passing urine by using abdominal straining without simultaneous sphincter relaxation to empty their bladder (b).

In order to study the efficacy of low-frequency electrotherapy (LFE) for female patients with an early stage DUA due to neuromuscular deficiency, we have conducted a conservative treatment program to patients with DUA. Between April 2008 and April 2010, a total of 35 female patients with urodynamically confirmed DUA were subjected to LFE using an electrical stimulator (ES-420, Ito CO, Ltd. Tokyo, Japan). Patients received two treatment sessions (each lasting for 70 min) daily for two weeks. Patients were divided into DUA-NC (n=20, DUA with normal compliance) or DUA-LC (n=15, DUA with low compliance). Comprehensive urodynamic evaluations were performed in each patient prior to the LFE as the baseline and at 4 weeks following the procedure. At last, of the 20 patients with DUA-NC, 18 (90%) regained detrusor contractility after LFE (Fig. 12). The pattern of their detrusor contraction changed from low sustained contraction (in 5 cases), or wave-like contraction (13 cases) to normal parabola contraction. The percent of patients with DUA-NC who relied on catheterization for bladder emptying decreased by 40% (from 50% to 10%, P<0.001). Those with DUA-LC decreased by only 6.7% (from 86.7% to 80%, P>0.05) and none regained detrusor contractility following LFE. LFE was more effective for patients with DUA-NC than for those with DUA-LC. Patients with DUA-NC due to an early stage neuromuscular deficiency benefited from LFE but those with DUA-LC did not benefit from this procedure

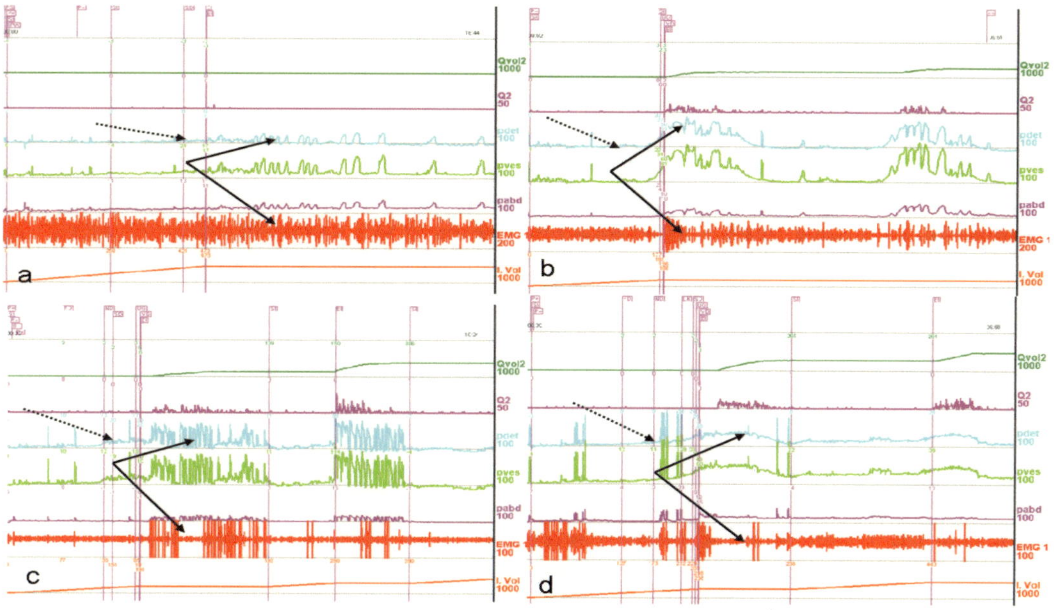

Fig. 12. Comprehensive urodynamic tracings of female patients with DUA-NC and the efficacy of LFE were displayed. The dashed arrows indicate normal compliance and solid arrows indicate the state of the detrusor contractility and the sphincter relaxing ability during voiding phase. (a) A women aged 32 years old, complained of chronic retention for 2 weeks due to iatrogenic reason, and her detrusor was still underactive when more than 500 ml saline was infused into the bladder. (b) After LFE, her detrusor function recovered, sphincter overactivity improved and got rid of catheterization thereafter. (c) A female patient, 52 years old, complained of urgency and frequency for two months, urodynamic study showed DUA and sphincter overactivity before LFE. (d) After the procedure, detrusor became contractile and sphincter overactivity still remained. EMG, electromyogram; I. Vol, infused volume; Pabd, abdominal pressure; Pdet, detrusor pressure; Pves, vesical pressure; Q, flow rate; Qvol, uro volume.

2.2.7 Significance of symptoms and existing discrepancy between symptomatic and laboratory findings, and between symptomatic location and investigative location

There exists discrepancy between symptomatic and urodynamic findings in patients with LUTD. It is generally known that most epidemiological studies have relied on questionnaires to obtain widespread information about prevalence, symptoms, treatment usage and compliance; however, the results of such surveys must be interpreted with caution. So we should not let this prevent us from furthering our disease awareness via the use of physiological tests including urodynamics combined with sphincter EMG (Agur et al., 2009). In October 2006 The National Institute for Health and Clinical Excellence (NICE) published guidance on the management of urinary incontinence in women. (NICE, 2006). The guideline states that "the use of multichannel cystometry is not routinely recommended before surgery in women with a clearly defined clinical diagnosis of pure SUI". However, in a retrospective study of 6276 women with urinary incontinence, Agur W et al found that only 324 (5.2%) women had pure SUI; moreover, a quarter of those with pure SUI symptoms ultimately had urodynamic diagnoses other than urodynamic SUI, that could affect the outcome of continence surgery. These findings indicated that only a small group of women fulfiled the NICE criteria of pure SUI. These strict criteria did not ensure that all women with potentially important urodynamic findings were evaluated accordingly. The symptomatic assessment had a sensitivity of only 11.4%, and specificity of 98%. There were 1866 false negative cases with a negative predictive value of 69%, including voiding dysfunction (506 cases, 24.0%), overactive bladder wet (OAB wet) (1209 cases, 57.4%), OAB dry (151 cases, 7.2%) and 83 false positive cases with a positive predictive value of 74%, including normal (35 cases, 10.8%), voiding dysfunction (4 cases, 1.2%), and detrusor overactivity (44 cases, 13.6%). (Agur et al., 2009). Furthermore, even the symptom location of the patients is usually very factitious and sometimes vague and so clinical investigation is necessary. What characteristics of the pain caused patients with interstitial cystitis/painful bladder syndrome to perceive that it involved the bladder was wondered by many surgeons. Recently, preliminary work for a RAND (Santa Monica, CA) prevalence study of interstitial cystitis/painful bladder syndrome revealed difficulty in finding a single symptom-based definition of interstitial cystitis/painful bladder syndrome with both sufficient sensitivity and specificity to separate patients with interstitial cystitis/painful bladder syndrome from those with physician-diagnosed OAB, vulvodynia, or endometriosis. (Berry, et al., 2010, as cited in Warren et al., 2011). The symptoms of other syndromes, for example, irritable bowel syndrome, and systemic syndromes, such as fibromyalgia, do overlap those of interstitial cystitis/painful bladder syndrome. (Warren et al., 2009, as cited in Warren et al., 2011). Symptoms are the heralds of a disease that prompt a patient to seek medical care. It then is the task of the patient and clinician to reveal a sufficient description of the symptoms to prompt an appropriate diagnosis of the disease. If symptoms overlap to a large degree, it would imply that the distinction among these various syndromes is rather arbitrary. An extrapolation of this logic to the pelvic and systemic syndromes we have noted suggests that a similarity of symptoms might have only nosologic implications; if boundaries cannot be identified between syndromes, are they different diseases? Based on above-mentioned data, in order to locate the origin of symptoms and to validate the nature of the disease, necessary examination, including urodynamics and EMG, had to be carried out.

3. Conclusion

Anal sphincter EMG is an indispensable parameter for diagnosis and treatment option for patients with LUTD or pelvic floor dysfunction. It could present functional state of the urethral sphincter, and further replace urethral sphincter EMG thereafter. According to our experience, nearly 70%-80% so-called "artifacts" or bad recordings of EMG came actually from an open circuit, not from a closed circuit, of the electrocircuit system. We must make every effort to record an excellent EMG trace for the purpose of developing evidence-based medicine as well as performance-based medicine, not only based on experience-based medicine.

4. Acknowledgment

The authors wish to express appreciation to Youhua Zhu, Zhilian Min, Changlin Mei, Yiyong Liu, Jun Zhou, Juan Du, Chunlin Hou, Haodong Lin, Junjie Zou, Xuehua Ding and Shen Zhang for their outstanding efforts in data management; to Hong Meng and Bing He for statistical help; and to Yi Ge, Cheng Zhong, Bing He and Xingwei Liu for their constant support.

5. References

Abrams, P.; Blaivas, J.G.; Stanton, S.L.; & Andersen, J.T. (1988). The Standardization of Terminology of Lower Urinary Tract Function. *Scand J Urol Nephrol,* Vol.114, No.Suppl, pp.5-19

Agur, W.; Housami, F.; Drake M.; & Abrams P. (2009). Could the National Institute for Health and Clinical Excellence Guidelines on Urodynamics in Urinary Incontinence Put Some Women at Risk of a Bad Outcome from Stress Incontinence Surgery? *BJU International*, Vol.103, No.5, (March 2009), pp. 635-639

Akkad, T.; Pelzer, A.; Mitterberger, M.; et al. (2007). Influence of Intravesical Potassium on Pelvic Floor Activity in Women with Overactive Bladder Syndrome: Comparative Urodynamics Might Provide better Detection of Dysfunctional Voiding. *BJU International*, Vol.100, No.4, (October 2007), pp. 830-834

Aminoff, M.J. (2007). Electrophysiology, In: Textbook of Clinical Neurology, 3rd ed., Goetz (Ed.), 477-497, Saunders, ISBN, Philadelphia, USA

Blaivas, J.; Chancellor, M.; Weins, J.; & Verhaaren, M. (2007). *Atlas of Urodynamics.* 2nd edition, 69-82, Blackwell Publishing, ISBN: 978-1-4051-4625-8, Oxford, UK

Carlson, K.V.; Rome S.; Nitti, V.W. (2001). Dysfunctional Voiding in Women. *Journal of Urology,* Vol.165, No.1, (January 2001), pp. 143–148

Chancellor, M.; & Kaufman, J. (2008). Case for Pharmacotherapy Development for Underactive Bladder. *Urology*, Vol.75, pp. 966-967

Che, J.P; Xu, D.F.; Cui, X.G.; Liu, Y.S.; Gao, Y.; Chen, J.; & Qu, C.Y. (2009). Lower Compliance at

Second-half Storage Phase as Main Cause of Hydroureteronephrosis in Patients with Diabetes Insipidus. *Urology*, Vol.74 No.suppl 4A, (October 2009), pp. S294.

Chen, K.J.; Peng, H.Y.; Cheng, C.L.; et al. (2007). Acute Unilateral Ureteral Distension Inhibits Glutamate-dependent Spinal Pelvic-Urethra Reflex Potentiation via GABAergic Neurotransmission in Anesthetized Rats. *American Journal of Physiology-Renal Physiology,* Vol.292, pp. F1007–F1015

Chen, S.L.; Huang, Y.H.; Kao, Y.L.; et al. (2008). Acute Anal Stretch Inhibits NMDA-Dependent Pelvic-urethra Reflex Potentiation via Spinal GABAergic Inhibition in Anesthetized Rats. *American Journal of Physiology-Renal Physiology*, Vol.295, pp.F923-F931

Cho, S.Y.; Yi, J.S.; & Oh, S.J. (2009). The Clinical Significance of Poor Bladder Compliance. *Neurourology & Urodynamics*, Vol.28, pp. 1010–1014

Chuang, F.C.; & Kuo, H.C. (2007). Correlation of Bladder Base Elevation with Pelvic Floor Hypertonicity in Women with Lower Urinary Tract Symptoms. *Neurourology & Urodynamics*, Vol.26, No.4, (July 2007), pp. 502–506

Cui, X.G.; Xu, D.F.; Zhu, F.Y.; Jiang, H.H.; Lv, C.; & Qu, C.Y. (2009). Radian of the Wire-Electrodes and its Influence on the Amplitude and Quality of Electromyogram for Patients with Detrusor Stable Lower Urinary Tract Dysfunction. *Urology*, Vol.74, No.suppl 4A, (October 2009), pp. S293

Deindl, F.M.; Vodusek D.B.; Bischoff CH.; Hofmann R. & Hartung R. (1998). Dysfunctional Voiding in Women: Which Muscles are Responsible? *British Journal of Urology*, Vol. 82, No.6, (December 1998), pp. 814–819

Finsterer, J. EMG-Interference Pattern Analysis. (2001). *Journal of Electromyography & Kinesiology*, Vol.11, pp. 231–246

Fowler, C.J.; Christmas, T.J.; Chapple, C.R.; Parkhouse, H.F.; Kirby, R.S.; & Jacobs, H.S. (1988). Abnormal Eelectromyographic Activity of the Urethral Sphincter, Voiding Dysfunction, and Polycystic Ovaries: a New Syndrome? *British Medical Journal*, Vol.297, pp. 1436–1438

Fowler CJ. Urinary retention in women. (2003). *BJU International*, Vol.91: pp. 463–464

Goldman, H.B.; & Zimmern, P.E. (2006). The Treatment of Female Bladder Outlet Obstruction. *BJU International*, Vol.98, No.2, (August 2006), pp. 359-366

Griffiths, D.; Hofner, K.; van Mastrigt, R.; Rollema, H.J.; Spamgberg, A.; & Gleason, D. (1997). Standardisation of Terminology of Lower Urinary Tract Function: Pressure-Flow Studies of Voiding, Urethral Resisitance and Urethral Obstruction. International Continence Society Subcommittee on Standardization of Terminology of Pressure-Flow Studies. *Neurourology & Urodynamics*, Vol.16, No.1, (January 1997), pp. 1–18

Hinman, F.Jr. (1986). Nonneurogenic Neurogenic Bladder (the Hinman Syndrome)--15 Years later. *Journal of Urology*, Vol.136, pp. 769-777

Jiang, H.H.; Gustilo-Ashby, A.M.; Salcedo, L.B.; et al. (2009). Electrophysiological Function during Voiding after Simulated Childbirth Injuries. *Experimental Neurology*, Vol. 215, No.2, (February 2009), pp. 342-348

Jiang, H.H.; Pan, H.Q.; Gustilo-Ashby, M.A.; et al. (2009). Dual Simulated Childbirth Injuries Result in Slowed Recovery of Pudendal Nerve and Urethral Function. *Neurourology & Urodynamics*, Vol.28, No.3, (March 2009), pp. 229-235

Jiang, H.H.; Salcedo, L.B.; Song, B.; & Damaser, M.S. (2010). Pelvic Floor Muscles and the External Urethral Sphincter Have Different Responses to Applied Bladder Pressure during Continence. *Urology*, Vol.75, No.6, (June 2010), pp. 1515.e1–1515.e7

Kamo, I., Cannon, T.W.; Conway, D.A.; Torimoto, K.; Chancellor, M.B.; de Groat, W.C.; & Yoshimura, N. (2004). The Role of Bladder-to-Urethral Reflexes in Urinary Continence Mechanisms in Rats. *American Journal of Physiology-Renal Physioogy*, Vol.287, pp. F434-F441

Kavia, R; DasGupta, R.; Critchley H.; Fowler C. & Griffiths D. (2010). A Functional Magnetic Resonance Imaging Study of the Effect of Sacral Neuromodulation on Brain Responses in Women with Fowler's Syndrome. *BJU International*, Vol.105, No.3, (February 2010), pp. 366–372

Kuo, H.C. Dysfunctional Voiding and Bladder Neck Dysfunction. (2010). *Incontinence & Pelvic Floor*

Dysfunction. Vol.4, No.4, (December 2010), pp.115, ISSN 1994-568X

Lin, H.D.; Hou, C.L.; Zhen, X.Y.; et al. (2009). Clinical Study of Reconstructed Bladder Innervation below the Level of Spinal Cord Injury to Produce Urination by Achilles Tendon to Bladder Reflex Contractions. *Journal of Neurosurgery of Spine*, Vol.10, pp. 452-457

Lin, H.D.; Hou, C.L.; Zhong, G.; et al. (2008). Reconstruction of Reflex Pathways to the Atonic Bladder after Conus Medullaris Injury: Preliminary Clinical Results. *Microsurgery*, Vol.28, pp. 429-435

Lin, H.D.; Hou, C.L.; Chen, A.M.; & Xu, Z. (2010). Innervation of Reconstructed Bladder above the Level of Spinal Cord Injury for Inducing Micturition by Contractions of the Abdomen-to-Bladder Reflex Arc. *Neurosurgery* Vol.66, pp. 948-952,

Lin, H.D.; Hou, C.L.; & Zhen XY. (2008). Bypassing Spinal Cord Injury: Surgical Reconstruction of Afferent and Efferent Pathways to the Urinary Bladder after Conus Medullaris Injury in a Rat Model. *Journal of Reconstructive Microsurgery*. Vol.24, No.8, pp. 575-581

Mahajan, S.T.; Fitzgerald, M.P.; Kenton, K., et al. (2006). Concentric Needle Electrodes Are Superior to Perineal Surface-patch Electrodes for Electromyographic Documentation of Urethral Sphincter Relaxation during Voiding. *BJU International*, Vol.97, No.1, (January 2006), pp. 117-120

Nandedkar, S.D.; Sanders, D.B.; & Stalberg, E.V. (1986). Simulation and Analysis of the Electromyographic Interference Pattern in Normal Muscle. Part II: Activity, Upper Centile Amplitude, and Number of Small Segments. *Muscle Nerve*, Vol.9, pp. 486-90

NICE. Urinary Incontinence. The Management of Urinary Incontinence in Women. NICE Clinical Guidline 40, 2006; 40. Available at: http://www.nice.org.uk/nicemedia/pdf/CG40NICEguideline.pdf. Accessed 4 November 2008

Park W.H. (2010). Management of Low Compliant Bladder in Spinal Cord Injured Patients. *Lower Urinary Tract Symptoms*, Vol.2, No.2, (September 2010), pp. 61 - 70, ISSN: 1757-5664

Podnar, S. (2007). Neurophysiology of the Neurogenic Lower Urinary Tract Disorders. *Clinical Neurophysiology*, Vol.118, No.7, (July 2007), pp. 1423–1437

Podnar, S.; Vodusek, D.B.; & Stalberg, E. (2000). Standardization of Anal Sphincter Electromyography: Normative Data. *Clinical Neurophysiology*, Vol.111, No.13, (December 2000), pp. 2200-2207

Rudy, E.; & Woodside, J. (1991). Non-neurogenic Neurogenic Bladder: The Relationship between Intravesical Pressure and the External Sphincter Electromyogram. *Neurourology & Urodynamics*, Vol.10, No.2, (April 1991), pp169-176

Stöhrer, M.; Blok, B.; Castro-Diaz, D.; Chartier-Kastler, E.; et al. (2009). EAU Guidelines on Neurogenic Lower Urinary Tract Dysfunction. *European Urology*, Vol.56, No.1, (July 2009), pp. 81-88

Takahash, S.; Homma, Y.; Fujishiro, T.; Hosaka, Y.; Kitamura, T.; & Kawabe K. (2000). Electromyographic Study of the Striated Urethral Sphincter in type 3 Stress Incontinence: Evidence of Myogenic-Dominant Damages. *Urology*, Vol.56, No.6, (December 2000), pp. 946–950

Thomas, A.W.; Cannon, A.; Bartlett, E.; Ellis-Jones, J.; & Abrams, P. (2005). The Natural History of Lower Urinary Tract Dysfunction in Men: Minimum 10-year

Urodynamic Follow-up of Untreated Detrusor Underactivity. *BJU International*, Vol.96, pp. 1295-1300

van Koeveringe, G.A.; Rahnama'I, M.S.; & Berghmans B.C.M. (2009). The Additional Value of Ambulatory Urodynamic Measurements Compared with Conventional urodynamic measurements. *BJU International*, Vol.105, pp.508-513

Wang, A.C.; & Chen, M.C. (2003). The Correlation between Preoperative Voiding Mechanism and Surgical Outcome of the Tension-Free Vaginal Tape Procedure, with Reference to Quality of Life. *BJU International*, Vol.91, No.6, (January 2003), pp. 502-506

Warren, J.W.; Diggs, C.; Horne L.; & Greenberg, P. (2011). Interstitial Cystitis/Painful Bladder Syndrome: What Do Patients Mean by "Perceived" Bladder Pain?. *Urology*, Vol.xx, No.X, (XXX 2011), pp.XX-XX doi:10.1016/j.urology.2010.08.030

Webster, G.D. & Guralnick, M.D. (2002). The Neurourologic Evaluation, In: *Walsh:Campbell's Urology*, 8th ed., P.C. Walsh (Ed.), 905-925, Saunders Elsevier, ISBN 13: 978-0-8089-2353-4, Philadelphia, USA

Wiseman, O.J.; Swinn, M.; Brady, C.; & Fowler, C.J. (2001). Urethral Sphincter Volume and Maximum Urethral Closure Pressure in Women with Urinary Retention. *BJU International*, Vol.88, pp. 286–287

Xiao, C.G. (2006). Reinnervation for Neurogenic Bladder: Historic Review and Introduction of a Somatic-autonomic Reflex Pathway Procedure for Patients with Spinal Cord Injury or Spina Bifida. *European Urology*, Vol.49, No.1, (January 2006), pp. 22–29

Xiao, C.G.; Du, M.X.; Li, B. ; et al. (2005). An Artificial Somatic-Autonomic Reflex Pathway Procedure for Bladder Control in Children with Spinal Bifida. *Journal of Urology*, Vol.173, No.6, (June 2005), pp. 2112-2116

Xu, D.F.; Qu, C.Y.; Meng, H.; Ren, J.Z.; Zhu, Y.H.; Min, Z.L.; Kong, Y.L. (2007). Dysfunctional Voiding Confirmed by Transdermal Perineal Electromyography, and Its Effective Treatment with Baclofen in Women with Lower Urinary Tract Symptoms: a Randomized Double-Blind Placebo-Controlled Crossover Trial. *BJU International*, Vol.100, No.3, (September 2007), PP. 588-592

Xu, D.F.; Qu, C.Y.; Ren, J.Z.; et al. (2010). Impact of Tension-Free Vaginal Tape Procedure on Dysfunctional Voiding in Women with Stress Urinary Incontinence. *International Journal of Urology*, Vol.17, No.4, (April 2010) pp. 346-352

Xu, D.F.; Lu L.; Cui, X.G.; Wang, R.Y.; & Qu, C.Y. (2009). A Long-term Observation on Technique Remoulding and Accessory Modification for Gaining Precise High Quality Results in Urodynamic Examination. *Urology*, Vol.74, No.suppl 4A, (October 2009), pp. S293-S294

Xu, D.F.; Che J.P.; Cui X.G.; Gao, Y.; Yao, Y.; Ren, J.Z.; Chen, M.; Chen, J.; & Qu, C.Y. (2009). Timely Selection of Necessary Surgical Intervention for Obstructed patients with Decreased Bladder Compliance and Intact Detrusor Contractility. *Urology*, Vol.74, No.suppl 4A, (October 2009), pp. S32

Zhang, S.C. & Zhao, J. (1993). Gatism Treated with Neuroanastomosis. *J Neurol Orthop Med Surg*, Vol.14, pp. 37-38.

10

Electromyography of Pelvic Floor Muscles in Rats

Yolanda Cruz Gómez[1], Hai-Hong Jiang[2,3], Paul Zaszczurynski[4], Raúl Juárez[5], César Pastelin[6] and Margot S. Damaser[2,3,4]
[1]*Centro Tlaxcala de Biología de la Conducta, Universidad Autónoma de Tlaxcala, Tlax.*
[2]*Glickman Urological & Kidney Institute, the Cleveland Clinic, Cleveland, OH*
[3]*Department of Biomedical Engineering, the Cleveland Clinic, Cleveland, OH*
[4]*Advanced Platform Technology Rehabilitation Research & Development Center Louis Stokes VA Medical Center, Cleveland, OH*
[5]*Maestría en Ciencias Biológicas, Universidad Autónoma de Tlaxcala,Tlax.*
[6]*Doctorado en Neuroetología, Universidad Veracruzana, Ver.*
[1,5,6]*México*
[2,3,4]*USA*

1. Introduction

The pelvic floor muscles (PFM) form a hammock-like structure that closes the pelvic outlet and supports the pelvic viscera to maintain their position (Ashton-Miller et al. 2001). As such, they are important for maintenance of continence, both urinary and fecal, particularly in women, since women have a smaller external urethral sphincter (EUS). Dysfunction of these muscles is clinically related to female pelvic floor disorders, a spectrum of conditions that include pelvic organ prolapse as well as both urinary and fecal incontinence (Ashton-Miller & Delancey 2009; Shafik 2000; Thor & de Groat 2010).

Electromyography (EMG) is commonly used clinically to assess the integrity of the PFM, which include the coccygeus, iliococcygeus, and pubococcygeus (Ashton-Miller & Delancey 2009; Thor & de Groat 2010; Weidner et al. 2000; Weidner et al. 2000). Muscle activity is usually recorded through the anus or vagina using needle or surface electrodes during voluntary contraction of the PFM, during micturition, or during abdominal Credé maneuvers (Ashton-Miller & Delancey 2009; Chantraine & de 1978; Thor & de Groat 2010; Weidner et al. 2000a; Weidner et al. 2000b). This technique assumes that the pelvic floor behaves as a single unit and EMG recordings are comparable regardless of the recording location or the methods used. However, the PFM is not a single muscle. For example, only a limited number of PFM fibers are in close anatomical relation to the urethra, and therefore are more likely to play a greater role in maintaining urinary continence. We do not know whether, independent of their position, all fibers discharge simultaneously or have differentiated responses for maintaining continence.

Rats are the animal model most commonly utilized to study the mechanisms of continence and for preclinical testing of treatments since they are readily available and, despite their quadruped status, their PFM anatomy and innervation bears a distinct similarity to humans

(Bremer et al. 2003; Jiang et al. 2010; Poortmans & Wyndaele 1998; Poortmans & Wyndaele 2002; Thor & de Groat 2010). The pelvic muscles form a bowl-shaped support attached to the pelvis, the coccyx, the pelvic ligaments and supports the vesical organs (Ashton-Miller et al. 2001; Wall 1993). Anatomic landmarks for these muscles in female rats are generally similar to those in women except for the lack of a puborectalis muscle in rats and the coccyx which controls the well-developed tail in the rat (Barber et al. 2002; Borirakchanyavat et al. 1997; Pacheco et al. 1989). In female rats the pubococcygeus and iliococcygeus are primarily innervated by the levator ani nerve from the L6-S1 trunk (Figure 1) (Bremer et al. 2003; Jiang et al. 2010)

The levator ani nerve travels into the pelvic floor from the ventromedial surface and the nerve roots are generally more proximal in female rats compared to women (Barber et al. 2002; Jiang et al. 2010). However, the course and innervation of the levator ani nerve are similar between female rats and women (Barber et al. 2002; Jiang et al. 2010). Some reports have debated if the pudendal nerve also innervates the pelvic floor muscle both in rats and women (Barber et al. 2002; Erdogru 2008; Grigorescu et al. 2008; Strohbehn 1998; Wall 1993; Wallner et al. 2008). However, most of the anatomic and functional studies support the idea that the pudendal nerve does not contribute to the innervations of these muscles (Jiang et al. 2010; Thor & de Groat 2010).

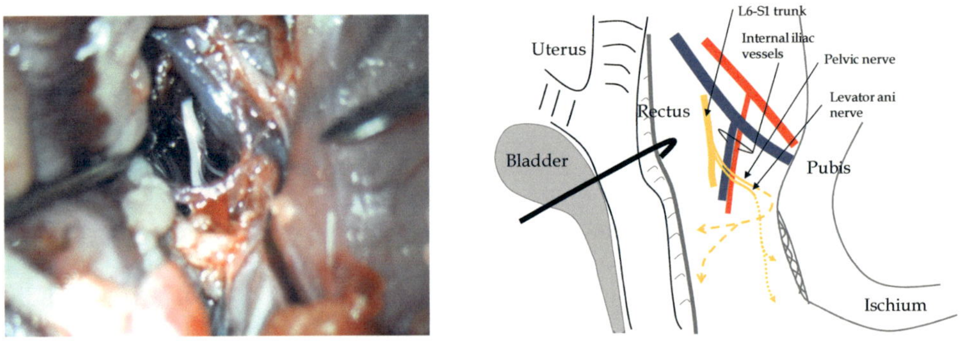

Fig. 1. Exposure of the levator ani nerve (left) in a female rat. The nerve branches from the L6-S1 trunk and enters the pelvic floor along with the pelvic nerve from its ventromedial surface.

The goal of this chapter is to review the literature regarding measurement of PFM EMGs in laboratory rats, focusing on methods and results to date and to present original data utilizing EMG measurement to determine if these muscles act as a single unit or act individually during micturition.

2. Electrodes and techniques used to measure PFM EMGs in laboratory rats

Several different electrodes have been utilized to study EMGs of pelvic and perineal muscles in rats, including concentric electrodes (Kerns et al. 2000), parallel electrodes (Jiang et al. 2009a, 2009b), and wire electrodes (Chang & Havton 2008; Cruz & Downie 2006; Peng et al. 2006; Yang et al. 2010). Several muscles in or close to the pelvic floor have been studied in rats, including the pubococcygeus, iliococcygeus, EUS, and external anal sphincter (EAS) muscles (Manzo et al. 1997; Salcedo et al. 2010; Thor & de Groat 2010). EUS EMG in female rats has been investigated more often than EMGs of the other pelvic or perineal muscles because of the clinical relevance to stress incontinence and urodynamic testing (Jiang et al. 2009b; Kerns et al. 2000; Peng et al. 2006; Thor & de Groat 2010).

2.1 Techniques for recording EMG of pelvic floor muscles in rats

Rats are usually anesthetized with urethane or ketamine and xylazine intraperitoneally for EMG recordings (Chang et al. 2007; Chang & Havton 2008; Jiang et al. 2009a, 2009b; Pikov et al. 1998). Sometimes isoflurane is used to supplement anesthesia during surgical preparation for the recording (Miyazato et al. 2008). To access pelvic and perineal muscles, the pubic symphysis is exposed with the rat in a supine position and after a hypogastric midline incision. The rectus muscles are then transected and the Retzius space is exposed after opening the pubic symphysis with mosquito forceps. To avoid unexpected bleeding, the bilateral inferior epigastric vessels are ligated and cut before opening the pubic symphysis (Jiang et al. 2010). Using wire electrodes, the EUS can be approached ventromedially by inserting a 30-gauge needle (Jiang et al. 2010).

If a caudal approach is needed, the pubococcygeus and iliococcygeus muscles can be partly exposed by bluntly separating the pubic symphysis to the ischiorectal fossa. The ischiorectal fossa is then opened slightly to approach the pubococcygeus and iliococcygeus muscles. The needle can be inserted through the ischiorectal fossa to the muscles (Figure 2, blue arrow in panel A). Parallel electrodes have been used to measure pelvic floor muscle EMGs by touching the electrodes to the muscles through the muscle surface nearest the pelvis (Jiang et al. 2010). If a survival procedure for the PFM EMG is necessary, the PFM may be approached without opening the pubic symphysis or via a dorsal approach after opening the ischiorectal fossa.

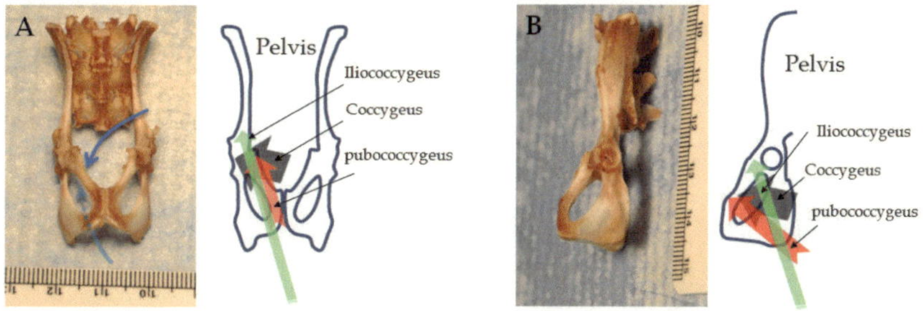

Fig. 2. Illustration of pelvic floor muscle attachments showing the direction of muscle contraction (arrows in right panels). A: vertical view of a female rat pelvis (blue arrows in left panel show the different approaches for recording pelvic floor muscles). B: lateral view of the same pelvis.

2.2 Techniques for recording EUS EMG in rats

EUS EMG in rats has been extensively studied for evaluation of lower urinary tract function and dysfunction (Jiang et al. 2009b; Kerns et al. 2000; Peng et al. 2006; Steward et al. 2010; Thor & de Groat 2010). The recording is usually performed simultaneous with recording bladder pressure during cystometry (CMG) or leak point pressure (LPP) testing to test the urinary continence reflex and coordination between the bladder and urethra (Jiang et al. 2009a; Peng et al. 2006; Steward et al. 2010; Yang et al. 2010). Several approaches to the EUS using concentric electrodes, parallel electrodes, and wire electrodes have been utilized (Figure 3) (Steward et al. 2010). An end-point recording under urethane anaesthesia is one of most commonly used techniques to record EUS EMG (Peng et al. 2006). To obtain better quality recordings, the pubic symphysis can be bluntly separated during the procedure to enable visualization of the mid-urethra.

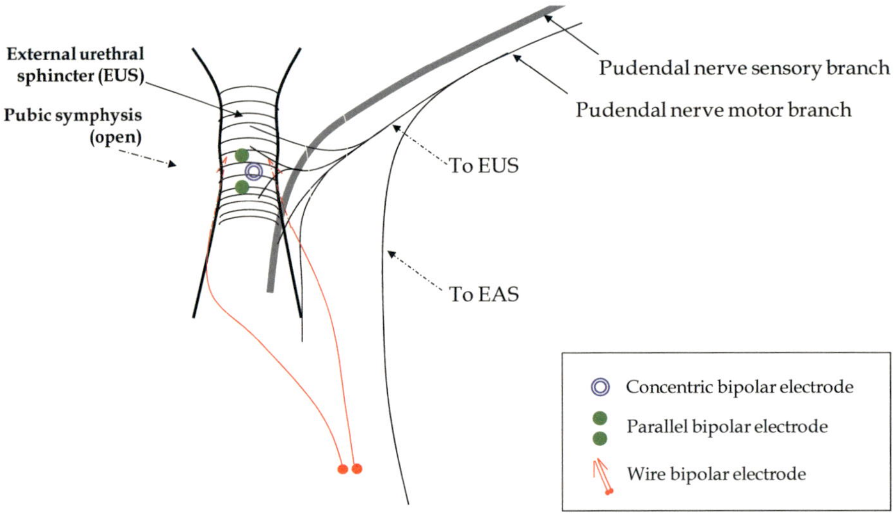

Fig. 3. Placement of different electrodes after opening the pubic symphysis for EUS EMG recording (adapted with permission from Steward et al. 2010).

If repeat EUS EMG recording is necessary, the EUS can be accessed with wire electrodes via a retropubic approach, a perineal approach, or through the anterior vaginal wall as a survival procedure under ketamine/xylazine anesthesia (Steinmetz et al. 2008). A female rat is placed in a supine position and a catheter (PE50) is inserted into the bladder via the urethral orifice to help locate the urethra for wire electrode insertion into the EUS (Figure 4). An audio monitor can be utilized to guide electrode insertion.

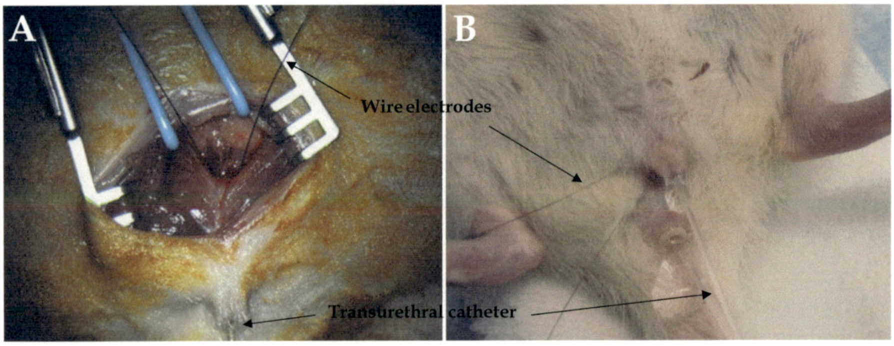

Fig. 4. Different approaches for repeat EUS EMG recording. A: retropubic approach. B: perineal or anterior vaginal wall approach.

In some animal models, such as spinal cord injury, EUS EMG may be recorded with the rat conscious but restrained. Wire electrodes are inserted via a perineal approach under isoflurane anaesthesia. Before awakening, the rats are placed in a restrainer (Figure 5) and then wakened from the anesthesia to make EMG recordings.

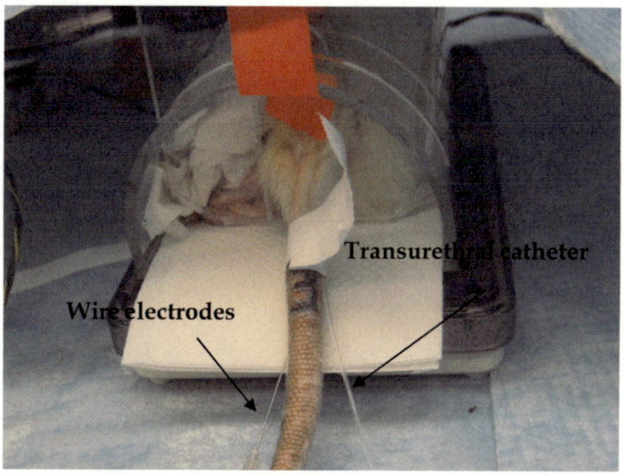

Fig. 5. A conscious spinal cord injured rat in a restrainer to make recordings of EUS EMG and bladder pressure.

2.3 Techniques for recording the external anal sphincter EMG in rats

EAS EMG has been well studied clinically as a substitute for EUS EMG during clinical urodynamics testing (Blaivas 1984), but is unlike the EUS EMG in rats (Salcedo et al. 2010). The anatomic location of the anus is a relatively longer distance from the urethra and vagina in rats (relative to body size) compared to women. The EAS is smaller and has reduced activity compare to the EUS in rats. In addition, the motoneurons innervating the EUS and EAS in rats are anatomically separated in the spinal cord (McKenna & Nadelhaft 1986).

Nonetheless, EAS EMG has been studied in rats for specific purposes (Holmes et al. 1998; Salcedo et al. 2010), such as for development of an animal model of fecal incontinence (Zutshi et al. 2009). EAS EMG is recorded using a 30 G concentric monopolar needle after inserting it into the EAS. Ketamine/xylazine anesthesia is used whether the procedure is a survival or terminal procedure, since urethane decreases anal sphincter contraction (Salcedo et al. 2010; Zutshi et al. 2009).

3. Rat PFM EMG signal processing and analysis methods

The majority of studies in rats involving EMG of the PFM, the EUS, or the EAS are analyzed qualitatively (Thor & de Groat 2010). However, with the development of EMG analysis methods, quantitative analysis of the EMG has become an effective method of quantifying the continence reflex, functional recovery, and the pattern of reinnervation of these muscles (Jiang et al. 2009b; Jiang et al. 2010; Liu et al. 2008; Peng et al. 2006; Steward et al. 2010; Zutshi et al. 2009).

3.1 EMG Signal collection and correction

A high quality EMG signal is critical for quantitative analysis. A segmental interval is chosen, usually one to several seconds, from a stable EMG recording or at a required time point, such as at the peak of LPP testing. The segment of the EMG is then filtered for 60 Hz noise (power supply frequency) using a notch filter (Jiang et al. 2009a, 2009b; Steward et al. 2010). To correct for a travelling baseline in the signal, it can be smoothed using a triangular Bartlett window to obtain a signal consisting only of baseline changes (Ritter et al. 2005). This smoothed signal is then subtracted from the original signal to create a corrected signal

(Figure 6). The resultant signal has a flattened baseline and is more appropriate for thresholding. The relative amount of baseline correction needed for each signal can be expressed as the sum of the amplitude spectrum normalized to the sum of the amplitude spectrum of the raw signal (Steward et al. 2010).

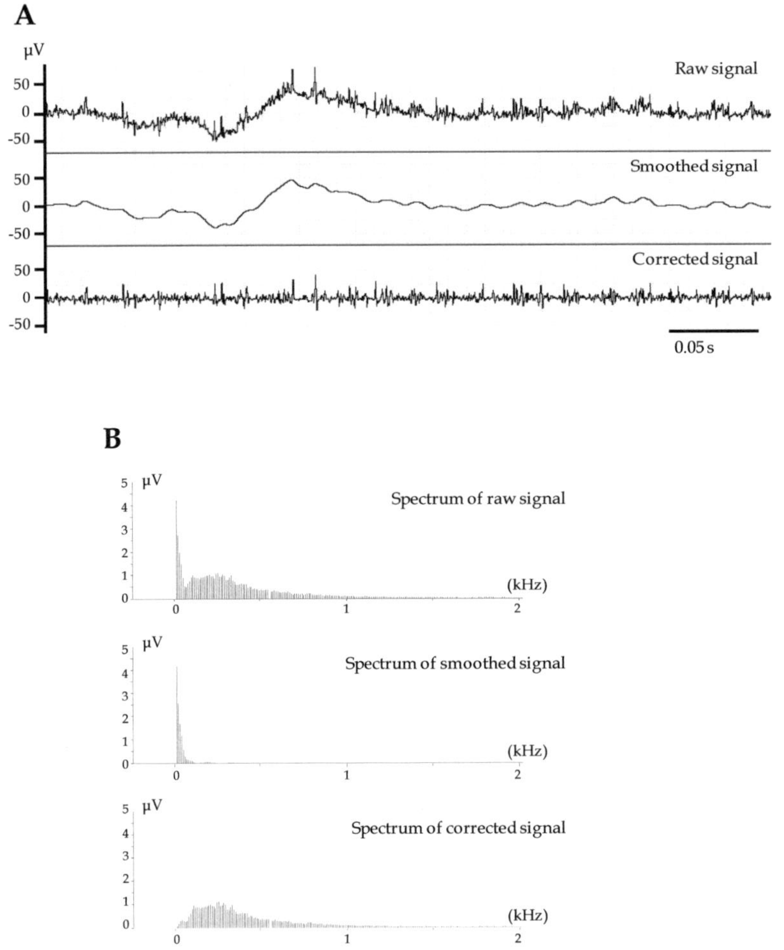

Fig. 6. Baseline correction of EMG recording. A: Example of EUS EMG during leak point pressure testing corrected by smoothing the baseline. B: Amplitude spectrums for the signal in panel A (adapted with permission from Steward et al, 2010).

3.2 Mean amplitude and firing rate calculation

EMG signals are then balanced by setting mean amplitude to zero to remove any offset. The signals are then rectified (Figure 7) and mean amplitude is calculated. To calculate mean firing rate of the EMG signal (previously termed "mean frequency" in Jiang et al. 2009a, 2009b; Salcedo et al. 2010; Steward et al. 2010), a threshold for differentiating noise from neuromuscular activity is set at a certain voltage (such as 0.25 μV), depending on the amplitude of noise in a particular situation. The mean firing rate is calculated by counting the number of peaks above the threshold per second (Steward et al. 2010).

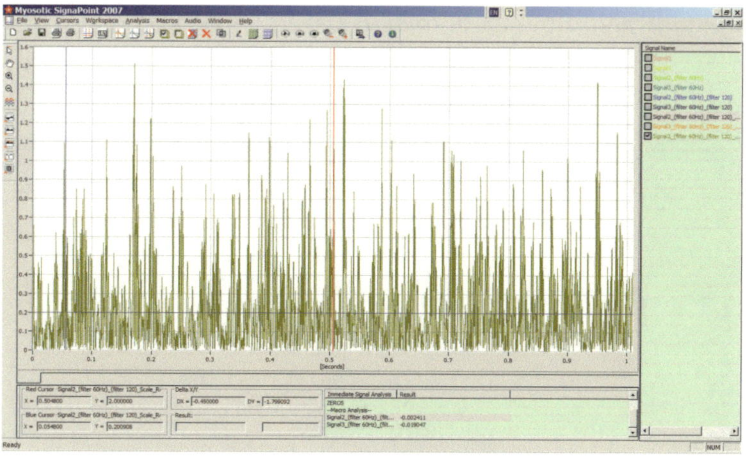

Fig. 7. Example of EMG rectification after offset. Mean amplitude and firing rate are calculated after setting a noise threshold (Myosotic SignPoint 2007).

3.3 Individual motor unit potential (MUP) quantitative assessment

Quantitative assessment of EMG signals can also be performed by decomposing the EMG signals to obtain individual motor unit potentials (MUPs) (Nandedkar et al. 1995; Stashuk 2001; Stålberg et al. 1996). In an example during LPP testing (Figure 8), a two-second sample of tonic baseline activity and peak activity during the pressure peak of LPP testing were identified and archived.

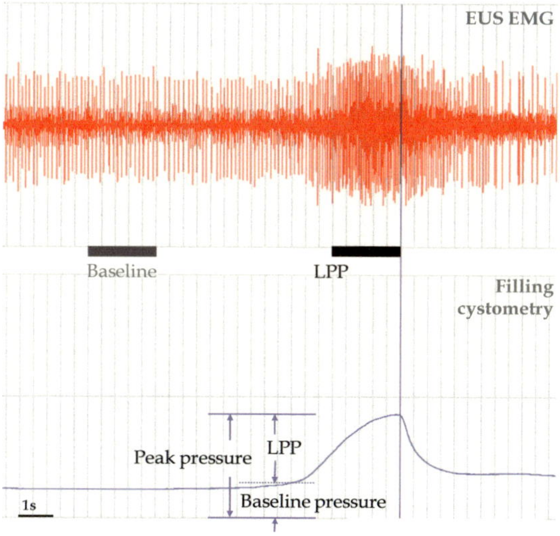

Fig. 8. Example of EUS EMG during filling CMG and LPP testing in a rat model of simulated childbirth injury, indicating recovery of continence.

Raw signals are first baseline corrected as described above. Power supply interference (60 Hz) is then filtered with a digital notch filter. Each two-second sample is then decomposed using an EMG decomposition program and the averaged MUP templates are archived. The total number of MUPs and the firing rate of each MUP can be determined for each sample

(Figure 9). Amplitude and duration of each averaged template can also be calculated, for example by using a custom Matlab code (Stålberg et al. 1996).

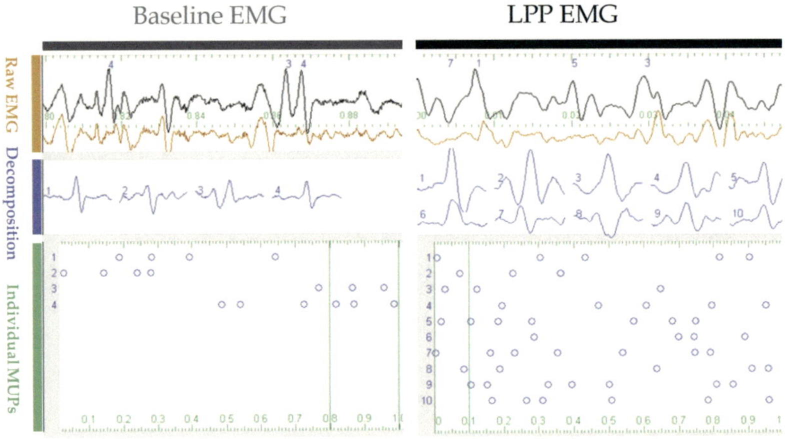

Fig. 9. EUS EMG during baseline recording and during LPP testing decomposed for individual motor unit potentials (MUPs). Increased number of MUPs in the EUS during LPP represents a guarding reflex to prevent leakage.

4. External urethral sphincter EMG in female rats

4.1 Anatomy of the EUS

The EUS, also called the rabdosphincter, consists of the striated muscle fibers surrounding the urethra (Bierinx & Sebille 2006; RJ Kim et al. 2007; Lehtoranta et al. 2006). The fibers do not have dedicated attachments to skeletal structures and thus act as true sphincters (Cruz & Downie 2005; RJ Kim et al. 2007; Thor & de Groat 2010). The EUS has two peaks, one in the middle of the urethra and the other distally (RJ Kim et al. 2007).

The characteristics of the EUS are sexually dimorphic since it is thinner in females than males (Cruz & Downie 2005). Sexual dimorphism is also observed in perineal muscles such as the bulbocavernosus and ischiocavernosus (McKenna & Nadelhaft 1986). These muscles are well developed in males but in females are vestigial, suggesting a male sexual function (McKenna & Nadelhaft 1986). Perineal muscles and their motoneurons degenerate after birth in females since their preservation depends on testosterone and perineal cutaneous stimulation as a neonate (Breedlove & Arnold 1981; Moore et al. 1992; Nordeen et al. 1985). We are aware of no studies analyzing if hormonal and sensory stimuli during the neonatal window could improve development, or avoid degeneration, of the EUS in females.

4.2 Innervation of the EUS

EUS motoneurons are located in the dorsolateral nuclei, in L6-S1 spinal cord segments, and the axons travel through the motor branch of the sacral plexus, also called the motor branch of the pudendal nerve, to reach their target (Cruz et al. 2004; de Groat et al. 2001; Kane et al. 2002; McKenna & Nadelhaft 1986; Pacheco et al. 1997; Schroder 1980). The motor branch of the sacral plexus (Mb in Figure 10) emerges from a loop of the nerve, the sacral plexus (SP in Figure 10). The plexus is made up of two anastomotic branches: one (ap in Figure 10) arises from the pudendal nerve and the other (als in Figure 10) from the lumbosacral trunk (Ls-T in Figure 10).

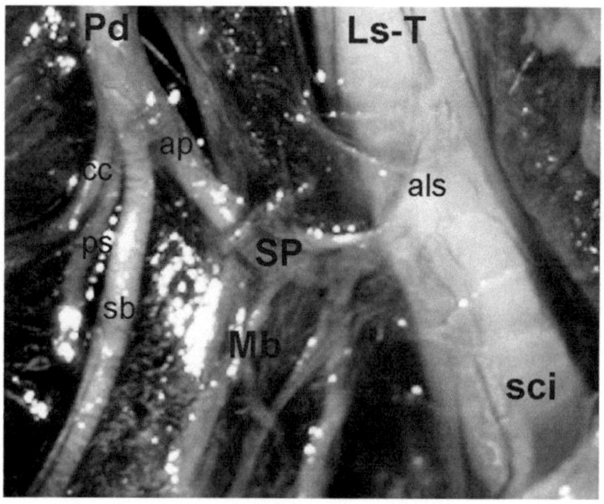

Fig. 10. Ventral view of the right sacral plexus in the female rat. Note that from the sacral plexus (SP) forms the source of innervation of the EUS (Mb, motor branch of the sacral plexus), and from the pudendal nerve (Pd), the sensory branch of the pudendal nerve (sb), and the branches to the coccygeus muscle (cc), and the perineal skin (ps). The sciatic nerve (Sci) originates from the lumbosacral trunk (Ls-T) below the sacral plexus; ap and als indicate anastomotic branches. Nerves from the sacral plexus to the perineal skin or to the internal obturator muscle are not labeled.

Knowledge of the pathways of peripheral innervation is an important tool to study EUS function in preclinical studies (Cruz & Downie 2005; Jiang & Damaser 2011; Jiang et al. 2009a, 2009b; Jiang et al. 2011; Kamo & Hashimoto 2007; Kamo et al. 2009; Kamo et al. 2003; Kerns et al. 2000; Lee et al. 2003; Peng et al. 2008a, 2008b). Animal models have been used to estimate the damage to nerves during simulated childbirth and to test pharmacological and neuromodulation strategies to promote neuroregeneration and recovery of EUS function (Cannon & Chancellor 2003; Cannon et al. 2002; Jiang & Damaser 2011; Jiang et al. 2009a, 2009b; Peng et al. 2008a; Streng et al. 2001; Thor 2003; Thor et al. 1989; Thor et al. 2007; Vera & Nadelhaft 2001). EMG EUS activity, or contraction, is usually measured along with bladder pressure, urethral pressure, leak point pressure and/or voiding frequency before and after a lesion to or stimulation of one or more of the nerves that innervate the EUS (Cruz & Downie 2005; Jiang & Damaser 2011; Jiang et al. 2009b; Peng et al. 2006; Peng et al. 2008a, 2008b). However, it is difficult to compare results because some studies do not describe the site of the nerve lesion and the dissection procedures to access the nerves differ between studies (Cruz & Downie 2005; Damaser et al. 2007; Furuta et al. 2008; Kamo et al. 2003; Kim et al. 2009; Peng et al. 2006; Wai et al. 2004).

A procedure commonly used to eliminate EUS activity is to make a lesion to the pudendal nerve. The pudendal nerve has been described as a nerve emerging from the L6-S1 trunk, the remaining one after the pelvic nerve leaves this trunk. As demonstrated in Figure 10, several branches emerge from the pudendal nerve: one provides innervation to the EUS and the others innervate the perigenital skin, the clitoris, and the coccygeus (Cruz et al. 2004; McKenna & Nadelhaft 1989; Pacheco et al. 1997; Pacheco et al. 1989). Some authors perform pudendal nerve lesion at the level of the iliac vein, cutting all branches, others lesion the nerve at the ischiorectal fossa, damaging the sensory branch of the pudendal nerve and the motor branch of the sacral plexus or only the motor branch of the sacral plexus (Cruz & Downie 2005; Damaser et al. 2007; Furuta et al. 2008; Kerns et al. 2000; Peng et al. 2006). Results of these studies are therefore not comparable.

Confusion is added with models of stress urinary incontinence created by lesioning the sciatic nerve to denervate the EUS (YT Kim et al. 2007; Kwon et al. 2006). A question arises whether the sciatic, as well as the pudendal nerve innervates the EUS. The authors probably lesioned the lumbosacral trunk (Ls-T in Figure 10). This would suggest that the axons of the EUS travel to the spinal cord through two pathways: the pudendal nerve and the lumbosacral trunk. Cutting either the pudendal nerve or the lumbosacral trunk would then not completely eliminate EUS activity. Because of this complexity of innervation, the exact site of a nerve lesion should be described in detail when presenting original studies.

4.3 EUS EMG activity

The activity of the EUS is related to urethral function. Simultaneous CMG and EMG recordings have shown EUS activity during high bladder pressure during effort that increases intra-abdominal pressure and during voiding (Cruz & Downie 2005; Jiang et al. 2010). In preclinical studies these conditions are imitated by the LPP test or by infusing saline to fill the bladder and induce reflex micturition (Jiang & Damaser 2011). LPP is associated with augmented EUS EMG activity (Jiang et al. 2010), as shown in Figure 8. This reflex muscle contraction closes the urethra to avoid urine leakage and has been recognized as a guarding reflex that relies on intact neural circuitry. Damage to nerves that innervate the EUS can weaken or eliminate the guarding reflex, decreasing urethral pressure and enabling urine leakage, similar to the clinical condition of stress urinary incontinence.

During the micturition cycle, activity of some motor units of the EUS maintains the muscular tone of the urethral sphincter during bladder filling, contributing to continence. With increasing bladder pressure, more EUS motor units are recruited and EUS EMG activity rises, one form of the guarding reflex (Jiang et al. 2010; Kenton et al. 2005; Thor & de Groat 2010). Unlike in humans, in rats EUS discharge reaches its maximum amplitude at the peak of bladder contraction during voiding and gradually decreases after bladder pressure returns to baseline (Cruz & Downie 2005; Streng et al. 2004; Streng et al. 2002) (Figure 11).

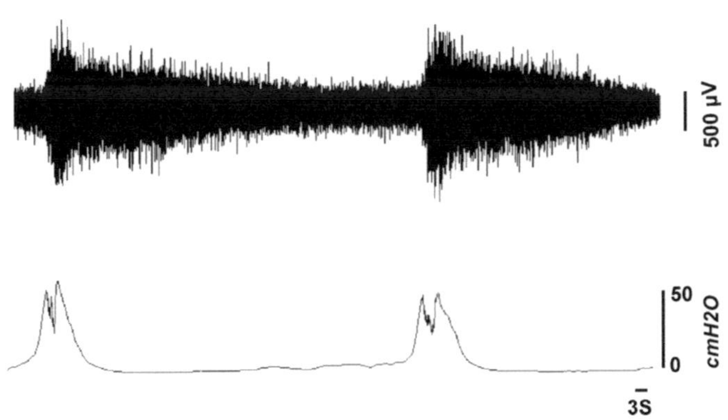

Fig. 11. EUS EMG and Bladder pressure recorded during continuous infusion of saline solution (5 ml/h). Voiding occurred between the two bladder pressure peaks.

During voiding in rats, the highest amplitude components of EUS EMG show a 6-10 Hz bursting pattern of activity concurrent with high frequency bladder oscillations and continued as tonic activity after the bladder contraction ends (Cruz & Downie 2005; Streng et al. 2004; Streng et al. 2002) (Figure 12A). This is in contrast to humans, in whom the EUS is quiet during voiding with little activity recorded on EMG (Yalla & Resnick 1997). A similar pattern is observed during LPP when urine leaks but with a smaller duration than during voiding and no bursting pattern (Figure 12B).

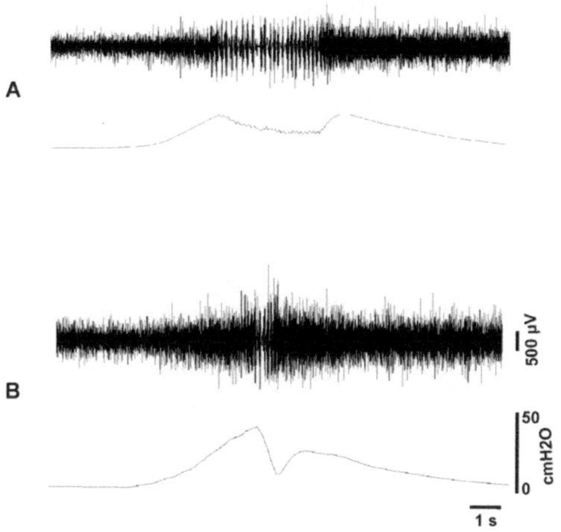

Fig. 12. EUS EMG and bladder pressure during voiding (A) and during leak point pressure testing (B). Note the bursting pattern in the EUS EMG during voiding. Scales apply to both figures.

It is not known whether the bursting pattern in EUS EMG activity results from temporally rhythmic inhibition of the EUS spinal motoneurons, since inhibition of the EUS is required for voiding in other species such as humans (Yalla & Resnick 1997), or from recruitment of motoneurons with a bursting pattern of firing. Nonetheless, the bursting activity of the striated sphincter during voiding is necessary for efficient bladder emptying (Cruz & Downie 2005). Voiding deficiency after spinal cord injury is correlated with decreased bursting and increased tonic activity during bladder contraction, described as bladder sphincter dyssinergia (Kruse et al. 1993).

The activity of the EUS is not only modulated by urethral and bladder afferents but also by other peripheral and central influences. In people, these reflexes mature during the first years of life since urinary continence appears postnatally. Mechanical stimulation of the genital and perineal skin increases EUS activity, suggesting that afferents from these regions also converge onto the L6-S1 segments and modulate activity of EUS motoneurons (Thor & de Groat 2010).

5. EMG of pelvic floor muscles in female rats

5.1 Coccygeal muscles in female rats

In rats, as in humans, a group of intrapelvic striated muscles extends from the ischial spines and pubic bone to the coccygeal vertebrae. According to their individual fiber distributions, the muscles have been classified as coccygeus, iliococcygeus, iliocaudalis, pubococcygeus, or pubocaudalis (Brink & Pfaff 1980; Pacheco et al. 1989; Poortmans & Wyndaele 1998). The last two are commonly referred as the levator ani muscles, although in rats this term can be confusing because levator ani is also used to name a sexually dimorphic striated muscle closely related to the rectum that is only present in males (Cihak et al. 1970; Poortmans & Wyndaele 1998).

The coccygeus is in a cranial-dorsal position (Cc in Figure 13) and its fibers arise from the medial face of the inominate bone, at a site just anterior to the obturator foramen. The fibers insert in the proximal tail bone, at the first and second coccygeal vertebral bone (Brink & Pfaff 1980; Pacheco et al. 1989; Poortmans & Wyndaele 1998). It is not directly related to the pelvic viscera.

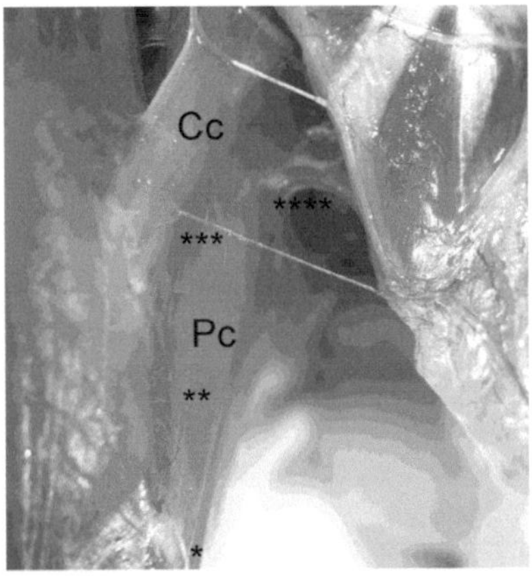

Fig. 13. Dorsal view of the pelvic floor muscles in the female rat. Cc, coccygeus muscle; Pc, pubococcygeus. Note that the iliococcygeus muscle is not observed in a dorsal view because it is ventral to the coccygeus muscle. *, **, ***, **** indicate sites of electrode placement for EMG recordings.

The fibers of the iliococcygeus originate in the ventromedial border of the ilial shaft, posterior to the gluteal notch and insert through tendons to the coccygeal vertebrae (Poortmans & Wyndaele 1998). The distal portions of its fibers run laterally to the rectum. The pubococcygeus is the largest muscle of the pelvic floor. Its fibers originate at the ventromedial border of the pubic bones at the level of the acetabulum and insert onto the ventromedial surface of the tail bone, at the third and fourth caudal vertebrae (Figure 13). Its ventromedial fibers have connective tissue that attach to the peritoneal surface of the ventral vaginal wall and run caudally, lateral to the rectum (Pacheco et al. 1989; Poortmans & Wyndaele 1998). The pubococcygeus and coccygeus are closely attached and are difficult to separate from each other (Poortmans & Wyndaele 1998).

5.2 Innervation of pelvic floor muscles

The motoneurons of pelvic floor muscles in rats are located in the ventral horn of the spinal cord. Tracer studies have shown that pubococcygeus motoneurons are located in a column approximately 2 mm in length in the central region of lamina IX of the sixth lumbar–first sacral spinal cord segments, with dendrites that project to the lateral, medial and ventral regions of the gray matter. Their morphometric characteristics are modulated by gonadal steroid hormones, as indicated by soma size and dendrite length and arborization reduction after ovariectomy and recovery after steroid treatment (Cuevas et al. 2006). In males it has been shown that the muscle fibers are also sensitive to gonadal steroids since castration reduces the cross-sectional area of the pubococcygeus muscle (Alvarado et al. 2008).

Afferents involved in induction of reflex activity of pelvic floor muscles travel through the pudendal and pelvic nerves (Pacheco et al. 1989). In contrast, the nomenclature for the peripheral motor innervation of the pelvic floor muscles remains controversial, with the pudendal nerve contribution to innervations of the pelvic floor muscles in question. Some studies claim that the efferent innervation of the pubococcygeus and iliococcygeus travels from the spinal cord via the somatomotor branch of the pelvic nerve, which arises from the L6-S1 trunk (Cruz et al. 2004; Pacheco et al. 1989). Others describe that these muscles are innervated by the levator ani nerve which has individual differences in the pattern of its origin (Bremer et al. 2003). In some rats the pelvic and levator ani nerves arise as distinct nerve fascicles from their origin at the L6-S1 trunk, but in most of rats (70%), a single nerve originates from the L6-S1 trunk (usually called the pelvic nerve) and divides into the levator ani and pelvic nerves as it enters the pelvic cavity (Bremer et al. 2003). Different authors may be describing the same nerve but have named it differently (Bremer et al. 2003; Cruz et al. 2004; Pacheco et al. 1989). In recent studies (unpublished observations) we have observed that in most cases, the pelvic nerve arises as a single fascicle that divides into two branches, one carrying axons to visceral and cutaneous structures (the viscerocutaneous branch of the pelvic nerve) through the major pelvic ganglion, and the other innervating the pubococcygeus and iliococcygeus muscles. Therefore, naming it the motor branch of the pelvic nerve seems to be most appropriate (Pacheco et al. 1989).

A similar nomenclature controversy is related to innervation of the coccygeus muscle, with some authors describing the coccygeal nerve as emerging from the L6-S2 trunk, 1-2 mm distal to the point where the pelvic nerve emerges, and without contribution from the pudendal nerve (Bremer et al. 2003; Thor & de Groat 2010). Others consider this nerve to be a branch of the pudendal nerve, as shown in Figure 10 (Cruz et al. 2004; Pacheco et al. 1989). Thus, the answer to the question of whether the pudendal nerve innervates pelvic floor muscles depends on where each investigator considers the origin of the pudendal nerve.

5.3 EMG activity of pelvic floor muscles

Reflex EMG activity of the iliococcygeus and pubococcygeus muscles can be induced by mechanically stimulating the perineum, clitoral sheath, or lower vagina (Martinez-Gomez et al. 1992; Pacheco et al. 1989). Contraction of this musculature, induced by electrical stimulation, produces movement of the vaginal orifice and wall, membranous urethra, tail and pelvis as well as increasing intravaginal pressure (Martinez-Gomez et al. 1992; Pacheco et al. 1989; Poortmans & Wyndaele 1998). Thus, the pelvic floor muscles might be activated by male stimulation during copulation and could increase penile stimulation to promote ejaculation, facilitate the retention of sperm and of the seminal plug, or enhance the quality of stimulation received by the female (Martinez-Gomez et al. 1992). Contraction of these muscles may also contribute to lordotic dorsiflexion, a stereotyped posture of female rat during copulation (Brink & Pfaff 1980; Martinez-Gomez et al. 1992).

Mechanical stimulation of the cervix inhibits the activity of pelvic floor muscles and induces reflex contraction of abdominal muscles, suggesting that the passage of the fetus through the cervix during parturition might reflexively relax the ilio- and pubococcygeus muscles, facilitating delivery (Martinez-Gomez et al. 1992; Pacheco et al. 1989). However, bilateral denervation of the iliococcygeus and pubococcygeus, by transection of the motor branch of the pelvic nerve, did not modify the temporal pattern of parturition (Martinez-Gomez et al. 1998). Considering that the pelvic floor muscles are inhibited during cervical stimulation, this musculature could be already inhibited during parturition such that denervation did not affect parturition.

In humans, pelvic floor muscles close the pelvic outlet and support pelvic viscera to maintain their position (Ashton-Miller & Delancey 2007). Visceral dysfunction, such as prolapse and fecal and urinary incontinence, are related to pelvic floor muscle disorders. However, to date there are only few preclinical studies focused on EMG activity of pelvic floor muscles during excretory function (Jiang et al. 2010; Kamo et al. 2006; Kamo et al. 2009; Kamo et al. 2003). The experimental conditions and results differ between studies. In male rats, the pubococcygeus muscle shows a bursting discharge during voiding (Manzo et al. 1997). In female rats, the pubococcygeus and iliococcygeus discharge during voiding only when filling rate is high (0.5 ml/min) and they do not show bursting activity (Thor & de Groat 2010). In contrast, in another study, the pelvic floor muscle of female rats did not demonstrate EMG activity during voiding or LPP testing (Jiang et al. 2010). Because pelvic floor muscles include several muscles, and the pubococcygeus is a large muscle, a possibility exists that this musculature does not behave as a single unit but has differential discharge. We tested this hypothesis in the following experiment.

6. Determination of individual action of pelvic floor muscles in female rats

6.1 Methods

Female virgin Sprague–Dawley rats (Harlan, Inc.) weighing 250–300 g underwent bladder filling with saline (5 ml/h) under urethane anesthesia (1.2 g/kg, i.p.) via a suprapubic polyethelene catheter connected to both a pressure transducer and a syringe pump to monitor intravesical pressure and fill the bladder, respectively. Air pressure was calibrated as zero at the level of the bladder. On continuous saline infusion, EMGs were recorded in animals in supine (n =5) or prone position (n = 3). In a supine position and under a microscope, a skin incision was made at the level of the pelvic bone and after cutting the pubic symphysis, the urethra was exposed. The ischium, the obturator internus muscle and the lateral perineal skin were removed to expose the pubococcygeus and iliococcygeus muscles. Care was taken to avoid cutting the perineal cutaneous innervation.

In a supine position, a pair of Teflon-coated platinum electrodes (0.002 in diameter, bared for 1 mm at the tip) were inserted in the EUS. Another pair of identical electrodes was placed in the iliococcygeus or pubococcygeus muscles. In a prone position, the skin and gluteal muscles were removed. The ischiorectal fossa was opened slightly to expose the coccygeus and pubococcygeus muscle as shown in Figure 13. The electrodes were inserted in the coccygeus or in the different sites (*, **, ***, ***) of the pubococcygeus muscle as indicated in Figure 13.

The electrodes were connected to an amplifier and an electrophysiological recording system to record the EMG signal (10 kHz) simultaneous with bladder pressure recording during continuous saline infusion. In the same animal the electrodes were moved to different sites of the pelvic floor muscle. LPP testing was performed only with animals in a supine position as follows (Jiang et al. 2010). The intravesical pressure was increased by placing gentle external pressure on the bladder at approximately half bladder capacity via a cotton applicator. The external pressure was quickly withdrawn as soon as a leak was observed at the urethral meatus. If no EMG activity was observed during micturition, the perineal skin was mechanically stimulated to induce activity and confirm appropriate electrode position and equipment functionality.

6.2 Results

In a supine position neither the iliococcygeus nor any site of the pubococcygeus muscle demonstrated activity during LPP testing (Figure 14). A little EMG activity was observed during voiding when the electrodes were placed in the ventromedial fibers of the pubococcygeus muscle (Figure 14).

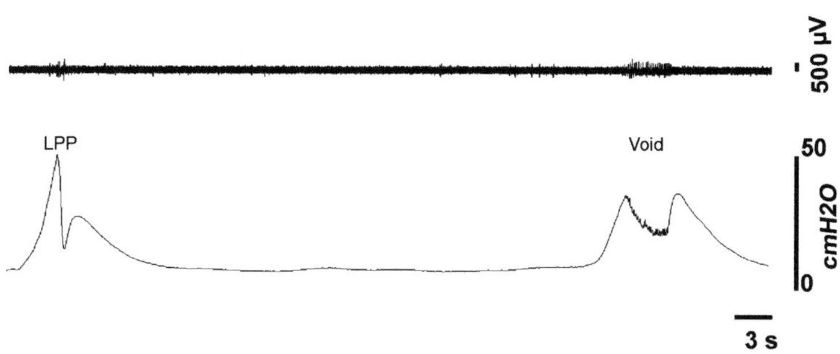

Fig. 14. EMG of the pubococcygeus muscle (upper trace) and simultaneous bladder pressure recording (bottom trace) during LPP testing and voiding in an anesthetized female rat.

Mechanical stimulation of the perigenital skin induced EMG activity of the iliococcygeus and all recording sites of the pubococcygeus muscles. The fibers of the caudal and lateral regions of the pubococcygeus demonstrated activity for the full duration of stimulus duration (Figure 15). Cutaneous stimulation failed to induce EMG activity when bladder pressure reached its maximum value and during voiding.

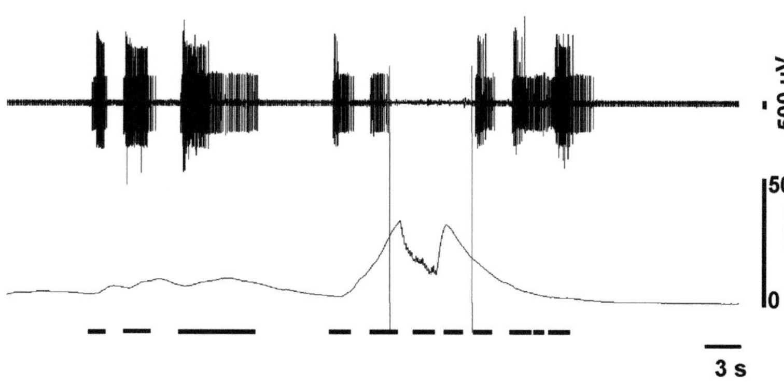

Fig. 15. EMG of the pubococcygeus muscle (upper trace) and simultaneous bladder pressure recording (bottom trace) during voiding in an anesthetized female rat. Activity of the pubococcygeus muscle was recorded close to its attachment to the coccygeal bone. Horizontal lines below the bladder pressure data indicate the duration of mechanical stimulation of the perineal skin. Note that during voiding, mechanical stimulation did not activate the pubococcygeus muscle.

The fibers of the iliococcygeus and those in the medial region of the pubococcygeus (close to the urethra) responded to perigenital stimulation with a long afterdischarge (Figure 16). Cutaneous stimulation-induced EMG activity of the pubococcygeus was completely inhibited during LPP testing and voiding (Figure 16A and B). The inhibition started before bursting in the EUS EMG and ended when the bladder pressure decreased after voiding and the EUS showed tonic activity. However, EMG activity of the iliococcygeus was inhibited only during voiding and for a shorter period (Figure 16C).

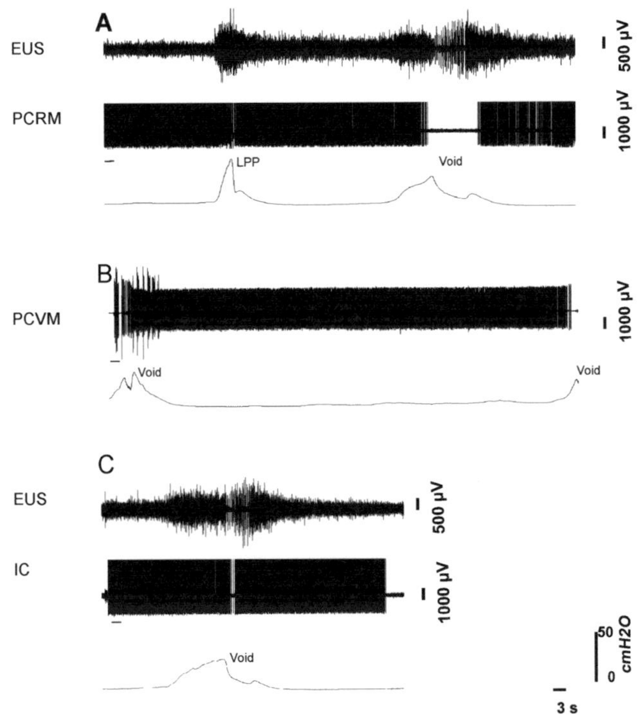

Fig. 16. EMG of the pubococcygeus muscle (middle trace in A and upper trace in B), external urethral sphincter (EUS: top trace in A & C), and iliococcygeus (IC; middle trace in C) as well as simultaneous bladder pressure recording (bottom trace) during LPP testing and voiding in an anesthetized female rat. PCRM, rostromedial fibers of the pubococcygeus; PCVM, ventromedial fibers of the pubococcygeus. The horizontal line below EMG data indicates the duration of mechanical stimulation of the perineal skin.

The iliococcygeus and pubococcygeus muscles discharged when the tail was held contralaterally (Figure 17). The discharge stopped when the tail was placed in the midline. Since muscle spindles have been described in the pubococcygeus muscle (Alvarado et al. 2008), the activity related to tail contralateral movement may be a reflex response with muscle spindles as afferents.

In a prone position, the coccygeus muscle and most of the pubococcygeus recording sites did demonstrate activity during micturition. However, when the electrodes were placed ventromedially (**** in Figure 13) a small discharge appeared to be measurable during voiding (A in Figure 18). However, with magnification of the signal, it seems to be an artifact, probably related to urethral movements induced by EUS contraction (B in Figure 18).

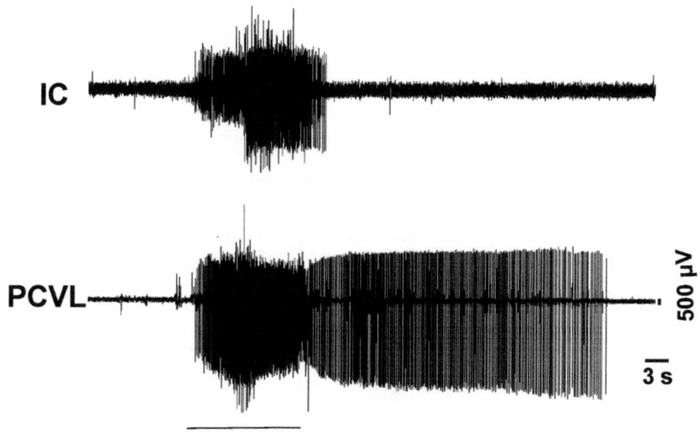

Fig. 17. EMG activity of the iliococcygeus (IC) and pubococcygeus (PCVL, ventrolateral fibers) during contralateral movement of the tail in an anesthetized female rat. The horizontal line below the EMG data indicates when the tail was held contralaterally.

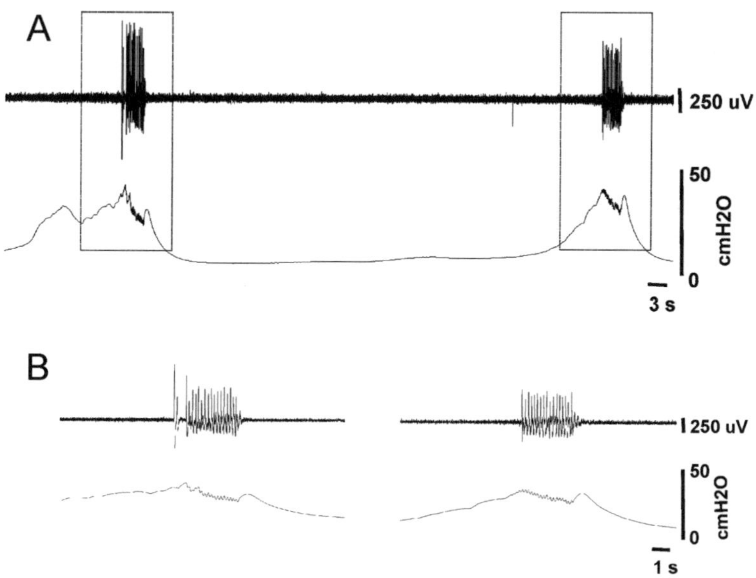

Fig. 18. EMG from the ventromedial region of the pubococcygeus muscle (upper trace) and simultaneous bladder pressure recording (bottom trace) during voiding in an anesthetized female rat. B shows the data indicated by the boxes in A on a magnified scale.

With the exception of the most distal region of the pubococcygeus (** in Figure 13), mechanical stimulation of the perigenital skin induced activity of this muscle consistently; although, in a supine position, the characteristics of the afterdischarge differed between recording sites. The dorsal fibers (*** in Figure 13) discharged only during mechanical stimulation (PCD, panel A in Figure 19) while the fibers closest to the viscera (**** in Figure 13) demonstrated an afterdischarge (PCV, panel B in Figure 19). Only some ventral fibers of the coccygeus muscle responded to perigenital stimulation with bursting potentials (CCV; Figure 19A).

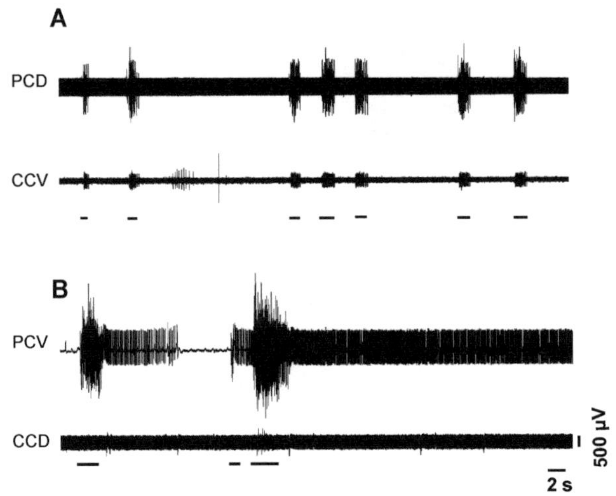

Fig. 19. Simultaneous EMG activity of the pubococcygeus and coccygeus muscle during mechanical stimulation of the perigenital skin in an anesthetized female rat. The electrodes were placed in the dorsal or ventral fibers of the pubococcygeus (PCD or PCV) or coccygeus (CCD or CCV). Horizontal lines below the EMG data indicate the duration of mechanical stimulation of the perineal skin

7. Conclusions

In female rats the EUS behaves as a true sphincter with anatomy and consistent reflex activity tightly linked to urethral pressure. Its responses to a suddenly increased bladder pressure represent a guarding reflex, preventing urine leakage. Its bursting potential during voiding ensures that the bladder empties efficiently (Cruz & Downie 2005; Peng et al. 2008b; Streng et al. 2004). Its response to cutaneous and genital stimulation could increase urethral resistance to prevent voiding during intercourse.

Anatomy and activity of the pelvic floor muscles suggests that they are postural muscles primarily related to sexual function in female rats. During copulation this musculature may be activated voluntarily or reflexively by pudendal nerve afferents. However, their contribution to visceral function is not fully undertood. Their contraction seems not to be necessary for voiding, but visceral afferents seem to be inhibitory in a graded manner, depending on the muscle. We conclude that the pelvic floor musculature does not act as a single unit, neither to visceral nor to perigenital stimulation. The site of EMG recording may also influence the results. Pelvic floor inhibition during voiding suggests similarities between rats and humans in the neural control of micturition.

Some studies in rats have shown that levator ani denervation decreases urethral pressure and that neurectomized rats leak at sneeze (Conway et al. 2005; Kamo et al. 2003). However, we could not demonstrate a pelvic floor response during a LPP test and the LPP value did not decrease after levator ani nerve transection (Jiang et al 2010). It is possible that these differences stem from different experimental conditions such as pump rate and anesthesia level, which should be considered in future studies.

Clinically, measurement of the EUS and pelvic floor muscle activity is an important test to determine their integrity, innervations, and recovery from injury. However, because the muscles are intrapelvic, it is difficult to access them and the electrodes are often placed blindly through the vagina or anus. Alternatively, the anal sphincter is recorded as a surrogate for urethral sphincter activity (Aanestad & Flink 1999; Chantraine & de 1978; Kenton et al. 2005; Weidner et al. 2000; Weidner et al. 2000; Weidner et al. 2009). However, it is important to consider that the pattern of the EUS activity is different from that of pelvic floor muscles and differential responses are observed according to their topography. Recognizing the site of recording and systematically recording in comparable sites will provide consistent and comparable investigations and may avoid misdiagnoses.

8. References

Aanestad, O. & Flink, R. 1999. Urinary stress incontinence. A urodynamic and quantitative electromyographic study of the perineal muscles. Acta Obstet. Gynecol. Scand., 78, 245-253.

Alvarado, M., Cuevas, E., Lara-Garcia, M., Camacho, M., Carrillo, P., Hudson, R. & Pacheco, P. (2008). Effect of gonadal hormones on the cross-sectional area of pubococcygeus muscle fibers in male rat. *Anat. Rec.* (Hoboken.), 291, 586-592.

Ashton-Miller, J.A. & Delancey, J.O. (2007). Functional anatomy of the female pelvic floor. *Ann. N. Y. Acad. Sci.*, 1101, 266-296.

Ashton-Miller, J.A. & Delancey, J.O. (2009). On the biomechanics of vaginal birth and common sequelae. *Annu. Rev. Biomed. Eng*, 11, 163-176.

Ashton-Miller, J.A., Howard, D. & Delancey, J.O. (2001). The functional anatomy of the female pelvic floor and stress continence control system. Scand. *J. Urol. Nephrol. Suppl*, 1-7.

Barber, M.D., Bremer, R.E., Thor, K.B., Dolber, P.C., Kuehl, T.J. & Coates, K.W. (2002). Innervation of the female levator ani muscles. *Am J Obstet. Gynecol.*, 187, 64-71.

Bierinx, A.S. & Sebille, A. (2006). The urethral striated sphincter in adult male rat. *Anatomy and Embryology*, 211, 435-441.

Blaivas, J. (1984). Multichannel urodynamic studies. *Urology*, 23, 421.

Borirakchanyavat, S., Aboseif, S.R., Carroll, P.R., Tanagho, E.A. & Lue, T.F. (1997). Continence mechanism of the isolated female urethra: an anatomical study of the intrapelvic somatic nerves. *J Urol.*, 158, 822-826.

Breedlove, S.M. & Arnold, A.P. (1981). Sexually dimorphic motor nucleus in the rat lumbar spinal cord: response to adult hormone manipulation, absence in androgen-insensitive rats. *Brain Res.*, 225, 297-307.

Bremer, R.E., Barber, M.D., Coates, K.W., Dolber, P.C. & Thor, K.B. (2003). Innervation of the levator ani and coccygeus muscles of the female rat. *Anat. Rec. A Discov. Mol. Cell Evol. Biol.*, 275, 1031-1041.

Brink, E.E. & Pfaff, D.W. (1980). Vertebral muscles of the back and tail of the albino rat (Rattus norvegicus albinus). *Brain Behav. Evol.*, 17, 1-47.

Cannon, T.W. & Chancellor, M.B. (2003). Pharmacotherapy for stress urinary incontinence. *Rev. Urol.*, 5, 135-141.

Cannon, T.W., Wojcik, E.M., Ferguson, C.L., Saraga, S., Thomas, C. & Damaser, M.S. (2002). Effects of vaginal distension on urethral anatomy and function. *BJU. Int.*, 90, 403-407.

Chang, H.Y., Cheng, C.L., Chen, J.J.J. & de Groat, W.C. (2007). Serotonergic drugs and spinal cord transections indicate that different spinal circuits are involved in external

urethral sphincter activity in rats. American journal of physiology. *Renal physiology,* 292, F1044.
Chang, H.Y. & Havton, L.A. (2008). Differential effects of urethane and isoflurane on external urethral sphincter electromyography and cystometry in rats. *Am. J. Physiol Renal Physiol,* 295, F1248-F1253.
Chantraine, A. & de, L.J. (1978). [Electromyography in usual urology (author's transl)]. J. Belge *Med. Phys. Rehabil.,* 1, 29-34.
Cihak, R., Gutmann, E. & Hanzlikova, V. (1970). Involution and hormone-induced persistence of the M. sphincter (levator) ani in female rats. *J. Anat.,* 106, 93-110.
Conway, D.A., Kamo, I., Yoshimura, N., Chancellor, M.B. & Cannon, T.W. (2005). Comparison of leak point pressure methods in an animal model of stress urinary incontinence. *Int. Urogynecol. J. Pelvic. Floor. Dysfunct.,* 16, 359-363.
Cruz, Y. & Downie, J.W. (2005). Sexually dimorphic micturition in rats: relationship of perineal muscle activity to voiding pattern. *American Journal of Physiology-Regulatory Integrative and Comparative Physiology,* 289, R1307-R1318.
Cruz, Y. & Downie, J.W. (2006). Abdominal muscle activity during voiding in female rats with normal or irritated bladder. *American journal of physiology. Regulatory, integrative and comparative physiology,* 290, R1436.
Cruz, Y., Zempoalteca, R., Angelica, L.R., Pacheco, P., Hudson, R. & Martinez-Gomez, M. (2004). Pattern of sensory innervation of the perineal skin in the female rat. *Brain Res.,* 1024, 97-103.
Cuevas, E., Camacho, M., Alvarado, M., Hudson, R. & Pacheco, P. (2006). Participation of estradiol and progesterone in the retrograde labeling of pubococcygeus motoneurons of the female rat. *Neuroscience,* 140, 1435-1442.
Damaser, M.S., Samplaski, M.K., Parikh, M., Lin, D.L., Rao, S. & Kerns, J.M. (2007). Time course of neuroanatomical and functional recovery after bilateral pudendal nerve injury in female rats. *American Journal of Physiology-Renal Physiology,* 293, F1614-F1621.
de Groat, W.C., Fraser, M.O., Yoshiyama, M., Smerin, S., Tai, C., Chancellor, M.B., Yoshimura, N. & Roppolo, J.R. (2001). Neural control of the urethra. Scand. *J. Urol. Nephrol. Suppl,* 35-43.
Erdogru, T. (2008). Editorial comment on: the contribution of the levator ani nerve and the pudendal nerve to the innervation of the levator ani muscles: a study in human fetuses. *Eur. Urol.,* 54, 1143-1144.
Furuta, A., Jankowski, R.J., Pruchnic, R., Egawa, S., Yoshimura, N. & Chancellor, M.B. (2008). Physiological effects of human muscle-derived stem cell implantation on urethral smooth muscle function. *Int. Urogynecol. J. Pelvic. Floor. Dysfunct.,* 19, 1229-1234.
Grigorescu, B.A., Lazarou, G., Olson, T.R., Downie, S.A., Powers, K., Greston, W.M. & Mikhail, M.S. (2008). Innervation of the levator ani muscles: description of the nerve branches to the pubococcygeus, iliococcygeus, and puborectalis muscles. *Int. Urogynecol. J. Pelvic. Floor. Dysfunct.,* 19, 107-116.
Holmes, G.M., Rogers, R.C., Bresnahan, J.C. & Beattie, M.S. (1998). External anal sphincter hyperreflexia following spinal transection in the rat. *Journal of neurotrauma,* 15, 451.
Jiang, H.H. & Damaser, M.S. (2011). Animal models of stress urinary incontinence. *Handb. Exp. Pharmacol.,* 45-67.

Jiang, H.H., Gustilo-Ashby, A.M., Salcedo, L.B., Pan, H.Q., Sypert, D.F., Butler, R.S. & Damaser, M.S. (2009a). Electrophysiological function during voiding after simulated childbirth injuries. *Exp. Neurol.*, 215, 342-348.

Jiang, H.H., Pan, H.Q., Gustilo-Ashby, M.A., Gill, B., Glaab, J., Zaszczurynski, P. & Damaser, M. (2009b). Dual simulated childbirth injuries result in slowed recovery of pudendal nerve and urethral function. *Neurourol. Urodyn.*, 28, 229-235.

Jiang, H.H., Salcedo, L.B. & Damaser, M.S. (2011). Quantification of neurological and other contributors to continence in female rats. *Brain Res.*, 1382, 198-205.

Jiang, H.H., Salcedo, L.B., Song, B. & Damaser, M.S. (2010). Pelvic floor muscles and the external urethral sphincter have different responses to applied bladder pressure during continence. *Urology*, 75, 1515-1517.

Kamo, I. & Hashimoto, T. (2007). Involvement of reflex urethral closure mechanisms in urethral resistance under momentary stress condition induced by electrical stimulation of rat abdomen. *Am. J. Physiol Renal Physiol*, 293, F920-F926.

Kamo, I., Kaiho, Y., Canon, T.W., Chancellor, M.B., de Groat, W.C., Prantil, R.L., Vorp, D.A. & Yoshimura, N. (2006). Functional analysis of active urethral closure mechanisms under sneeze induced stress condition in a rat model of birth trauma. *J. Urol.*, 176, 2711-2715.

Kamo, I., Kaiho, Y., Miyazato, M., Torimoto, K. & Yoshimura, N. (2009). Two kinds of urinary continence reflexes during abrupt elevation of intravesical pressure in rats. *Low Urin. Tract. Symptoms.*, 1, S40-S43.

Kamo, I., Torimoto, K., Chancellor, M.B., de Groat, W.C. & Yoshimura, N. (2003). Urethral closure mechanisms under sneeze-induced stress condition in rats: a new animal model for evaluation of stress urinary incontinence. *Am. J. Physiol Regul. Integr. Comp Physiol*, 285, R356-R365.

Kane, D.D., Shott, S., Hughes, W.F. & Kerns, J.M. (2002). Motor pudendal nerve characterization in the female rat. *Anat. Rec.*, 266, 21-29.

Kenton, K., Fitzgerald, M.P. & Brubaker, L. (2005). Striated urethral sphincter activity does not alter urethral pressure during filling cystometry. *Am. J. Obstet. Gynecol.*, 192, 55-59.

Kerns, J.M., Damaser, M.S., Kane, J.M., Sakamoto, K., Benson, J.T., Shott, S. & Brubaker, L. (2000). Effects of pudendal nerve injury in the female rat. *Neurourol. Urodyn.*, 19, 53-69.

Kim, D.K., Jankowski, R.J., Pruchnic, R., de, M.F., Yoshimura, N., Honda, M., Furuta, A. & Chancellor, M.B. (2009). In vitro and in vivo effect of lidocaine on rat muscle-derived cells for treatment of stress urinary incontinence. *Urology*, 73, 437-441.

Kim, R.J., Kerns, J.M., Liu, S., Nagel, T., Zaszczurynski, P., Lin, D.L. & Damaser, M.S. (2007). Striated muscle and nerve fascicle distribution in the female rat urethral sphincter. *Anat. Rec.* (Hoboken.), 290, 145-154.

Kim, Y.T., Kim, D.K., Jankowski, R.J., Pruchnic, R., Usiene, I., de, M.F. & Chancellor, M.B. (2007). Human muscle-derived cell injection in a rat model of stress urinary incontinence. *Muscle Nerve*, 36, 391-393.

Kruse, M.N., Belton, A.L. & de Groat, W.C. (1993). Changes in bladder and external urethral sphincter function after spinal cord injury in the rat. *Am. J. Physiol*, 264, R1157-R1163.

Kwon, D., Kim, Y., Pruchnic, R., Jankowski, R., Usiene, I., de, M.F., Huard, J. & Chancellor, M.B. (2006). Periurethral cellular injection: comparison of muscle-derived progenitor cells and fibroblasts with regard to efficacy and tissue contractility in an animal model of stress urinary incontinence. *Urology*, 68, 449-454.

Lee, J.Y., Cannon, T.W., Pruchnic, R., Fraser, M.O., Huard, J. & Chancellor, M.B. (2003). The effects of periurethral muscle-derived stem cell injection on leak point pressure in a rat model of stress urinary incontinence. *Int. Urogynecol. J. Pelvic. Floor. Dysfunct.*, 14, 31-37.

Lehtoranta, M., Streng, T., Yatkin, E., Paranko, J., Kolts, I., Talo, A. & Santti, R. (2006). Division of the male rat rhabdosphincter into structurally and functionally differentiated parts. *Anat. Rec. A Discov. Mol. Cell Evol. Biol.*, 288, 536-542.

Liu, G., Lin, Y.H., Yamada, Y. & Daneshgari, F. (2008). External urethral sphincter activity in diabetic rats. *Neurourol. Urodyn.*, 27, 429-434.

Manzo, J., Esquivel, A., Hernandez, M.E., Carrillo, P., Martinez-Gomez, M. & Pacheco, P. (1997). The role of pubococcygeus muscle in urinary continence in the male rat. J. *Urol.*, 157, 2402-2406.

Martinez-Gomez, M., Chirino, R., Beyer, C., Komisaruk, B.R. & Pacheco, P. (1992). Visceral and postural reflexes evoked by genital stimulation in urethane-anesthetized female rats. *Brain Res.*, 575, 279-284.

Martinez-Gomez, M., Cruz, Y., Pacheco, P., Aguilar-Roblero, R. & Hudson, R. (1998). The sensory but not muscular pelvic nerve branch is necessary for parturition in the rat. *Physiol Behav.*, 63, 929-932.

McKenna, K.E. & Nadelhaft, I. (1986). The organization of the pudendal nerve in the male and female rat. *J. Comp Neurol.*, 248, 532-549.

McKenna, K.E. & Nadelhaft, I. (1989). The pudendo-pudendal reflex in male and female rats. *J. Auton. Nerv. Syst.*, 27, 67-77.

Miyazato, M., Sasatomi, K., Hiragata, S., Sugaya, K., Chancellor, M.B., de Groat, W.C. & Yoshimura, N. (2008). GABA receptor activation in the lumbosacral spinal cord decreases detrusor overactivity in spinal cord injured rats. *The Journal of urology*, 179, 1178.

Moore, C.L., Dou, H. & Juraska, J.M. (1992). Maternal stimulation affects the number of motor neurons in a sexually dimorphic nucleus of the lumbar spinal cord. *Brain Res.*, 572, 52-56.

Nandedkar, S.D., Barkhaus, P.E. & Charles, A. (1995). Multi-motor unit action potential analysis (MMA). *Muscle & nerve*, 18, 1155.

Nordeen, E.J., Nordeen, K.W., Sengelaub, D.R. & Arnold, A.P. (1985). Androgens prevent normally occurring cell death in a sexually dimorphic spinal nucleus. *Science*, 229, 671-673.

Pacheco, P., Camacho, M.A., Garcia, L.I., Hernandez, M.E., Carrillo, P. & Manzo, J. (1997). Electrophysiological evidence for the nomenclature of the pudendal nerve and sacral plexus in the male rat. *Brain Res.*, 763, 202-208.

Pacheco, P., Martinez-Gomez, M., Whipple, B., Beyer, C. & Komisaruk, B.R. (1989). Somato-motor components of the pelvic and pudendal nerves of the female rat. *Brain Res.*, 490, 85-94.

Peng, C.W., Chen, J.J., Chang, H.Y., de Groat, W.C. & Cheng, C.L. (2006). External urethral sphincter activity in a rat model of pudendal nerve injury. *Neurourol. Urodyn.*, 25, 388-396.

Peng, C.W., Chen, J.J., Cheng, C.L. & Grill, W.M. (2008a). Improved bladder emptying in urinary retention by electrical stimulation of pudendal afferents. *J. Neural Eng*, 5, 144-154.

Peng, C.W., Chen, J.J., Cheng, C.L. & Grill, W.M. (2008b). Role of pudendal afferents in voiding efficiency in the rat. *Am. J. Physiol Regul. Integr. Comp Physiol*, 294, R660-R672.

Pikov, V., Gillis, R.A., Jasmin, L. & Wrathall, J.R. (1998). Assessment of lower urinary tract functional deficit in rats with contusive spinal cord injury. *Journal of neurotrauma*, 15, 375.

Poortmans, A. & Wyndaele, J.J. (1998). M. levator ani in the rat: does it really lift the anus? *Anat. Rec.*, 251, 20-27.

Poortmans, A. & Wyndaele, J.J. (2002). Preventing fatigue of fast striated muscles of the pelvic floor and slow striated muscles of the limb by manipulating the on-off time of electric stimulation. *Arch. Phys. Med. Rehabil.*, 83, 550-554.

Ritter, A.B., Reisman, S. & Michniak, B.B. (2005). Signal Acquisition and Processing. In: *Biomedical Engineering Principles*, pp. 265-289. CRC Press.

Salcedo, L., Damaser, M., Butler, R., Jiang, H.H., Hull, T. & Zutshi, M. (2010). Long-term effects on pressure and electromyography in a rat model of anal sphincter injury. *Dis. Colon Rectum*, 53, 1209-1217.

Schroder, H.D. (1980). Organization of the motoneurons innervating the pelvic muscles of the male rat. *J. Comp Neurol.*, 192, 567-587.

Shafik, A. (2000). The role of the levator ani muscle in evacuation, sexual performance and pelvic floor disorders. *Int. Urogynecol. J. Pelvic. Floor. Dysfunct.*, 11, 361-376.

Stashuk, D. (2001). EMG signal decomposition: how can it be accomplished and used? Journal of electromyography and kinesiology: official journal of the *International Society of Electrophysiological Kinesiology*, 11, 151.

Steinmetz, M.P., Alilain, W., Horn, K., Jiang, H.H., Fletter, P., Damaser, M.S. & Silver, J. (2008). Light induced alteration of external urethral function through the activation of channelrodopsin-2. Poster; Washington. Society for Neuroscience. 2008. Society for Neuroscience 469.14/MM19..

Steward, J.E., Clemons, J.D., Zaszczurynski, P.J., Butler, R.S., Damaser, M.S. & Jiang, H.H. (2010). Quantitative evaluation of electrodes for external urethral sphincter electromyography during bladder-to-urethral guarding reflex. *World journal of urology*, 28, 365.

Streng, T., Launonen, A., Salmi, S., Saarinen, N., Talo, A., Makela, S. & Santti, R. (2001). Nontraumatic urethral dyssynergia in neonatally estrogenized male rats. *J. Urol.*, 165, 1305-1309.

Streng, T., Santti, R., Andersson, K.E. & Talo, A. (2004). The role of the rhabdosphincter in female rat voiding. *BJU. Int.*, 94, 138-142.

Streng, T., Santti, R. & Talo, A. (2002). Similarities and differences in female and male rat voiding. *Neurourol. Urodyn.*, 21, 136-141.

Strohbehn, K. (1998). Normal pelvic floor anatomy. *Obstet. Gynecol. Clin. North Am*, 25, 683-705.

Stålberg, E., Nandedkar, S.D., Sanders, D.B. & Falck, B. (1996). Quantitative motor unit potential analysis. Journal of clinical neurophysiology: official publication of the *American Electroencephalographic Society*, 13, 401.

Thor, K.B. (2003). Serotonin and norepinephrine involvement in efferent pathways to the urethral rhabdosphincter: implications for treating stress urinary incontinence. *Urology*, 62, 3-9.

Thor, K.B. & de Groat, W.C. (2010). Neural control of the female urethral and anal rhabdosphincters and pelvic floor muscles. *Am. J. Physiol Regul. Integr. Comp Physiol*, 299, R416-R438.

Thor, K.B., Hisamitsu, T., Roppolo, J.R., Tuttle, P., Nagel, J. & Degroat, W.C. (1989). Selective inhibitory effects of ethylketocyclazocine on reflex pathways to the external urethral sphincter of the cat. *J. Pharmacol. Exp. Ther.*, 248, 1018-1025.

Thor, K.B., Kirby, M. & Viktrup, L. (2007). Serotonin and noradrenaline involvement in urinary incontinence, depression and pain: scientific basis for overlapping clinical efficacy from a single drug, duloxetine. *Int. J. Clin. Pract.*, 61, 1349-1355.

Vera, P.L. & Nadelhaft, I. (2001). Effects of the atypical neuroleptic clozapine on micturition parameters in anesthetized rats. *Neurourol. Urodyn.*, 20, 623-639.

Wai, C.Y., Liehr, P., Boreham, M.K., Schaffer, J.I. & Word, R.A. (2004). Effect of periurethral denervation on smooth muscles of the lower urinary tract. *Am. J. Obstet. Gynecol.*, 191, 1950-1960.

Wall, L.L. (1993). The muscles of the pelvic floor. *Clin. Obstet. Gynecol.*, 36, 910-925.

Wallner, C., van, W.J., Maas, C.P., Dabhoiwala, N.F., DeRuiter, M.C. & Lamers, W.H. (2008). The contribution of the levator ani nerve and the pudendal nerve to the innervation of the levator ani muscles; a study in human fetuses. *Eur. Urol.*, 54, 1136-1142.

Weidner, A.C., Barber, M.D., Visco, A.G., Bump, R.C. & Sanders, D.B. (2000a). Pelvic muscle electromyography of levator ani and external anal sphincter in nulliparous women and women with pelvic floor dysfunction. *Am. J. Obstet. Gynecol.*, 183, 1390-1399.

Weidner, A.C., Sanders, D.B., Nandedkar, S.D. & Bump, R.C. (2000b). Quantitative electromyographic analysis of levator ani and external anal sphincter muscles of nulliparous women. *Am. J. Obstet. Gynecol.*, 183, 1249-1256.

Weidner, A.C., South, M.M., Sanders, D.B. & Stinnett, S.S. (2009). Change in urethral sphincter neuromuscular function during pregnancy persists after delivery. *Am. J. Obstet. Gynecol.*, 201, 529-6.

Yalla, S.V. & Resnick, N.M. (1997). Initiation of voiding in humans: the nature and temporal relationship of urethral sphincter responses. *J. Urol.*, 157, 590-595.

Yang, Z., Dolber, P.C. & Fraser, M.O. (2010). Differential vulnerabilities of urethral afferents in diabetes and discovery of a novel urethra-to-urethra reflex. *Am. J. Physiol Renal Physiol*, 298, F118-F124.

Zutshi, M., Salcedo, L.B., Zaszczurynski, P.J., Hull, T.L., Butler, R.S. & Damaser, M.S. (2009). Effects of sphincterotomy and pudendal nerve transection on the anal sphincter in a rat model. *Dis. Colon Rectum*, 52, 1321-1329.